NEPHROLOGY RESEARCH AND CLINICAL DEVELOPMENTS

ADVANCES IN PATHOGENESIS OF DIABETIC NEPHROPATHY

NEPHROLOGY RESEARCH AND CLINICAL DEVELOPMENTS

Additional books in this series can be found on Nova's website under the Series tab.

Additional E-books in this series can be found on Nova's website under the E-book tab.

NEPHROLOGY RESEARCH AND CLINICAL DEVELOPMENTS

ADVANCES IN PATHOGENESIS OF DIABETIC NEPHROPATHY

SHARMA S. PRABHAKAR
EDITOR

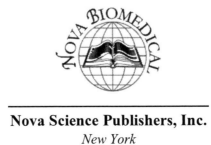

Nova Science Publishers, Inc.
New York

Copyright © 2012 by Nova Science Publishers, Inc.

All rights reserved. No part of this book may be reproduced, stored in a retrieval system or transmitted in any form or by any means: electronic, electrostatic, magnetic, tape, mechanical photocopying, recording or otherwise without the written permission of the Publisher.

For permission to use material from this book please contact us:
Telephone 631-231-7269; Fax 631-231-8175
Web Site: http://www.novapublishers.com

NOTICE TO THE READER

The Publisher has taken reasonable care in the preparation of this book, but makes no expressed or implied warranty of any kind and assumes no responsibility for any errors or omissions. No liability is assumed for incidental or consequential damages in connection with or arising out of information contained in this book. The Publisher shall not be liable for any special, consequential, or exemplary damages resulting, in whole or in part, from the readers' use of, or reliance upon, this material. Any parts of this book based on government reports are so indicated and copyright is claimed for those parts to the extent applicable to compilations of such works.

Independent verification should be sought for any data, advice or recommendations contained in this book. In addition, no responsibility is assumed by the publisher for any injury and/or damage to persons or property arising from any methods, products, instructions, ideas or otherwise contained in this publication.

This publication is designed to provide accurate and authoritative information with regard to the subject matter covered herein. It is sold with the clear understanding that the Publisher is not engaged in rendering legal or any other professional services. If legal or any other expert assistance is required, the services of a competent person should be sought. FROM A DECLARATION OF PARTICIPANTS JOINTLY ADOPTED BY A COMMITTEE OF THE AMERICAN BAR ASSOCIATION AND A COMMITTEE OF PUBLISHERS.

Additional color graphics may be available in the e-book version of this book.

Library of Congress Cataloging-in-Publication Data
Advances in pathogenesis of diabetic nephropathy / editor, Sharma S. Prabhakar.
    p. ; cm.
 Includes bibliographical references and index.
 ISBN 978-1-61122-134-3 (hardcover)
 1. Diabetic nephropathies. I. Prabhakar, Sharma S.
 [DNLM: 1. Diabetic Nephropathies--etiology. WK 835]
 RC918.D53A38 2010
 616.6'1--dc22
                    2010041333

Published by Nova Science Publishers, Inc. † New York

Contents

Preface		vii
Foreword		xi
Chapter I	Diabetic Nephropathy: An Overview *Sharma S Prabhakar*	1
Chapter II	Histopathologic Aspects of Diabetic Nephropathy *Irfan Warraich and Ruc Tan*	5
Chapter III	Role of Hyperfiltration in the Pathogenesis of Diabetic Nephropathy *Sandra Sabatini and Neil Kurtzman*	21
Chapter IV	Experimental Approaches to Investigate the Pathogenesis of Diabetic Nephropathy *Sharma S Prabhakar*	49
Chapter V	Role of Hyperglycemia and its Metabolic Effects in the Pathogenesis of Diabetic Nephropathy *Philip Abraham and Howard Trachtman*	69
Chapter VI	Advanced Glycation End Products and Diabetic Nephropathy *Jaime Uribarri*	93
Chapter VII	Growth Factors in the Pathogenesis of Diabetic Nephropathy *Charbel C. Khoury and Fuad N. Ziyadeh*	111
Chapter VIII	Role of Activated Renin-Angiotensin System in the Pathogenesis of Diabetic Nephropathy *Hiroyuki Kobori, Lisa M. Harrison-Bernard and L. Gabriel Navar*	161
Chapter IX	Role of Oxidative Stress in Diabetic Nephropathy *Josephine M. Forbes, Melinda T. Coughlan and Mark E. Cooper*	199
Chapter X	Role of Vaso-Active Factors in Diabetic Nephropathy *Sharma S. Prabhakar*	219
Chapter XI	Endothelial Dysfunction in Diabetic Nephropathy *Takamune Takahashi and Raymond C. Harris*	239

Chapter XII	Recent Advances on Cell Biology of Podocytes and their Contribution to the Pathogenesis of Diabetic Glomerulosclerosis *Sandeep Magoon, Hitesh Shah, Saul Teichberg and Pravin C. Singhal*	**273**
Chapter XIII	Role of Translational Dysregulation in Diabetic Nephropathy *Denis Feliers and B. S. Kasinath*	**289**
Chapter XIV	Genetics of Diabetic Nephropathy *Barbara C. Pence and Wyatt McMahon*	**315**
Index		**337**

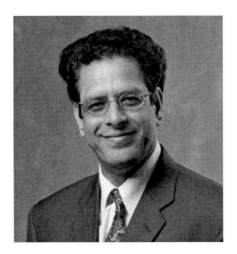

Preface

Over the past two decades, diabetic nephropathy has emerged as the most frequent cause of end stage renal disease needing renal replacement therapy is the western hemisphere. The developing nations and the Eastern countries are fast catching up with the trend and the most recent statistics reveal that diabetes is the leading cause of end stage kidney failure globally. Slowing the development and progression of nephropathy in diabetes was accomplished hitherto predominantly by controlling hyperglycemia and hypertension and inhibiting renin angiotensin system. However the currently available preventive and therapeutic interventions for diabetic nephropathy are obviously sub-optimal since the incidence and prevalence continues to increase. Such trends prompted intense search for other pathogenic factors that lead to renal structural and functional damage in diabetes. The past three decades witnessed a plethora of scientific investigation into pathogenesis of diabetic nephropathy, which attempt to seek the role of several potential cytokines, growth factors, second messengers, vasoactive factors, and candidate genes in leading to structural and functional demise of the kidneys in diabetes. Establishing more extensive knowledge of pathogenesis is crucial to expand the therapeutic options for diabetic nephropathy. While there are a few monographs dealing with the subject of diabetic nephropathy, this book is an exclusive treatise on the current knowledge about the pathogenesis of this condition.

The book is designed to offer the most current data on the pathogenic factors incriminated in the nephropathy of diabetes. Accordingly the list of contributors includes some of the most respected authorities in their own field in the broad area of diabetic nephropathy.

The initial chapter is an overview of diabetic nephropathy that serves as a foundation to understand more intricate aspects of the pathogenesis. There have been significant advances in the understanding the natural history and association with other vascular complications of diabetes. A short description of epidemiology, pathophysiology together with a broad outline of the current treatment strategies forms the main contents of this chapter. This is followed by a chapter on pathology of diabetic nephropathy, which is necessary to understand the connection between pathogenesis, pathophysiology and functional correlates of diabetic nephropathy. Warraich and Tran provide an excellent review of the histopathological aspects of the diabetic nephropathy with very representative illustrations. The sections on differential diagnosis and the differences between nephropathy of type I and II diabetes are particularly useful from the clinical standpoint. This is followed by an exciting chapter on the role of glomerular hyperfiltration which is conventionally believed to predispose to development of microalbuminuria and overt nephropathy. Kurtzman and Sabatini provide a very critical review of this topic with extensive review of seminal articles in this area.

Hyperglycemia, the main culprit in initiating several distal pathogenic events in diabetic nephropathy, is the focus of the chapter written by Trachtman and Abraham. This very well organized review divides the contents into basic studies that describe the general effects, signaling effects and clinical studies that relate to the role of hyperglycemia in the pathogenesis of diabetic nephropathy. Uribari provides an extensive discussion in his chapter on the role of advanced glycosylation end products, which are now considered to be pathogenic not only in diabetic nephopathy but all micro- and macro-vascular complications of diabetes.

Khory and Ziyadeh discuss the role of growth factors, one of the most exciting areas in the pathogenesis of diabetic nephropathy. The role of TGF-β and VEGF, which stimulated great interest in translational research in diabetic nephropathy is the main focus of this chapter although there is adequate discussion on the role of CCN2 (CTGF), PDGF, BMP-7 and others. Kabori, Harrison-Bernard and Navar provide a comprehensive discussion on the role of activated rennin angiotensin system, a very crucial factor in the pathogenesis of diabetic nephropathy. The sections of intra renal RAS and the potential role of urinary angiotensinogen as a biomarker in diabetic nephropathy are strong features of this chapter.

The role of oxidative stress in diabetic nephropathy has been a very highly debated topic in this field. Forbes, Coughlan and Cooper offer a very balanced and critical yet comprehensive discussion of this subject in an outstanding review. Over the past two decades, the focus of my laboratory has been to understand the pathogenesis of nephropathy in diabetes (particularly type II) and we investigated specifically the role of nitric oxide both in vitro and in vivo studies. These studies along with the angiotensin-nitric oxide interactions, role of endothelins and prostaglandins are the theme of an exciting chapter on the role of vaso-active factors in diabetic nephropathy. A closely related but pathophysiologically very important subject is endothelial dysfunction which is the focus of a superb review in a chapter written by Takahashi and Harris.

Recent years have witnessed major advances in understanding the physiologic and pathophysiologic significance of podocytes in renal health and disease. The role of podocyte biology in diabetic nephropathy is very explicitly described by Magoon et al. while Feliers and Kasinath contributed an excellent review on the role of translation dysregulation, a fascinating topic in diabetic nephropathy. Finally Pence and McMahon discuss the role of genetics in diabetic nephropathy, a highly complex topic that is gaining tremendous momentum in the recent years.

In summary, while this book is written with intent of serving primarily as a reference book for investigators in the field, we hope it will be a valuable resource for a broad range of professionals including nephrologists, endocrinologists, pathophysiologists and basic and traslational scientists.

Sharma S. Prabhakar MD MBA FACP FASN
Texas Tech University Health Sciences Center

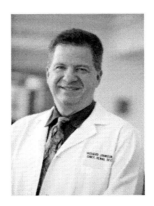

Foreword

Diabetic nephropathy is the most common cause of chronic kidney disease throughout the world. A key to both prevention and treatment is a solid understanding of the mechanisms driving diabetic kidney disease. In this elegant textbook, Dr Sharma Prabhakar has brought together leading experts in the field to give us the state of the art on the pathogenesis of this important disease. Dr Prabhakar takes us on a tour of the major systems thought to be driving the disease, including the effects of hyperglycemia, the role of the renin angiotensin system, and the importance of genetics. A discussion of the pathophysiological and hemodynamic responses is also provided, as well as the interplay of oxidative stress, endothelial dysfunction, and the effects of growth factors and other vasoactive mediators. The book is a delight to read, and brings together in one volume all of the major factors that are thought to be contributing to the disease. The book will be of interest not only to scientists and researchers, but also clinicians interested in diabetic renal disease.

Richard J Johnson, M.D.
Temple Hoyne Buell and NKF of Colorado Endowed Professor of Medicine
Chief, Division of Renal Diseases and Hypertension
University of Colorado, Denver

In: Advances in Pathogenesis of Diabetic Nephropathy
Editor: Sharma S. Prabhakar

ISBN: 978-1-61122-134-3
© 2012 Nova Science Publishers, Inc.

Chapter I

Diabetic Nephropathy: An Overview

Sharma S. Prabhakar
Department of Medicine, Texas Tech University Health Sciences Center,
Lubbock, TX 79430, US

Diabetic nephropathy has emerged as the leading cause of end stage renal disease worldwide and continues to increase in many parts of the world. This is predominantly initiated by the global explosion in incidence of diabetes which is reaching epidemic proportions. While the exact figures are unknown, it is estimated that there are over 150 million people affected with diabetes in the world and the prevalence of diabetes is expected to more than double in the next 20 years especially in countries like India and China and reach the 400 million by the year 2030. Nephropathy is a serious and major complication of diabetes and hence the reason for concern. Management of diabetes with nephropathy remains complex and challenging.

Nephropathy develops in about 30-35% of all diabetics with a trend towards declining prevalence in type I diabetics and a wider prevalence range in type 2 diabetes. The reasons for a decline in nephropathy in type 1 diabetes currently remain largely unknown. Development of albuminuria is the clinical hallmark of onest of nephropathy in diabetes. The cumulative incidence of microalbuminuria is 28-34 % and 25-31% in a 25 year period in type I and type 2 diabetes respectively. The highest prevalence is seen in Native Americans followed by Asians, Hispanics, Blacks and Caucasians in that order. Apart from the racial and genetic factors, male sex, obesity, environmental factors such as smoking influence the development of nephropathy in diabetes.

The etio-pathogenesis of nephropathy in diabetes remains unclear and complicated. While uncontrolled hyperglycemia, hypertension and genetic factors account to some extent, it is unknown why only about a third develop renal disease. The natural history of the disease, which is derived from largely studies from type I diabetes is immensely useful in understanding the pathophysiology and to relate to etio-pathogenesis. Glomerular hyperfiltration occurs in large number of diabetics and correlates with uncontrolled hyperglycemia. Longitudinal studies suggest that hyperfiltration is a strong risk factor for development of micoalbuminuria and diabetic nephropathy especially in type I diabetes. The prognostic significance of hyperfiltration continues to be controversial in type II diabetics. Several studies have documented that 5- 15 years of poor glycemic control, together with hyperfiltration, hypertension and smoking predispose diabetics to develop persistent microalbuminuria and overt nephropathy. Once overt nephropathy onsets with macroalbuminuria, the course is often relentless with progressive azotemia, hypertension and nephritic syndrome. Most patient develop end stage renal disease in five years from the time overt nephropathy onsets. The development of other cardiovascular complications of diabetes particularly coronary artery disease, stroke and peripheral artery disease compounds the morbidity and mortality of diabetic patients with nephropathy.

The pathogenesis of diabetic nephropathy was believed to be largely from poor glycemic and blood pressure control. Many clinical studies including the DCCT study (NEJM 1993) supported this theory. However it was the ACE inhibitor trial led by Lewis et al. (NEJM 1993) along with many other subsequent clinical studies that established the therapeutic potential of inhibition of RAAS in diabetic nephropathy. The role of diet particularly protein restriction in slowing the progression of diabetic nephropathy remains controversial, although most authorities recommend protein restriction to 0.8 g/day. These measures slow the progression of nephropathy but the fact the disease continues to march towrch towards ESRD albeit at a slower pace, strongly hints other unknown pathogenic mediators of this condition.

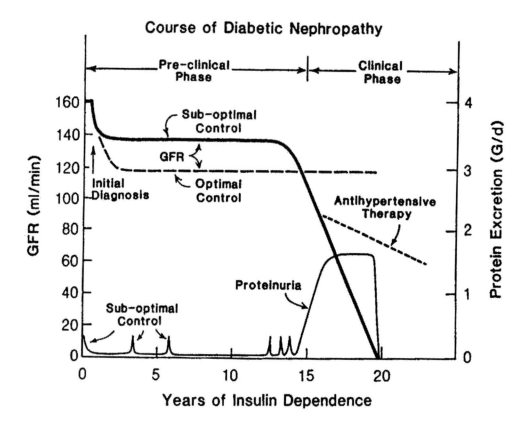

The last two decades has witnessed a major effort in investigating other pathogenic mediators which included growth factors, cytokines, signaling pathways and candidate genes amongst many others. The various chapters presented in this book reflect a systematic effort to elaborate the major research findings pertaining to most of such putative pathogenic mediators of diabetic nephropathy. Notwithstanding the fact that represents most current sate of knowledge in this field, as with most rapidly advancing and evolving fields of medicine, we expect many more developments in the near future. As such the reader is advised to supplement the information presented in this monograph with the most recent journals.

Despite major advances in the therapeutic strategies, diabetic nephropathy is on the increase, which is predominantly due to major gaps in understanding the pathogenesis of this condition. Currently the preventive and therapeutic interventions are directed against the obvious contributory factors which include systemic hypertension, uncontrolled hypertension and inhibition of rennin angiotensin system. When ESRD develops in these patients, all the optons that are offered to non-diabetic ESRD patienst are very acceptable and well tolerated in this population. While morbidity and mortality is somewhat higher in diabetics with ESRD compared to non-diabetics, the outcomes continue to improve both with dialytic therapies and renal transplantation With the evolution of additional pathogenic mediators with strong translational potential, we expect new therapeutic options becoming available in the very near future.

In: Advances in Pathogenesis of Diabetic Nephropathy
Editor: Sharma S. Prabhakar

ISBN: 978-1-61122-134-3
© 2012 Nova Science Publishers, Inc.

Chapter II

Histopathologic Aspects of Diabetic Nephropathy

Irfan Warraich and Ruc Tan
Texas Tech University Health Sciences Center, Lubbock, TX 79430, US

Abstract

As a general rule, patients with known diabetes mellitus and albuminuria usually have diabetic nephropathy. However, they may have some other non diabetic renal disease, either alone or superimposed on diabetic nephropathy. The value of renal biopsy is in confirming whether the patient has diabetic nephropathy or another disorder requiring a different management. Additionally, renal biopsy establishes the extent of chronic damage that determines the prognosis for the patient.

Constellation of morphologic findings for a typical diabetic nephropathy includes a diffuse form with an increase in mesangial matrix and uniform thickening of capillary walls and a nodular form. These lesions are sometimes accompanied by microaneurysms and hyalinosis lesions.

When well developed, the nodular lesion with hyaline arteriolosclerosis is considered virtually pathognomonic of diabetes. However, a few mimicking disorders like renal amyloidosis, light chain deposition disease, immunotactoid glomerulonephritis, and membranoproliferative glomerulonephritis need to be ruled out. In biopsies with absence of the typical nodular lesion, the presence of diffuse mesangiosclerosis, typical linear immunofluorescence staining of glomerular capillary walls with IgG and albumin, and thickening of the GBM on electron microscopy is typical of diabetic glomerulopathy.

Diabetes has two types; insulin-dependent diabetes mellitus (IDDM) or type 1 and non-insulin dependent diabetes mellitus (NIDIM) or type 2. The pathologic features in these two forms are quite similar but not identical as patients with type 2 diabetes have been reported to have a more heterogeneous morphology.

Pathologic Findings

Gross Appearance

The kidney of the diabetic patient may be increased, decreased, or normal in size. At early stages, the kidneys may be diffusely and symmetrically enlarged; particularly in patients with hyperfiltration [1]. Later in disease course, kidney size may be variable. When diabetic glomerulosclerosis progresses, along with scarring and loss of parenchyma, a reduction in the size of the kidney can be seen, but the end-stage kidney of the diabetic patient does not commonly show significant decrease in size. This difference in size variably depends on the presence or absence of superimposed vascular or infectious diseases. Papillary necrosis may be present resulting in loss of pyramids.

Light Microscopy

Glomeruli

Early in the disease course the glomeruli may appear enlarged, especially in patients with IDDM [2]. The mesangial expansion may be seen and capillary walls may be slightly thickened, but these changes are better identified by electron microscopy. At later stages, the glomeruli show a constellation of findings. These include a diffuse form with mesangial sclerosis with uniform thickening of capillary walls, a nodular lesion (Kimmelstiel-Wilson nodules), microaneurysms, hyalinosis lesions, and the capsular drop.

Diffuse Lesion

The diffuse lesion which is found in almost all cases of diabetic glomerulopathy consists of diffuse and global expansion of the mesangium with eosinophilic, periodic acid Schiff (PAS)-positive material. Glomerular capillary basement membranes are uniformly and diffusely thickened (Figure 1). The increase in capillary basement membrane thickness may be seen as early as 2 years after the onset of diabetes mellitus, and usually does not manifest clinical evidence of renal dysfunction [3,4]. The Glomerular basement membranes are thickened and mesangial matrix is increased by the time microalbuminuria appears clinically [5,6]. Mesangial cellularity is variable; usually normal but may be increased. Mesangial expansion progressively increases, resulting in compromised capillary lumina and decreased filtration surface area. As the glomerular sclerosis progress, they do not contract to the degree seen in other diseases resulting in solidified glomeruli.

Nodular Lesion

The most characteristic lesion of diabetic glomerulonephropathy is nodular intercapillary glonneruloselerosis (Kimmelstiel–Wilson nodule) (Figure2).

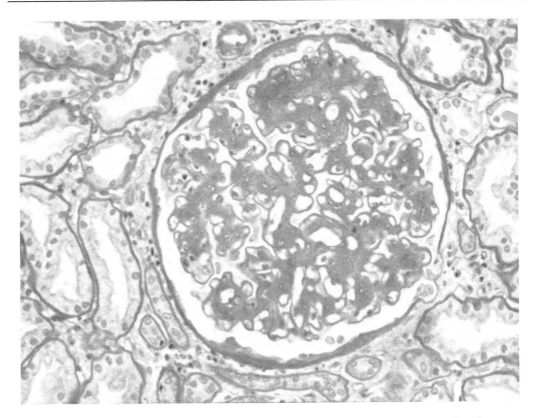

Figure 1. Diffuse Lesion. Glomerulus showing global uniform thickening of capillary wall and mesangial expansion (PAS). (Courtesy of Dr. Ruc Tran Department of Pathology, Texas Tech Health sciences Center, Lubbock, TX).

Typically, these nodules are eosinophilic and round; the center of the nodule is largely acellular, but cells may be seen at the periphery. If multiple, these nodules tend to vary in size. Microaneurysms appear to precede the development of large nodules [7]. The nodules are PAS-positive and stain green with Masson's trichrome, and black with silver stains (Figures 2 and 3). The nodules may appear laminated on silver stains. Although Kimmelstiel–Wilson nodules are considered pathognomonic of diabetic glomerulonephropathy (except for a few mimics), they are found in only a quarter of diabetic cases. In one literature review only 27% to 46% of diabetic patients had nodular lesions [8]. Diffuse glomerulosclerosis frequently coexists with nodular lesions. Presence of the nodular lesion often suggests a more serious diabetic nephropathy corresponding well with the clinical signs and symptoms [9,10].

Hyalinosis Lesions

The hyalinosis lesion or fibrin cap, is often present in diabetic nephropathy. It is located between the glomerular capillary endothelial cells and the glomerular basement membrane. This lesion consists of a homogeneous, eosinophilic, hyaline appearing nodule that may represent insudation of plasma proteins (Figure4). As the lesion evolves, the material eventually occludes the capillary lumen. Sometimes, lipid droplets or lipid-laden macrophages may be seen within the lesion.

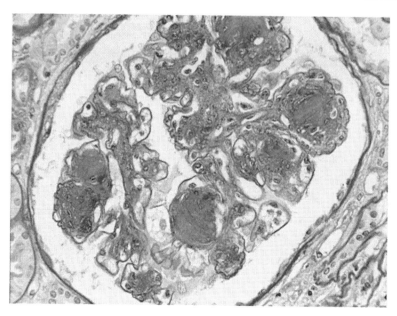

Figure 2. Kimmelstiel-Wilson nodules. Glomerulus with well-developed Kimmelstiel-Wilson nodules. (PAS). (Courtesy of Dr. Ruc Tran Department of Pathology, Texas Tech Health sciences Center, Lubbock, TX).

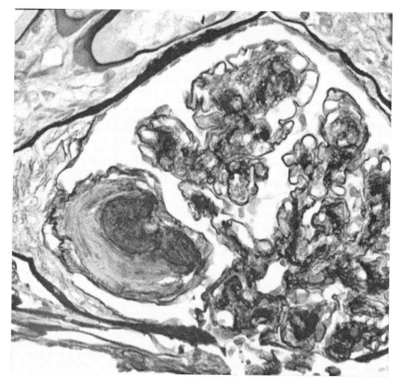

Figure 3. Kimmelstiel-Wilson nodule. Glomerulus with a nodule displaying laminations on silver stain. (Periodic acid methenamine silver). (Courtesy of Dr. Ruc Tran Department of Pathology, Texas Tech Health sciences Center, Lubbock, TX).

Adhesions are often observed between the glomerular lobule containing such a lesion and nearby Bowman's capsule. The material within the capillary lumen stains intensely pink with PAS.

Although it is seen in approximately 60% of diabetic kidneys [7], fibrin caps are not specific for diabetic nephropathy. Similar lesions are seen in other diseases including focal segmental glomerulosclerosis, reflux nephropathy, and arteriolosclerosis.

Another characteristic lesion of diabetic glomerulonephropathy is the capsular drop. It is identified as a round, eosinophilic accumulation of material located within Bowman's capsule (Figure 5). Capsular drops do not stain with silver stains. Capsular drops are considered strongly suggestive, but not quite pathognomonic of diabetic glomerulonephropathy as it may be seen in other conditions [11].

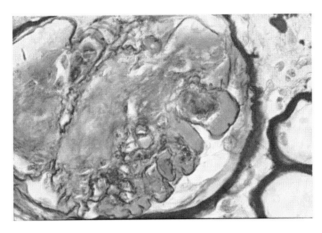

Figure 4. Fibrin cap (hyalinosis). Fibrin cap appears as homogeneous, eosinophilic, hyaline appearing nodule (Periodic acid methenamine silver). (Courtesy of Dr. Ruc Tran Department of Pathology, Texas Tech Health sciences Center, Lubbock, TX).

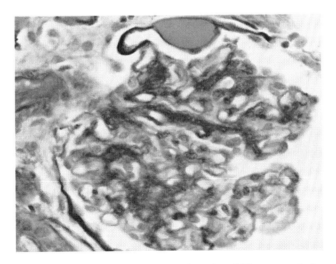

Figure 5. Capsular drop. Capsular drop appears as round, eosinophilic accumulation of material located within Bowman's capsule. (Courtesy of Dr. Ruc Tran Department of Pathology, Texas Tech Health sciences Center, Lubbock, TX).

Microaneurysms of glomerular capillaries are another characteristic lesion. It manifests as capillary loop dilatation due to mesangiolysis.

Tubules

The tubules generally show changes that reflect the degree of glomerular alterations. Obsolescent glomeruli show atrophy of surrounding tubules and tubular basement membranes become progressively thickened. (Figure 6). Sometimes, proximal tubular epithelial cells exhibit fine vacuolation and contain lipid; this is usually seen in patients manifesting nephrotic syndrome. Collection of neutrophils in tubular lumina suggests superimposed pyelonephritis.

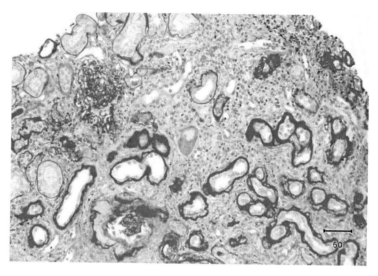

Figure 6. Tubular atrophy. Tubular loss and thickening of tubular basement membrane along with interstitial inflammation is seen. (PAS).

Blood Vessels

Both arteries and arterioles invariably exhibit the changes of arteriosclerosis and arteriolosclerosis, respectively. In arteries, this type of injury is manifested by varying degrees of intimal thickening accompanied by reduplication of elastic lamina. However, it is difficult to distinguish the effects of diabetes from those of hypertension. Hyaline arteriolosclerosis is a frequent and early manifestation of diabetic nephropathy. It is manifests as prominent hyalin deposition in arterioles (Figure7), and both afferent and efferent arterioles may be affected. However this finding is only seen if pathologist is fortunate enough to have a biopsy section that has both afferent and efferent arterioles present. Intimal hyaline thickening of arterioles is the most characteristic change; the presence of marked hyaline arteriolosclerosis, especially in a young patient, should alert the pathologist to look for other changes of diabetes.

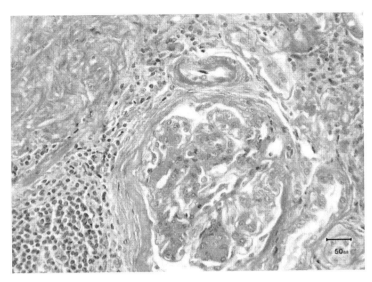

Figure 7. Hyaline arteriolosclerosis. Hyaline arteriolosclerosis manifests as prominent hyalin deposition. (Arteriole above the glomerulus at 12 o' clock).

Interstitium

Interstitial fibrosis is commonly seen in the diabetic kidney and is usually proportional to the degree of vascular change. The interstitial fibrosis, especially when accompanied by inflammatory infiltrate (Figure 6), has been reported to correlate with renal survival [12]. Moreover, some authors have reported that the degree of interstitial fibrosis correlates inversely with the GFR [13]. Interstitial inflammation may sometimes be due to superimposed infection or be caused by chronic renal failure.

Immunofluorescence Microscopy

The most characteristic finding is linear staining along the glomerular capillary walls with immunoglobulin G (IgG) (Figure 8). This staining represents nonspecific adhesion to the GBM rather than a specific immunologic reaction. Linear staining of capillary walls has also been seen with IgM, the third component of complement (C3), fibrinogen, and albumin. Linear GBM staining in diabetes may be confused with anti-GBM antibody disease; however, the coexistence of staining for albumin and IgG is consistent with diabetes rather than anti-GBM antibodies. The term pseudolinear staining has been suggested to avoid confusion with anti-GBM antibody disease.

Hyalinosis lesions usually demonstrate staining for IgM and C3. This finding is similar to the identical lesions found in focal segmental glomerular sclerosis. Hyaline arteriolosclerosis in diabetes stain with IgM and C3 as well as in vessels showing hypertensive changes. Hyalinosis lesions may also exhibit staining for fibrinogen and IgG.

Tubular basement membranes may also show linear staining for IgG and albumin.

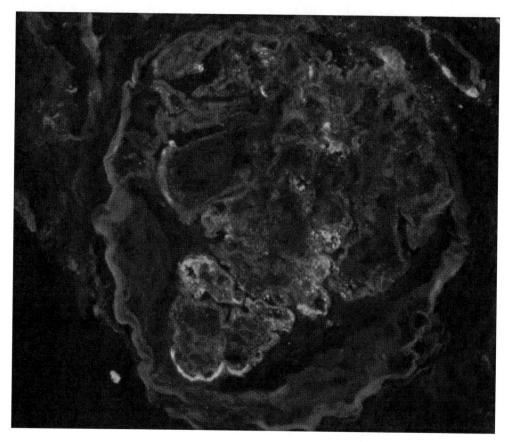

Figure 8. Pseudolinear IgG staining. Immunofluorescence study picture exhibits a linear (pseudolinear) IgG staining along capillary basement membrane in a glomerulus with diabetic nephropathy (at 6 o' clock).

Electron Microscopy

Glomerular Capillary Wall

Glomerular basement membrane (GBM) in the adult human ranges in thickness from 300 to 350 nm [14]. Glomerular capillary basement membranes become progressively thickened in diabetic nephropathy with variable effacement of foot process in epithelial cells (Figure 9). This increase in the thickness of the GBM is considered the earliest change [5].

The isolated finding of thickened GBM has been reported as a possible manifestation of early diabetes in patients who presented with proteinuria greater than 0.5 g/day but without clinical evidence of diabetes [15].

Mesangium

The glomerular mesangium is expanded because of extracellular matrix material, which appears amorphous or granular. This material may appear relatively electron dense, although not as intense as seen in immune complex deposits. Similarly Kimmelstiel-Wilson nodules appear amorphous or granular.

Hyalinosis

Hyalinosis lesions are seen as amorphous, electron-dense material. This distinction of hyalinosis accumulations from immune deposits may sometimes be difficult.

Tubules

Tubular basement membranes also exhibit thickening similar to those seen in GBMs.

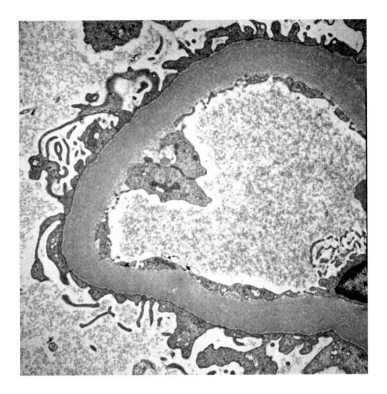

Figure 9. Increase in the thickness of the GBM in diabetic nephropathy. Electron micrograph is showing uniform thickening (920nm) in a patient with diabetic nephropathy.

Non Diabetic Renal Lesions in Diabetic Patients

Diabetic patients can develop nondiabetic renal diseases either superimposed on diabetic nephropathy or independently. This scenario is more commonly observed in type 2 diabetes.

These patients are often biopsied because of unusual clinical features [16]. In an autopsy study, 7% of diabetic patients had nondiabetic renal disease [17].

Glomerular Lesions

Diabetic nephropathy is the most common renal disease to be complicated by another form of glomerular disease. The frequency of nondiabetic glomerular lesions ranges from 5% to 71% in different reports [18]. The second disorder is usually suspected in patients with rapid worsening of renal function, persistent hematuria, or sudden onset of nephrotic syndrome, especially before 8 years' duration of diabetes or in the absence of retinopathy [19,20].

In a retrospective analysis by Tone A, et al., sensitivity and specificity of four clinical parameters (duration of diabetes, presence or absence of diabetic retinopathy, microscopic hematuria and granular casts for the prediction of non diabetic renal disease (NDRD) was evaluated in 97 Japanese patients. Absence of retinopathy had the highest sensitivity (87%) and specificity (93%) followed by diabetes duration of less than 5 years (sensitivity of 75% and specificity of 70%). The authors concluded that that the absence of retinopathy and short duration of diabetes are useful clinical indications for renal biopsy in diabetic patients with overt proteinuria [20].

Any form of glomerulonephritis may superimpose on diabetic nephropathy, however, the most common is membranous glomerulonephropathy.

Other nondiabetic glomerular lesions described in diabetic patients either superimposed or independent include acute postinfectious glomerulonephritis, IgA nephropathy, crescentic glomerulonephritis, focal proliferative glomerulonephritis, membranoproliferative glomerulonephritis, lupus nephritis, and amyloid [14].

Moreover, minimal change disease and focal segmental glomerular sclerosis have also been reported [18]. However, the diagnosis of these two entities can be established only in the absence of diabetic nephropathy.

Renal and Urinary Tract Infections

There is increased incidence of complications of acute infection such as renal and perirenal abscesses, and xanthogranulomatous pyelonephritis in diabetic patients [21, 22].

Papillary Necrosis

Papillary necrosis occurs more frequently in diabetic patients (2.7% to 7.2%) compared with nondiabetic patients (0.6% to 1.4%) [21,22]. Diabetes was present in 22% to 27% of cases in two large studies [22,23]. This increase incidence with diabetes has been attributed to ischemia because of vascular disease and infections [24,25]. However, possibility of other etiologies associated with papillary necrosis such as analgesic abuse, urinary tract obstruction, and sickle cell disease also needs to be considered.

Post Renal Transplantation Diabetic Nephropathy

Recurrence of diabetic nephropathy has been reported in the transplanted kidneys [26]; however, this occurrence usually does not result in graft failure. The earliest change in kidneys from nondiabetic donors when transplanted into patients with diabetes is the hyaline arteriolosclerosis [26]. Nodular glomerulosclerosis has been reported. Diabetic nephropathy has also been seen in patients who develop diabetes after transplant (secondary to non diabetic disorder) [27].

Interestingly, regression of diabetic nephropathy has also been seen when kidneys from diabetic donors are transplanted into nondiabetic patients [28].

Differential Diagnosis

By clinical presentation, the differential diagnosis includes any cause of proteinuria or the nephrotic syndrome. This includes disorders like minimal change disease, membranous glomerulonephropathy, focal segmental glomerulosclerosis, and amyloidosis.

Histologically, the differential diagnosis can vary depending on which feature of the constellation of diabetic nephropathy is predominant. Some lesions in diabetic nephropathy, when present in isolation are not specific at all. This can be an important consideration in situations when there is no clinical evidence of diabetes mellitus [29]. For example, the hyalinosis lesions are not specific for the diagnosis of diabetic nephropathy as it may be seen in focal segmental glomerular sclerosis as well.

The nodular form of diabetic glomerulosclerosis, when well developed is fairly diagnostic but can bring a few other conditions in differential diagnosis. These conditions are amyloidosis, light chain deposition disease, immunotactoid glomerulonephritis, and membranoproliferative glomerulonephritis.

Amyloidosis

Amyloidosis has a nodular appearance resembling Kimmelstiel-Wilson nodules. However, amyloid nodules tend to stain poorly with PAS and do not stain with silver stains at all. Moreover, they stain with Congo red and exhibit the characteristic "apple green" birefringence under polarized light. Ultrastructural study shows nonbranching fibrils measuring 8 to 10 nm in diameter.

Light Chain Deposition

Light-chain deposition disease (LCDD) may cause nodular lesions similar to Kimmelstiel-Wilson nodules. However, unlike diabetic nodules, the nodules in LCDD are often uniform in size, both within single glomerulus and between different glomeruli in the biopsy. The finding of light chain restriction on immunofluorescence studies for kappa and lambda is fairly diagnostic for LCDD.

Immunotactoid Glomerulonephritis

Early in this disease course, capillary loops are thickened, resembling diffuse lesion of diabetes. However, this thickening is variable unlike uniform thickening typical of diabetes. Sometimes, nodule formation is also observed. The lesion stains with PAS but does not with the silver stain. Ultrastructural study confirms the diagnosis with the characteristic fibrils measuring between 15 and 60.

Membranoproliferative Glomerulonephritis

The mesangial nodules, which in advance cases may have sclerosis, may resemble diabetic glomerulosclerosis. However, membranoproliferative glomerulonephritis (MPGN) uniformly affects all glomeruli to a similar degree, unlike the nodular change of diabetic glomerulosclerosis, which usually manifests in only some of the glomeruli. Additionally, MPGN lesions are typically hypercellular, unlike diabetic nodules, which show only a mild increase in cells, characteristically arranged at the periphery of the nodule. Silver stains highlight a double contour in MPGN. Electron microscopy confirms the presence of subendothelial and mesangial immune deposits in type I MPGN and intramembranous deposits in the type II MPGN.

Hypertension

Diabetic nephropathy if not well developed, can be difficult to differentiate from hypertensive renal disease because of the similar morphologic features (thickened GBM) and often coexistence of the two disorders. Hyaline arteriolosclerosis is a common in both diseases, and although the presence of hyaline change involving both afferent and efferent arterioles strongly favors diabetic nephropathy, this feature often cannot be demonstrated on needle biopsies.

Diabetic Nephropathy in Type 2 Diabetes Mellitus

The earlier reports for morphologic findings in diabetic nephropathy were mostly from patients with type 1 diabetes. However, more recently, reports with main focus on type 2 diabetes have surfaced. The common indications for biopsy in type 2 diabetes mellitus are rapid onset of acute or chronic renal insufficiency and nephrotic syndrome relative to the known duration of the diabetes or a normal hemoglobin-A1C. Overall, studies have reported many similarities in morphologic appearance with type 1 diabetes mellitus. Both types of diabetes exhibit increased GBM thickness, mesangial sclerosis with nodules, hyalinosis, and hyaline arteriolosclerosis in [18,30,31,]. However, some reports have concluded that the renal biopsies with type 2 diabetes exhibit more heterogeneous morphology compared to biopsies from type 1 diabetes [18, 30]. These authors have described higher incidence of nondiabetic glomerular disease, more severe interstitial fibrosis, and arteriosclerosis and arteriolosclerosis.

Dalla Vestra et al. report that only 30% of Type 2 diabetes patients had typical diabetic glomerulopathy, while 40% had more advanced tubulo-interstitial and/or vascular lesions and 30% had normal renal structure [32].

Fioretto P in their work have concluded that although tubular, interstitial, and arteriolar lesions are present in type 1 diabetes, the most important structural changes are seen in the glomerulus [33]. This is in contrast to type 2 diabetic patients where a significant proportion of type 2 patients, despite the presence of microalbuminuria or proteinuria, have normal glomerular morphology with or without tubulointerstitial and/or arteriolar abnormalities.

In a comprehensive review, a more heterogeneous morphologic pattern of renal lesions in type 2 diabetes has been documented [18]. The prevalence for different lesions is variable in different studies. This variability has been attributed to various factors, including small number of cases investigated in some studies, different policies for performing renal biopsies, geographic and/or ethnic factors.

Based on their study, Mazzucco G, et al. suggest that diabetic nephropathy alone affects only approximately one third of patients with type 2 diabetes, and non-diabetic glomerular changes (superimposed or isolated) are the most frequent findings [18].

Conclusion

The clinical picture of diabetic nephropathy in type 1 and type 2 diabetic patients is fairly similar. This similarity also extends to histopathologic features; as both types may exhibit a diffuse form with mesangial sclerosis with uniform thickening of capillary walls, a nodular lesion, hyalinosis lesions, along with tubulointerstitial and vascular manifestations. However, the frequency of these different renal lesions in the two conditions may differ. It appears that the predominant histopathologic changes in type 1 diabetes, involve the glomerulus. On the other hand, a significant proportion of type 2 diabetic patients, do not have glomerular lesions but have significant tubulo-interstitial and/or arteriolar changes.

References

[1] Mogensen CE, Christensen CK, Vittinghus E. The stages in diabetic renal disease: With emphasis on the stage of incipient diabetic nephropathy. *Diabetes* 1983;32(Suppl 2):64.

[2] Ã˜sterby R. Structural changes in the diabetic kidney. *Clin. Endocrinol. Metab.* 1986;15:733.

[3] Mauer SM, et al. Long-term study of normal kidneys transplanted into patients with type I diabetes. *Diabetes* 1989;38:516.

[4] Ã˜sterby R, et al. Diabetic glomerulopathy. Structural characteristics of the early and advanced stages. *Diabetes 1983*;32(Suppl 2):79.

[5] Drummond K, Mauer M. The early natural history of nephropathy in type 1 diabetes. II. Early renal structural changes in type 1 diabetes. *Diabetes* 2002;51:1580.

[6] Bangstad HJ, et al. Early glomerulopathy is present in young, type 1 (insulin-dependent) diabetic patients with microalbuminuria. *Diabetologia* 1993;36:523.

[7] Bloodworth JM Jr. A re-evaluation of diabetic glomerulosclerosis 50 years after the discovery of insulin. *Hum. Pathol.* 1978;9:439.
[8] Hennigar GR, et al. Nodular glomerulosclerosis: Clinico-pathological correlation of 40 advanced cases. Am J Med 1961;241:89.
[9] Stout LC, Kumar S, Whorton EB. Focal mesangiolysis and the pathogenesis of the Kimmelstiel-Wilson nodule. *Hum. Pathol.* 1993;24:77.
[10] Paueksakon P, et al. Microangiopathic injury and augmented PAI-1 in human diabetic nephropathy. *Kidney Int.* 2002;61:2142.
[11] Stout LC, Kumar S, Whorton EB. Insudative lesions: Their pathogenesis and association with glomerular obsolescence in diabetes: A dynamic hypothesis based on single views of advancing human diabetic nephropathy. *Hum. Pathol.* 1994;25:1213.
[12] Bohle A, et al. The pathogenesis of chronic renal failure in diabetic nephropathy. Investigation of 488 cases of diabetic glomerulosclerosis. *Pathol. Res. Pract.* 1991;187:251.
[13] Taft JL, et al. Clinical and histological correlations of decline in renal function in diabetic patients with proteinuria. *Diabetes* 1994;43:1046.
[14] Hepinstall's Pathology of the Kidney, 6th Edition 2007 Lippincott Williams and Wilkins
[15] Mac-Moune Lai F, et al. Isolate diffuse thickening of glomerular capillary basement membrane: A renal lesion in prediabetes? *Mod. Pathol.* 2004;17:1506.
[16] Mazzucco G, et al. The prognostic value of renal biopsy in type 2 diabetes mellitus patients affected by diabetic glomerulosclerosis. *J. Nephrol.* 2005;18:696.
[17] Carpenter AM, et al. Glomerulosclerosis in type 2 (non-insulin-dependent) diabetes mellitus: Relationship to glycaemia in the University Group Diabetes Program (UGDP). Diabetologia 1993;36:1057.
[18] Mazzucco G, et al. Different patterns of renal damage in type 2 diabetes mellitus: A
[19] multicentric study on 393 biopsies. *Am. J. Kidney Dis.* 2002;39:713.
[20] Ibrahim HN, Hostetter TH. Diabetic nephropathy. J Am Soc Nephrol 1997;8:487.
[21] Tone A, et al. Clinical features of non-diabetic renal diseases in patients with type 2 diabetes. Diabetes *Res. Clin. Pract.*2005;69:237.
[22] Nicolle LE. Urinary tract infection in diabetes. Curr Opin Infect Dis 2005;18:49.
[23] Tseng CC, et al. Host and bacterial virulence factors predisposing to emphysematous pyelonephritis. *Am. J. Kidney Dis.* 2005;46:432.
[24] Groop L, Laasonen L, Edgren J. Renal papillary necrosis in patients with IDDM. *Diabetes Care* 1989;12:198.
[25] Ronald A, Ludwig E. Urinary tract infections in adults with diabetes. *Int. J. Antimicrob. Agents* 2001;17:287.
[26] Griffin MD, Bergstralhn EJ, Larson TS. Renal papillary necrosis: A sixteen-year clinical experience. *J. Am. Soc. Nephrol.* 1995;6:248.
[27] Mauer SM, et al. Development of diabetic vascular lesions in normal kidneys transplanted into patients with diabetes mellitus. *N. Engl. J. Med.* 1976;295:916.
[28] Bhalla V, et al. Recurrent and de novo diabetic nephropathy in renal allografts. *Transplantation* 2003;75:66.
[29] van Goor H, et al. Results of transplantation of kidneys from diabetic donors. *Proc. Eur. Dial Transplant Assoc. Eur. Ren. Assoc.* 1985;21:655.

[30] Strauss FG, Argy WP Jr, Schreiner GE. Diabetic glomerulosclerosis in the absence of glucose intolerance. *Ann. Intern .Med.* 1971;75:239.

[31] Gambara V, et al. Heterogeneous nature of renal lesions in type II diabetes. *J. Am. Soc. Nephrol.* 1993;3:1458.

[32] Schwartz MM, et al. Renal clinicopathology of type II diabetes mellitus. *J. Am. Soc. Nephrol.* 1996;1364.

[33] Dalla Vestra M, et al. Structural involvement in type 1 and type 2 diabetic nephropathy. *Diabetes Metab.* 2000 Jul;26 Suppl 4:8-14.

[34] Fioretto P, et al. Histopathology of diabetic nephropathy. *Semin. Nephrol.* 2007 Mar;27(2):195-207.

In: Advances in Pathogenesis of Diabetic Nephropathy
Editor: Sharma S. Prabhakar

ISBN: 978-1-61122-134-3
© 2012 Nova Science Publishers, Inc.

Chapter III

Role of Hyperfiltration in the Pathogenesis of Diabetic Nephropathy

Sandra Sabatini and Neil Kurtzman
Department of Internal Medicine, Division of Nephrology,
Texas Tech University Health Sciences Center, Lubbock, TX 79430, US

Abstract

Diabetes mellitus, Type 1 and Type 2 combined, is the leading cause of end stage renal disease in the United States. While the disease is complex and mutifactorial, one of the major factors leading to diabetic nephropathy is glomerular hyperfiltration. Hyperfiltration and the rise in single nephron glomerular filtration are believed to occur during the first five years of the disease. In the 30-40% of susceptible individuals an increase in both mesangial matrix and microalbuminuria (20 to 200micrograms/min) heralds the onset of diabetic nephropathy. Of the hemodynamic factors involved in the rise in single nephron glomerular filtration rate increases in glomerular pressure as well as glomerular blood flow appear to be of critical importance. The cellular effects resulting from sheer stress (or stretch) may be the major cause for the rise in glomerular pressure although other factors are also involved. Inhibition of the renin-angiotensin-aldosterone axis appears to slow the progression of diabetic nephropathy as does good long term control of hyperglycemia. Many patients with diabetes mellitus have hyporeninemic-hypoaldosteronism. The pathogenesis and management of this interesting subdivision of diabetic nephropathy is also discussed.

Introduction

Diabetes mellitus has been known since antiquity, but it was not until the second half of the 20th century that we began to see the myriad of complications of this disease. In 1921, Banting and Best [1 for Review] at the University of Toronto showed that an extract of the pancreas lowered blood glucose in dogs with hyperglycemia. One year later, the very first diabetic patient was treated with insulin. In 1923, Banting and Macleod (the prize committee never did acknowledge Best) won the Nobel Prize in Medicine and Physiology for this monumental work.

In 2008, the Center of Communicable Diseases estimated that 24 million people in the United States have diabetes mellitus [2]. It is thought that about six million or 25% of these patients are not yet diagnosed. Approximately 57 million people in the United States are believed to be pre-diabetic because of risk factors such as family history, ethnicity, body habitus, and age. The vast majority of diagnosed patients (i.e., 90%) have Type 2 diabetes (insulin resistance). In the United States 13% of Type 2 diabetics are black, 15% are Amerindian, and 10% are Hispanic [2]. Of the patients with Type 2 diabetes mellitus 30-40% will develop diabetic nephropathy [3, 4].

Only a small percentage of diabetic patients (i.e., 5-10%) have Type 1 diabetes mellitus. This form of the disease is associated with insulin deficiency, typically the result of autoimmune destruction of the β-cells of the pancreas. Type 1 diabetics are usually young and Caucasian. It has long been thought that 30-40% of these patients will develop nephropathy after 10 years of the disease. A recently published prospective report (The Oxford Regional Prospective Study) has cast doubt on these numbers [5]. The Oxford Study showed that 51% of these patients developed microalbuminuria and 14% had macroalbuminiuria by 10 years after diagnosis and that more females than males developed diabetic nephropathy. The patients in this study were recruited within 3 months of developing Type 1 diabetes mellitus and were an average of 8.8 years of age. They were followed prospectively for 10 years and most were on no medications other than insulin. The mean Hemoglobin A_1C of these patients was 9.8% [5]. Good glycemic control is considered to be less than 7.0%. This report of 527 patients documents a much higher cumulative incidence of albuminuria than the 30-40% that has been previously reported. It further suggests that even at the young age of 9, most of these patients should be on renoprotective therapy and have tighter blood glucose control.

Increasingly, we have recognized the importance of gestational diabetes mellitus. This disorder affects 2 to 5% of all pregnancies. It is estimated that 20-50% of these women will develop diabetes mellitus later in life [6, 7]. Most will have the Type 2 form of the disease.

The medical cost for managing diabetes mellitus in the United States now exceeds $132 billion annually [1]. It is the leading cause of chronic renal failure, blindness in adults, and amputation of limbs in the United States. It is one of the major factors contributing to cardiovascular morbidity and mortality. According to the Centers for Medicare and Medicaid, in 2009, there were 18 million people diagnosed as having some degree of chronic kidney disease; more the 410,000 of these patients are now receiving renal replacement therapy (i.e., dialysis or kidney transplant) [7]. As stated above, diabetic nephropathy is the leading cause of renal failure in the United States, accounting for >50% of cases (hypertension is the second most common cause of chronic renal failure).

In 1975, three years after the End Stage Renal Disease program was started, patients with diabetes mellitus comprised less than 5% of dialysis patients. In the intervening time there has been an explosion of Type 2 diabetes mellitus, due in part to obesity, easy access to food, and lack of exercise. Also, we have not restricted dialysis or renal transplant to people with the disease. We both remember the "death boards," weekly meetings deciding who would be able to receive dialysis and who would not (i.e., those who would live and those who would die). In the 1970's, patients with diabetes mellitus (as well as the aged) were in the latter group.

Diabetic Nephropathy in Humans

Renal biopsies of patients with diabetes mellitus reveal both macrovascular as well as microvascular disease. This has been noted in a large number of cases, even in the absence of abnormal renal function. Much of our understanding of the natural course of diabetic nephropathy comes from the original observations of young adults with Type 1 diabetes. Prior to 1922, virtually all of these patients died from severe ketoacidosis with hyperglycemia and hyperkalemia. Chronic renal failure or uremia by and large was not seen because of the short duration of the disease. In the mid-1930s, by contrast, approximately 15 years after insulin first had been administered clinically, it became clear that the disease affected many organs, including the kidney. Cardiovascular disease, retinopathy, peripheral vascular disease, and autonomic dysfunction (gastroparesis, cystopathy, and peripheral polyneuropathy) are the rule rather than the exception in diabetes mellitus [8]. Upwards of 75% of these patients will die from cardiovascular disease whether they have nephropathy or not.

Renal histology in these early patients showed nodular glomerulosclerosis, first described at autopsy by Kimmelsteil and Wilson [9] at Harvard. It is now apparent that this lesion is but one of several abnormalities which occur in the diabetic kidney. The most common glomerular lesion is diffuse intercapillary glomerulosclerosis, characterized by an eosinophilic deposition of matrix in the mesangium and thickening of the glomerular basement membrane. Nodules are invariably found in diffuse intercapillary glomerulosclerosis due to deposition of mesangial matrix. The only pathognomonic tubular change noted and one we rarely see today is the Armani-Ebstein lesion. This is characterized by pale glycogen-filled cells of the *pars recta* of the proximal tubule. There is also hyaline deposition in the afferent and efferent arterioles. In advanced diabetic nephropathy, the tubules atrophy and one often sees interstitial edema, fibrosis, and cellular inflammation with macrophages and polymorphonuclear leukocytes [8]. The various factors involved in the development of nephropathy as well as those interventions which may alter the progression to renal failure are the subject of this book.

The time course for untreated diabetes mellitus in those individuals susceptible to developing diabetic nephropathy may be divided into two stages [8, 10].

1. Early Changes

The early stage (less than 10 years) of diabetic nephropathy is associated with a greater than 30 % increase in glomerular filtration rate (GFR)). There is also a lesser rise in PAH (para-aminohippuric acid) measured effective renal plasma flow such that the filtration fraction (the ratio of GFR to renal plasma flow) increases significantly from a normal of about 18% to 26%. Renal size and the tubular maximum glucose reabsorbtive rate (Tm glucose) are both increased. At this stage hypertension is not often found. Microalbuminuria, perhaps the most important early measure of abnormal renal function, is present and unless treated, heralds subsequent azotemia and chronic renal failure. Urinary albumin excretion is typically in the range of 30 to 300microgm/24hr (normal is <30microgm/24hr). If renal biopsy is performed at this stage, one sees expansion of the mesangium, an increase in the size of mesangial cells, and thickening of the glomerular basement membrane.

2. Late Changes

The late stage (about 10 to 15 years) of diabetic nephropathy is characterized by proteinuria (>300microgm/24hr), though not necessarily in the nephrotic range. After 30 years, fully one-half of patients with diabetes mellitus and microalbuminuria will develop overt proteinuria. If nephrotic range proteinuria (>3gm/24hrs) occurs, renal replacement therapy typically will be required within 3 years.

In this chapter we shall summarize the role that hemodynamic changes play in early diabetic nephropathy. We also shall discuss the mechanisms responsible for these hemodynamic changes as well as the effect of pharmacologic therapies on these hemodynamic abnormalities. Finally, as we have a long standing interest in the syndrome of hyporeninemic-hypoaldosteronism in diabetes, we shall conclude with a discussion of this disorder.

Determinants of Intrarenal Hemodynamics

In the 1970's the nephrology laboratory at the Peter Bent Brigham in Boston, led by the great renal physiologist, Dr Barry F Brenner, published a series of carefully performed micropuncture experiments [11-20]. The group studied, in superficial cortical nephrons of Munich-Wistar rats, the hemodynamic forces controlling filtration by the glomerulus. Figure 1 is a schematic of a single glomerulus with its afferent and efferent arterioles, the mesangium, the macula densa, the glomerular basement membrane, the urinary space, and the early proximal convoluted tubule [21]. We shall refer to Figure 1 again later in this chapter.

Brenner's group posited that intrarenal physical forces were etiologic in causing chronic renal failure (i.e., glomerulosclerosis) regardless of underlying disease. This hypothesis was based on the well known observation that when renal function decreased in humans to about ½ - ¼ of normal, with time, end stage renal failure inevitably occurred.

Brenner, Deane, Hostetter and colleagues [11-20] measured intrarenal pressures, afferent and efferent blood flow, single nephron glomerular filtration rate (SN_{GFR}), and then calculated the afferent/efferent arteriolar resistances and the filtration coefficient (K_f). After defining these parameters in normal animals, these investigators then characterized what occurred in the remnant kidney where renal function was decreased [16, 18]. These animals, even without an underlying disease such as diabetes mellitus, will follow an inexorable path to end stage renal failure and uremia. Humans behave similarly.

In the 1980's, Brenner's laboratory then concentrated on the intrarenal hemodynamic forces found in experimentally-induced Type 1 diabetes mellitus [22-24]. The effect of therapy on this model was also examined [25]. We shall discuss their findings as it relates to hyperfiltration of diabetes mellitus after a brief review of normal intrarenal hemodynamics.

Each normal human kidney contains approximately 1 million nephrons with 75-80% of these nephrons being in the superficial cortex. While it is not possible to study single nephron GFR in humans using micropuncture techniques, it is possible to do so in animals under a variety of conditions, including experimentally-induced diabetes mellitus. The Munich-Wistar rat has been the most extensively studied because it has easily accessible surface nephrons and the preparation is stable for many hours.

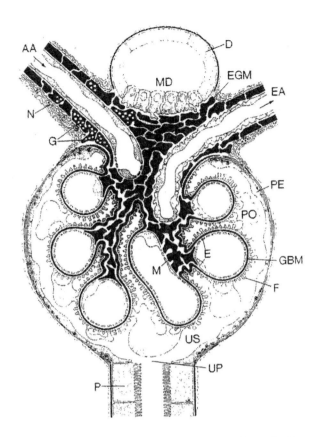

Figure 1. Anatomy of the glomerulus and juxtaglomerular apparatus. Schematic diagram of a section of a glomerulus and its juxtaglomerular apparatus. Structures shown are as follows: afferent arteriole (AA), efferent arteriole (EA), macula densa (MD) of the distal tubule, nerve endings (N), mesangial cell (M), extraglomerular mesangial cell (EGM), endothelial cell (E), epithelial podocyte (PO), with foot process (F), parietal epithelial cell (PE), glomerular basement membrane (GBM), urinary space (US), urinary pole (UP), and proximal tubule (P). G shows the renin containing granules of the juxtaglomerular apparatus. (Reprinted with permission of the National Kidney Foundation). [Ref 21]

There are four main determinants of single nephron glomerular filtration rate (SN_{GFR}):

1. Qa, glomerular plasma flow rate
2. ΔP, mean transmembrane hydraulic pressure difference
3. Πa and Πe, afferent and efferent arteriolar colloid osmotic pressures and
4. K_f, glomerular ultrafiltration coefficient, a parameter which considers the surface area of the glomerulus and its intrinsic permeability.

The first three determinants are measured experimentally and the 4th determinant (i.e., K_f) is calculated.

From the experimentally measured values one can then calculate the resistances of the afferent and efferent arterioles. The formula for SN_{GFR} is:

$$SN_{GFR} \; \alpha \; \frac{Q \cdot HP \cdot K_f}{\pi}$$

where,

Q = glomerular plasma flow rate
HP = transmembrane glomerular pressure
K_f = glomerular ultrafiltration coeffient
   = intrinsic permeability of the glomerulus • surface area
π = colloid osmotic pressure difference

The one hemodynamic variable which can change most dramatically is glomerular effective renal plasma flow. Compared to other capillary beds, flow to the glomerulus is continuous, not intermittent. Both the afferent and efferent arterioles can dilate or constrict. They do not necessarily do so in tandem, thus glomerular pressure and hence filtration rate may be decreased or increased markedly. In states of volume expansion as is seen in normal pregnancy, flow increases markedly. Such a rise subsequently increases SN_{GFR}, all other things being equal.

A small variation in the mean transmembrane hydrostatic pressure gradient (ΔP) alone is rarely a major factor altering SN_{GFR}. Filtration cannot begin until ΔP exceeds the colloid osmotic pressure at the afferent end of the glomerular capillary. Only then does SN_{GFR} rise as ΔP increases; it does not rise linearly, however. Vasoconstriction of the efferent arteriole will result in an increase in pressure which is transmitted back to the glomerulus. Solely changing colloid osmotic pressure, as by an increase in multiple myeloma proteins will affect the afferent arteriole so much that SN_{GFR} falls.

The ultrafiltration coefficient (K_f) is not a fixed value. Decreases have been reported in experimental glomerulonephritis, acute renal failure, and long standing protein calorie malnutrition. In general, at very low flow rates, K_f has little effect on SN_{GFR}. Angiotensin II (AngII) decreases K_f by decreasing the surface area available for filtration [4, 26]. The contractile elements in the mesangial cell and the afferent arteriole are the primary sites for AngII action. This effect of AngII is independent of its effect as a growth factor or any of its other actions [for in depth review of the renal circulation and glomerular hemodynamics, see also Refs # 8, 27-29].

Pathophsiology of Hyperfiltration (Increased SN_{GFR}) in Experimental Diabetes Mellitus

About one half century ago it was suggested that as nephrons failed, the remaining ones had to function at a higher level. Bricker and coworkers [30, 31] expanded and clarified this concept and coined the term "the intact nephron hypothesis". It was not until the 1970s, however, when Brenner's laboratory at the Peter Bent Brigham Hospital began their micropuncture studies in the rat following first unilateral nephrectomy and then more extensive renal ablation that we fully understood the changes in all of the hemodynamic parameters occurring in a single nephron with reduced nephron mass. Based on their results we can now describe the features of these remaining "super nephrons" and theorize on the consequences of single nephron hyperfiltration.

Following uninephrectomy, SN_{GFR} as well as whole kidney GFR increases by about 40% two weeks after surgery although significant increases in both parameters are detectable at 15 hours [16]. Glomerular capillary flow (Qa) rises because both afferent and efferent arteriolar resistances are decreased. Since the fall in the afferent arteriole is much greater, the hydraulic transmembrane pressure (ΔP) rises and SN_{GFR} increases. So the combination of glomerular hypertension and glomerular hyperperfusion explains the "hyperfiltration" which occurs in the remaining nephrons. These changes occur in the absence of uremia. When more extensive renal ablation is performed (i.e., uninephrectomy followed by infarction of the upper two-thirds of the remaining kidney and uremia developed, SN_{GFR} increased even further, by about 75% [18]. Under these conditions, Qa was about the same as seen with uninephrectomy alone, but the hydraulic transmembrane pressure (ΔP) was more markedly increased. With time, both proteinuria and focal segmental glomerulosclerosis were seen. Eventually the animals will die with uremia.

In the 1980's, the Brenner's group (22) published the first paper describing intrarenal hemodynamics in rats with drug-induced diabetes mellitus. The authors sought to answer the question why SN_{GFR} rises in early diabetes mellitus. In subsequent studies, they examined whether any drug intervention could ameliorate the progression of the renal disease [25].

A single injection of streptozotocin (STZ) destroys the β-cells of the pancreas and the animals develop Type 1 diabetes mellitus. The drug was isolated from a strain of *streptomyces* in the 1960s and is an alkylating agent. It is transported into the β-cells of the pancreas by the GLUT2 protein and has been used in the treatment of insulinoma. STZ-treated animals do not develop all the classical findings of diabetic nephropathy and they do not become uremic. The animals do, however, have an increase in kidney size early in the course of the disease; both proteinuria and mesangial cell proliferation also occur [32, 33].

Hostetter et al. [22] studied three groups of male Munich-Wistar rats 74 days after a single intravenous injection of 60mg/kg STZ, STZ plus 2 units NPH insulin sc each pm, or diluent-treated controls. On the morning of the micropuncture study, the animals were anesthetized, given an infusion of isoncotic plasma equal to 1% of body weight appropriate for each group; micropipettes were placed in the proximal tubules of surface nephrons for determination of flow rate and inulin concentration. Efferent arteriolar blood samples were obtained to measure total protein concentration. Hydraulic transmembrane pressure was measured in cortical tubules and vessels using the servo-null micropipette technique [27]. Thus, the 4 determinants of SN_{GFR} were measured and calculated. Afferent and efferent arteriolar resistances were also determined. Additionally, catheters were inserted in the femoral artery, the jugular vein, and the urinary bladder for measurements of whole kidney GFR, mean arterial pressure and hematocrit.

Note in Table 1 that at 18 weeks mean arterial pressure was the same in all groups, but whole kidney GFR in the STZ + insulin diabetic group was 50% higher than control. By contrast, in the STZ group where blood glucose was 5 times control and about two-fold higher than the diabetic animals receiving insulin, GFR was not elevated; it was, in fact, lower than the diluent injected controls (discussed subsequently).

Table 1. Experimental Type 1 Diabetes Mellitus in Rats

Group	N	Mean arterial P (mmHg)	pGlucose (mg/dL)	[a]Whole Kidney GFR(mL/min)
Control	8	103	115	1.10
Streptozotocin	7	102	565*	0.76**
Streptozotocin plus NPH insulin sc	6	114	375*	1.47**

[a]Inulin clearance; total blood volume (Cr51 RBC) between the 3 groups was NS
*P<0.001 from control and from each other
**P<0.02 from control and from each other
(Data from Ref. # 22)

A rise in GFR has been consistently noted in humans with early diabetes, be it Type 1 or Type 2 and it may last for 5 to 10 years during which time microalbuminuria begins in susceptible individuals.

When micropipettes were placed in the kidney to measure SN_{GFR} and the various parameters which regulate it, the following values were noted (Table 2): SN_{GFR} of the superficial cortical nephrons in the STZ + insulin group was increased by approximately 40%. The increase in SN_{GFR} was due directly to a doubling of glomerular capillary flow rate (Qa) and to a 25% increase in the transmembrane hydraulic pressure difference (ΔP). Because this group of animals was in filtration pressure disequilibrium (with the efferent arteriolar colloid osmotic pressure being less than ΔP), one could calculate Kf and compare it to the control group. When this was done, there was no difference noted between the two groups, a change in Kf could not explain the rise in SN_{GFR}.

While the afferent arteriolar protein concentration and therefore, its colloid osmotic pressure, was slightly higher than control, neither of these parameters could contribute to the rise in SN_{GFR}. If anything, these alterations would make SN_{GFR} fall, as may be seen in some patients with severe multiple myeloma.

The afferent arteriole was markedly vasodilated (i.e., its calculated resistance fell significantly by 36%) and while the efferent arteriolar resistance tended to fall, the value was not different from control at the P<0.05 level. Total renal vascular resistance fell by 30%. These results are qualitatively similar to those of the uremic renal ablation model described at the beginning of this section [18].

Table 2. Glomerular Hemodynamics in Rats with Early Type 1 Diabetes Mellitus in Rats

Group	N	SN_{GFR} (nL/min)	Q_A (nL/min)	ΔP (mmHg)	Colloid Osmotic Pressure afferent/efferent	R_t	K_f
Control	8	48.9	142	35	18/34	5.0	>0.095
Streptozotocin	7	28.8*	86**	36	[b]15/32	8.4*	>0.048
Streptozotocin plus NPH insulin sc	6	69.0*	240**	[a]44	[b]20/35	3.5*	0.080

SN_{GFR} = Single nephron glomerular filtration rate
Q_A = Flow
ΔP = Transmembrane hydraulic pressure difference
R_t = Total renal vascular resistance
K_f = Ultrafiltration coefficient

* $P<0.05$ from control and from each other

** $P<0.01$ from control and from each other

[a] $P<0.005$ from control and from each other

[b] $P<0.02$ from control and from each other

(Data from Ref # 22)

The significance of the changes noted in the afferent and efferent arterioles will become clear when we later examine the effect of therapy on the rate of progression of diabetic nephropathy.

In the severely hyperglycemic group (STZ) where blood glucose approached 600mg/dl, the story is quite different. These animals must have had severe ketoacidosis and been volume contracted as they lost weight and had an increase in urine output. This group also had a fall in whole kidney GFR and SN_{GFR}. Glomerular capillary pressure and ΔP were not different from control. By contrast, glomerular plasma flow rate (Qa) fell by 40% and this was the cause of the fall in SN_{GFR}. Both afferent and efferent arteriolar resistances both rose substantially, by 57% and 67%, respectively, suggesting there was marked intrarenal vasoconstriction. This vasoconstriction was likely the result of the release of AngII, norepinephrine, or some other vasoactive agent [26].

Critics have said that the STZ model is not a pure one as the animals do not develop all the features of human diabetic nephropathy and the alkylating agent may have direct toxic effects which substantially alter the results obtained [34,35]. The tremendous amount of data compiled using this model, however, has given us an important basic understanding of the sequence of events occurring in Type 1 diabetes mellitus. With some limitations we believe the findings noted in animals to be compatible with the disease in humans. In order to circumvent the limitations, however, an extensive search has been done over the past decade to develop better animal models. The mouse has proved particularly useful.

Breyer and colleagues [36] have reviewed in depth the mouse models of diabetic nephropathy. We summarize some of their data here. For Type 1 diabetes mellitus we now have several including low dose STZ (40-50mg/kg/d intraperitoneally for 5 days). A milder form of the disease is noted with low grade β-cell damage to the pancreatic islets. After 5 weeks, glomerular hypertrophy as well as albuminuria occurs; at 15-30 weeks some mice have arteriolar hyalinosis and nodular glomerulosclerosis. It is thought that low dose STZ mitigates the toxic effects of the drug, although this is not completely certain. The Insulin-2 Akita mouse also has β-cell failure of the pancreas with the heterozygotes developing hyperglycemia, polyuria, and polydypsia at approximately 3 months of age (the homozygotes die at 2 months and, therefore, cannot be studied). The Non-Obese Diabetic mouse (NOD) is a model in which there is spontaneous autoimmune destruction of the pancreas at 5 months of age. There is a 4:1 female predominance of the disease in this strain. The major problem with the NOD mouse is that there is no good control group to study in parallel.

Since Type 2 diabetes mellitus, that form of the disease associated with insulin resistance and obesity, accounts for 90% of the cases of human diabetes, finding a good animal model is particularly important. Now we have several strains of mice, both mutants and transgenics which should prove useful experimentally. It should be noted that all mouse models, be they Type 1 or Type 2, have the disadvantage of being far more fragile than the Munich-Wistar rat studied by Brenner's group. Mice also respond very poorly to long term anesthesia. These difficulties have been overcome in at least one of the mutant strain which we shall discuss shortly.

Some of the mice with Type 2 diabetes include the Agouti yellow obese mouse, the New Zealand mouse, and several transgenics. There are now mouse strains transgenic for GLUT-1, one for ApoE, and another for advanced glycosylation end products. There is also a transgenic strain having endothelial nitric oxide synthase polymorphism. As stated, Breyer et al. (36) have reviewed these and other mouse strains in detail. They specifically point out those strains that develop diabetic nephropathy similar to that seen clinically in humans. The reader is referred to this very important review containing over 200 references.

The most widely studied of the animals with Type 2 diabetes mellitus and the only one thus far which can be prepared for micropuncture, is the db/db mouse. The nomenclature for the db/db mouse has been changed recently but for purposes of clarity we shall use the term db/db for the homozygote and db/m for the heterozygote [36]. The diabetic gene in these animals is transmitted as a recessive trait resulting from a G-to-T point mutation of the leptin receptor.

The db/db mutant strain exhibits many histologic features of diabetic nephropathy. At 10 weeks of age the mice begin to develop hyperglycemia. At 2 to 4 months of age features of diabetic nephropathy appears with a three-fold increase in mesangial matrix. Albuminuria of 70 to 600 micrograms/24 hrs also has been documented. Arterial hyalinosis has been described, but there is not yet evidence of the tubulointerstitial fibrosis seen in humans with longstanding disease.

Recently, David Levine's laboratory at the University of Ottawa has developed a stable preparation in the db/db Type 2 diabetic mouse [37, 38]. They have performed very careful micropuncture studies looking at intrarenal glomerular hemodynamics in the db/db animals before [37] and after uninephrectomy [38]. They have compared the results to heterozygous littermates (db/m) as well as to the wild type (WT) control strain from which they were developed.

Levine et al. [37] studied the animals at 10-11 weeks of age performing whole animal clearance studies, microalbumin excretion, and micropuncture of the superficial cortical nephrons at two sites for proximal and distal SN_{GFR}. Histopathology was performed on a separate group of identically treated animals when they were 30-40 wks of age. At the time of the micropuncture study, the animals varied in weight from 34gm to 51gm, with the highest weight noted in the db/db mutant. Results of the whole animal data are shown in Table 3. Note that blood glucose was 266mg/dl in the db/db Type 2 diabetic mouse at the time of micropuncture. Urine flow was 3-fold higher in the homozygotes than the other two groups, being 10.5µl/min. Whole kidney GFR was almost two-fold higher in the db/db group than in either the heterozygotes or the WT while systolic pressure was identical in all three groups. Urine albumin excretion rate was highest in the db/db mouse measuring 303µg/24hr ($P<0.02$ from the other two groups). It was 83µgm/24 hr in the db/m group and 62µg/24hr in the WT controls. The micropuncture data are shown in Figure 2. Note first that the SN_{GFR} in the db/db group is significantly higher than either WT controls or the heterozygotes. In the db/db mouse SN_{GFR} was about 14nl/min proximally and 11.5nl/min distally.

It is possible to test tubuloglomerular (TG) feedback by subtracting the proximal SN_{GFR} minus distal SN_{GFR} in the same nephron [28, 37]. Proximal SN_{GFR} eliminates the TG feedback signal. Distal SN_{GFR} measured in the same nephron bypasses both the macula densa and the afferent arteriole and is a true steady state value. In WT control mice, proximal SN_{GFR} exceeds distal by approximately 16%. In the db/db mouse proximal minus distal SN_{GFR} was increased to about 25% ($P<0.05$ from the other two groups). The heterozygotes had a proximal minus distal SN_{GFR} value of about 11%, a value not different from their WT littermates. These results suggest that there was a "resetting" of feedback control in the diabetic mice. The mechanism involved in this resetting is not completely known.

Since alterations in nitric oxide release or action have been suggested to be involved in the pathogenesis of diabetic nephropathy, the group examined one aspect of the system. They gave an acute intravenous infusion of the specific neuronal nitric oxide synthase inhibitor (S-methylthiocitrulline) at a dose that had no effect on blood pressure (i.e., acute nitric oxide inhibition). There was a dramatic fall in proximal SN_{GFR} in the db/db mouse but distal SN_{GFR} in these animals did not change. In the heterozygous db/m and the WT control mice, both proximal and distal SNGFR were decreased significantly. One would expect such results if nitric oxide were of major importance in the hyperfiltration of early diabetes mellitus. However other studies including some of Levine et al. have underscored the importance of nitric oxide in the hyperfiltration of early diabetic nephropathy (A detailed discussion of nitric oxide dysfunction in diabetic nephropathy is provided in another chapter in this book).

Histopathology showed that mean glomerular diameter was significantly higher in the db/db group as compared the WT animals (95.4 microns vs. 75.6 microns, respectively, $P<0.001$). Glomerular diameter of the heterozygotes measured an intermediate value. Mesangial expansion was noted only in the db/db group, being two-fold higher than the heterozygotes ($P<0.001$); arteriolar hyalinosis and luminal narrowing were also noted.

Table 3. Type 2 Diabetes Mellitus in the db/db Mouse

Group	Blood glucose (mg/dL)	Body wt (g)	[+]GFR (μl/min)	Systolic BP (mmHg)	Urine flow (μl/min)
Homozygous (db/db)	266*	51*	422*	107	10.5*
Heterozygous (db/m)	100	25[a]	179[a]	95[a]	3.6
Wild Type (WT)	113	34	262	100	3.4

[+]Insulin clearance; N = >6 animals/group
*$P<0.02$ from heterozygous db/m or WT control
[a] $P<0.02$ from the other 2 groups
Microalbumin excretion, 303 μg/24 in db/db vs. 62 μg/h in db/m mice ($P<0.02$) @ 10-11 weeks old

(Data from Ref # 37)

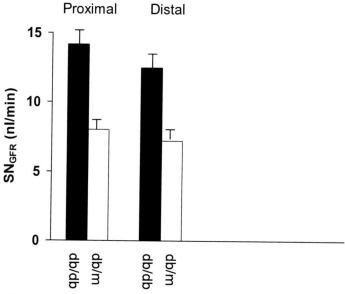

(Data from Ref # 37).

Figure 2. $SN_{GFR} \pm SE$ in db/db ■ homozygous and db/m □ heterozygous mice. The db/db mice were infused with 0.9% NaCl @ 4.0 mL/100g body weight/hr; the db/m mice were infused with 0.9% NaCl @ 3.3 mL/100g body weight/hr.

True nodules and interstitial fibrosis as seen in long standing human diabetic nephropathy, was not seen in these experiments.

In a second study Levine et al. [38] examined the effect of reduced renal mass in the db/db Type 2 diabetic mouse. The authors reasoned that a reduction in nephron mass would hasten the progression of diabetic renal disease, possibly by raising SN_{GFR} even further early on. The additional increase in SN_{GFR}, provoked by the loss of renal mass, would not be sustainable, however, and the glomerular hyperperfusion and hypertension would lead to an inexorable progression to renal failure. To decrease renal mass, right uninephrectomy (Nx) was performed in the db/db mouse at about 10 weeks of age. The animals were allowed to recover and were prepared for micropuncture 3 weeks later. Sham Nx was performed in a group of db/db littermates by only touching the right kidney intraoperatively. The results were compared to WT controls treated similarly. Detailed histopathology was performed in separate animals at 30 to 40 weeks of age.

The db/db Nx mice had an even higher whole kidney GFR and SN_{GFR} than did their db/db sham Nx littermates (Table 4). Histopathology showed a near linear increase in mean glomerular diameter at 15 to 30 weeks and an even higher value at 40 weeks. Glomerular diameter was greater in the db/db Nx group as compared to the WT Nx animals. While albumin excretion was not measured in this study, another early marker of diabetic nephropathy was — the mesangial matrix ratio. Mesangial matrix ratio was much higher in the db/db Nx than in the db/db sham group. These results suggest that a reduction of renal mass (i.e., uninephrectomy) exacerbated the progression of diabetic nephropathy.

Table 4. Uninephrectomy in the Type 2 Diabetes Mellitus db/db Mouse

Group	Blood Glucose (mg/dL)	Left Kidney GFR (μl/min)	SNGFR (nl/min)	Glomerular Diameter (μm)	Mesangial Ratio
db/dbNx (homozygous)	239	295**	17.9	95.8[c]	0.46[c]
db/db Sham	284	220	13.7[b]	NS	0.27*
Wild Type Nx	136[a]	269**	14.5	76.3	0.12
Wild Type Sham WT	151	177	12.3[b]	?	0.18

Nx = unilateral nephrectomy; inulin clearance for SNGFR (N = >6/group)
* P< 0.05 from WT sham
**P<0.02 from appropriate control
[a]P<0.05 from db/db Nx
[b]P<0.05 from appropriate control
[c]P<0.01 WT Nx
(Data from Ref # 38)

When neuronal nitric oxide synthase was inhibited chronically (by oral administration of S-methylthiocitrulline 24 μg/day for 2-3 weeks after Nx) there was no effect on SN_{GFR} or TG feedback. Thus, neither acute nor chronic inhibition of neuronal nitric oxide synthase altered TG feedback in the db/db Type 2 diabetic mouse. Schnermann [39] has shown recently that a knockout mouse for neuronal nitric oxide synthase in the macula densa had normal TG feedback activity. Similar findings have been reported in a thromboxane receptor knockout mouse. This is in marked contrast to knockouts for AT1 and ACE receptor where there is no TG feedback regulation [4, 39]. It may be that TG feedback is reset at a higher value in the hyperfiltration of early diabetes mellitus and that nitric oxide and Ang II are in some manner involved in the mechanism.

Possible Factors Leading to Hyperfiltration in Diabetic Nephropathy (Excluding RAA System)

A major question is whether the rise in SN_{GFR} in early diabetic nephropathy is the initiating factor leading the end stage renal disease or is it the final common pathway to chronic renal failure. If an elevated SN_{GFR} is the initiating factor, then what are the subsequent steps occurring at the cellular level which leads to end stage renal failure? If it is the final common pathway, what is initially turned on (or off) in the cell to cause the hyperfiltration?

When the "Hyperfiltration Theory" was first proposed by the Brenner laboratory, they felt it was the increase in glomerular pressure, which caused the rise in SN_{GFR} (Figure 3). This change, if left unabated, would overwhelm the remaining nephrons and lead to glomerulosclerosis by damaging the glomerular endothelial cells. An injury such as this would then cause an increase in flux of macromolecules especially to the mesangial cells (Figure 1). The enhanced flux, would in some manner, increase mesangial matrix and size. With time, nephrons would "drop out", the negative charge on the foot processes would be lost, and macromolecules (i.e., protein) would be lost in the urine. The combination of increased pressure and glomerular flow would only exacerbate this cascade.

The "Hyperfiltration Hypothesis" has been characterized as one broadly relating to physical or hemodynamic factors which will increase SN_{GFR}[40-44]. This is opposed to the many metabolic factors (i.e., uncontrolled hyperglycemia, advanced glycosylation end products, GLUT-1 activity, AngII, cytokines, growth factors) which may be involved in the rise in SN_{GFR}.

In this book there are separate chapters devoted to the role of various factors in the pathogenesis of diabetic nephropathy. These include the role of hyperglycemia and advanced glycosylation end products (Chapters 3 and 4) as well as the role of translational dysfunction (Chapter 5). In our view the role of the renin-angiotensin-aldosterone system (Chapter 6) is extremely important, very complex, and as yet not fully understood. Aspects relating to the role of growth factor activation (Chapter 8) could easily explain the rise in SN_{GFR}. Dysfunction of the nitric oxide system (Chapter 11) and oxidative stress (Chapter 10) are doubtless both crucial in the genesis of inflammation; an association with chronic inflammation and nephropathy has been recently advanced.

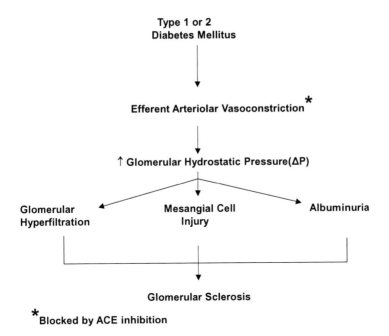

Figure 3. Schema whereby glomerular sclerosis could occur in diabetes mellitus. Once a certain degree occurs further renal injury would progress. Poor glycemic control would only aggravate intrarenal glomerular hemodynamics.

Any one or several of these factors in a genetically susceptible individual may be enough to tip the scale towards fulminate renal disease in diabetes mellitus.

We will concentrate on a physical process that increases flow and pressure on vessel walls and that is stretch or sheer stress. We believe this to affect growth factors and endothelial cell function and to be part of the pathogenesis of hyperfiltration.

Sheer Stress and Stretch

One of the major perturbations in blood vessels when there is an increase in pressure is a rise in wall tension and stretch. Such a rise may directly cause a cascade of events in each of the individual glomeruli and mesangial cells and this, in turn, may increase SN_{GFR} and affect matrix biosynthesis adversely. Narin's laboratory [45, 46] was one of the first groups to examine how pressure and stretch may be involved in the rise in SN_{GFR}. In rat mesangial cells in culture these investigators examined the effect of prolonged cyclic *in vitro* stretch on mesangial extracellular matrix (ECM) protein deposition Also examined was the effect of increasing perfusion pressure (from 0 to 200mmHg) on volume of isolated perfused rat cortical glomeruli. These authors found that, if one increased perfusion pressure *in vitro* from 60 to 100mmHg, values comparable to *in vivo* glomerular transcapillary pressures of 32 to 52mmHg, glomerular volume increased markedly from 8.3% to 17%, respectively($P<0.05$). Quantitatively similar effects were seen regardless of baseline glomerular volume.

When a stretch of 7% to 12% was applied to a cultured monolayer of human mesangial cells for 20 hours to 100 hours, a linear increase in total collagen synthesis occurred, indicating that the extracellular matrix was increased. When the specific components of the mesangial matrix were analyzed, enhanced production of collagen I, collagen IV, fibronectin and laminin was noted. While their studies did not examine the cellular mechanisms which may be involved, some of the possibilities include the generation of cyclic AMP or cyclic GMP, changes in cytosolic calcium, protein kinase C inhibition, and the enhanced release of specific growth factors.

Homma et al. [47] showed that *in vitro* stretch of 12% for 24 hours to cultured mesangial cells not only increased collagen production, but it enhanced non-collagen protein synthesis by 25%. Thus, not only did "stretch" increase synthesis of various components of the collagen family, it also caused the synthesis of new proteins. Addition of the growth factor AngII stimulated the synthesis of both protein fractions and did so even if the cells were not proliferating. Addition of epidermal growth factor was different as it increased only collagen production. Both growth factors stimulate phosphorylation of S6 kinase in mesangial cells when they are subjected to repeated mechanical stress. S6 kinase is the term used for a family of cyclic nucleotide serine/threonine kinases which act via protein kinase C mechanisms.

Both AngII and epidermal growth factor are important within the kidney [for reviews see Refs 4 and 48]. AngII stimulates EGF-dependent mitogenesis in the proximal tubule. In fact, the kidney is one of the major sites of epidermal growth factor biosynthesis. Receptors for this growth factor are found in mesangial cells, medullary interstitial cells, the basolateral membrane of the proximal tubule and the collecting duct. In early diabetes mellitus increases in epidermal growth factor may play a role in renal enlargement. Urinary excretion of this growth factor is increased 3-fold while its mRNA rises 4 to 8 times early in experimentally-induced disease [48]. The time course for changes in epidermal growth factor level may not be rapid enough to explain the early onset of hyperfiltration in early diabetic nephropathy.

Another growth factor thought etiologic in stimulating matrix protein synthesis in mesangial cells in response to repeated mechanical stretch is the cytokine transforming growth factor-beta (TGF-β) [4, 8, 42, 48]. There are several proteins in the TGF-β superfamily, including bone morphogenetic proteins, inhibins, and activins. These regulatory growth factors are unique in their broad effects on the extracellular matrix. They stimulate fibronectin, osteopontin, and thrombospondin production as well as inhibiting tissue collagenases. TGF-β actively modulates tissue repair and when present in excess leads to fibrosis. In addition to stretch there are a number of other stimulators of TGF-β which may be relevant to diabetes mellitus. They include AngII, uncontrolled hyperglycemia, advanced glycosylation end products, oxidative stress, and aging.

TGF-β 1 appears to be the isoform important in the kidney. All three of the isoforms and their specific receptors are present in the kidney[4]. If mesangial cells are subjected to *in vitro* stretch, first TGF-β 1 mRNA increases, then cellular TGF-β 1 rises, and finally mesangial matrix protein synthesis is stimulated [45]. When neutralizing TGF-β 1 antibody is added to the media the increase in matrix proteins does not occur [49]. While Yasuda et al. [49] also found an important role for enhanced TGF-β1 production in the proteinuria of diabetic nephropathy, they do not believe it to be the initiating factor primarily because the time course seems too long.

It seems clear that stretch (i.e., afferent arteriolar stretch), secondary to an increase in glomerular pressure results in one of the early findings of diabetic renal disease, that of mesangial expansion. It is likely that stretch, by increasing the size of the glomerulus results in damage to the foot processes. It would increase the space between the podocytes and decrease the efficacy of the negatively charged barrier of the glomerulus basement membrane, thus causing proteinuria.

Gruden et al. [50] indirectly examined the integrity of the negatively charged barrier by giving an infusion of vascular endothelial growth factor (VEGF) to rats and found that they developed proteinuria. These investigators also noted the presence of this growth factor in the plasma of patients with minimal change nephrotic syndrome. When human mesangial cells are exposed to stretch, VEGF mRNA more than doubled at 6 hours, findings much earlier than any effect of TGF-β 1 [50]. VEGF itself was tripled at 12 hours. Furthermore, when these "stretched" cells were preincubated with H7, an inhibitor of protein kinase C, VEGF levels fell by 75%. Preincubation with herbimycin A, a protein tyrosine-kinase blocker, caused VEGF levels to fall by 80%. These two inhibitors did not alter cell viability nor did they affect basal VEGF secretion. These results suggest that the VEGF system is extremely important in early diabetic renal disease. To further support a key role for this growth factor, if VEGF neutralizing antibodies are given to STZ-treated rats for 6 weeks diabetes associated hyperfiltration is fully abolished [52]. For reviews of VEGF biology, [see Refs 4, 48, 53]

Early in experimental diabetes mellitus, VEGF is up regulated. This growth factor is expressed in the mesangial cell and in the glomerular podocyte, as well as other parts of the kidney (54). It is also one of the most potent mitogenic factors known, and its activity is affected by many variables involved in diabetes mellitus. AngII stimulates its expression and biosynthesis in mesangial cells while preincubation with the A1 receptor blocker, losartan, prevents it. High glucose stimulates VEGF in vascular smooth muscle cells probably via a protein kinase C mechanism.

Genetics

Clearly, genetics affect the propensity to develop diabetic nephropathy. Genetics may predominate in the full expression of the disease or it may be a silent partner, contributing only when things begin to go awry [8, 55-57]. This seems to be true in either Type 1 (autoimmune destruction of the pancreas) or Type 2 (obesity, insulin resistance and aging) diabetes mellitus. Just as there are factors which make some individuals have the propensity to develop the disease and end organ damage, there must be factors which protect people as not all patients with the disease develop renal damage.

For Type 1 diabetes mellitus, there is evidence of genetic susceptibility on chromosome 3. For Type 2, susceptibility has been reported on chromosomes 10, 18, and 20 along with polymorphism to angiotensin converting enzyme. The genetic aspects of the disease and its relevance to nephropathy are discussed later in Chapter 12.

Understanding the genetics of diabetes mellitus is further complicated by the known strong association of the disease with that of "essential" hypertension. Furthermore, the extent of the interrelationships between activation genes and post-translational events are not known. The interactions may be so complicated that they can never be completely dissected. Because research in clinical medicine is so complex and diverse, those trained in one area may not have the expertise to attack a problem from varying and different perspectives. Thus, collaboration in clinical medicine is imperative so that a cohesive picture of the pathophysiology of this important disorder can be developed.

Hyperglycemia and Advanced Glycosylation Products

The role of tight control of blood glucose in the development of diabetic nephropathy continues to be debated. It appears that tight glucose control does not fully protect one against diabetic nephropathy in susceptible individuals. The advanced glycosylation end products resulting from prolonged hyperglycemia, however, may be important in mesangial expansion and loss of fusion of foot processes as these large molecules are continuously recycled and reabsorbed by the proximal tubule 54, 58). The topic is discussed later in this book.

Hypertension

A rise in glomerular pressure, even in the absence of hyperglycemia can lead to glomerulosclerosis and end stage renal disease. This was shown by Brenner's laboratory in the 1970s using the remnant kidney model (i.e., uninephrectomy followed 7 days later by infarction of the upper pole of the remaining kidney) [18]. When these Munich-Wistar rats were prepared for micropuncture 14 days later, clear differences in the glomerular hemodynamics of the remnant kidney model were noted as compared with the STZ-induced diabetic model [24]. Both models, with time, lead to proteinuria, nephrosclerosis, and chronic renal failure. Early, there is hyperfiltration with a significant increase in SN_{GFR} in the remnant kidney. This rise is due primarily to an increase in glomerular capillary pressure. Maneuvers which increase glomerular capillary pressure such as high protein diet or glucocorticoid administration lead to a further significant rise in SN_{GFR} and accelerate the rate of deterioration of renal function.

By contrast, maneuvers which decrease glomerular capillary pressure, such as chronic protein restriction or angiotensin converting enzyme inhibitors, protect the kidney from progressive damage.

Initially it was thought that any maneuver which lowered systemic blood pressure would automatically lower glomerular pressure (ΔP). Brenner's group (23, 59) addressed this issue in diabetic and non-diabetic animals. They gave another group of the remnant kidney animals hydralazine plus reserpine to lower mean arterial pressure to an equivalent degree. The measurements of glomerular hemodynamics were then repeated. The hydralazine/reserpine-treated animals were not protected because glomerular capillary pressure did not fall. Lowering the systemic blood pressure with these two pharmacologic agents vasodilated the afferent arteriole but they did *not* vasodilate the efferent renal arteriole. Consequently, the increased efferent pressure was transmitted back to the glomerulus. These results are very different from those obtained with captopril where systemic pressure falls to an equivalent degree. While captopril decreases afferent arteriolar pressure, it results in a *much larger* fall in the efferent arteriolar pressure, thus decreasing glomerular capillary pressure. It is this large fall in efferent arteriolar pressure which is unique to the angiotensin converting enzyme inhibitors and which may be the mechanism protective to the kidney.

Arguing against glomerular pressure causing the rise in SN_{GFR} and the subsequent cascade of pathologic events are results obtained with some drug models of nephrosclerosis. Fogo's group studied uninephrectomized rats given either puromycin or adriamycin for 2 months and showed that glomerular capillary pressure did not rise despite the development of proteinuria, nephrosclerosis, and renal failure [60]. In fact, with adriamycin administration, glomerular capillary pressure fell. Treating the animals with the angiotensin converting enzyme inhibitor, captopril, markedly decreased the severity of glomerulosclerosis without any change in glomerular capillary pressure. Fogo's group, well known for their precise morphometry, found that glomerular hypertrophy best correlated with the severity of glomerulosclerosis.

It would not be surprising if there were more than one important regulator of the rise in SN_{GFR}, i.e., not just increased glomerular capillary pressure. The more critical an event or factor is which sustains life, the more regulators there are to keep it within the normal physiologic range. Think of the many regulators there are which prevent lethal hyperkalemia, quickly shifting the ion inside cells as well as enhancing its excretion by the kidney.

Effect of Therapy on the Progression of Diabetic Nephropathy

Definitive therapy for reversal of diabetes mellitus and its myriad of complications, including nephropathy, is surgical. Unfortunately, pancreas transplantation is a viable option for only a minute number of patients now and this is not likely to change in the near future. In the United States in 2008, 705 kidney/pancreas transplants and only 307 pancreas transplants were performed [2]. By contrast, there were 13,743 kidney transplants done; a minority of kidney recipients had end stage renal disease due to diabetes mellitus. Recall that diabetic nephropathy is the leading cause of renal failure in the United States, accounting for more than 50% of patients, but most of these patients do not receive renal transplant; they remain on dialysis.

There is one study demonstrating the efficacy of pancreas transplant for diabetic nephropathy [61]. In this study, serial renal biopsies were performed for up to 10 years in 8 patients. Over this time period the authors found there was a gradual decrease in mesangial matrix and in the size of the mesangium. There was also a significant decrease in basement membrane thickness. Despite these optimistic results, pancreas transplantation as we know it today will never be a significant form of treatment for patients with diabetic renal disease.

Drug therapy will always be the mainstay of treatment for diabetic nephropathy. We include, but shall not discuss here the importance of weight loss and lipid control. Tight regulation of blood sugar, keeping hemoglobin A_1C to 6.5 or less is also obviously paramount.

Given the strong association of hypertension in diabetes mellitus and the huge pharmacologic armamentarium available, one has a wide variety of drugs from which to choose for patient treatment. The drugs, however, should be chosen carefully in the diabetic as some which prevent progression of nephropathy may not alone provide adequate blood pressure control. Moreover, drugs that effectively control blood pressure may not be "renoprotective." And finally, it may be necessary to use antihypertensive agents in diabetic patients who, by all criteria, have a normal blood pressure. In essence, we are saying that the drug chosen for both blood pressure control and protecting the kidney from further damage of diabetes mellitus may be the same initially, but added therapy may be required to achieve a desirable blood pressure of 120/70mmHg. We are also saying that one should treat normotensive patients with drugs that will lower blood pressure if certain markers of diabetic nephropathy are found.

The data in animals, and more importantly in humans, show that in order to prevent the progression of diabetic nephropathy and decrease microalbuminuria at the earliest clinical sign of nephropathy, drugs that inhibit the renin-angiotensin-aldosterone axis should be prescribed.

Currently we have four classes of drugs that fall into this category. They are the ACE inhibitors, the angiotensin receptor blockers (ARBs), and the anti-renin drugs. We also include the aldosterone receptor antagonists as an abnormally high aldosterone level appears to exert pathologic actions on certain cardiovascular/renal tissues, including the mesangium [62-65].

Very soon after Brenner's Laboratory published their results that controlling glomerular capillary pressure in rats with experimental diabetes, many small clinical studies appeared demonstrating that proteinuria and the rate of progression of diabetic nephropathy was ameliorated by the administration of ACE inhibitor therapy to patients. Brenner [44] has summarized some of them recently. Anecdotally, we know of a number of nephrologists who began using these drugs as first line therapy early in the 1980s in all their diabetic patients.

There are now many major clinical trials, both here and in Europe, examining the role of drug therapy in the prevention of the progression of diabetic nephropathy (two early landmark studies, one here and the other in the United Kingdom looked at the results of long term tight glycemic control) [66, 67]. While the role glucose control and renal disease continue to be debated there is no question it is important [68]. The initial large scale clinical trial using pharmacologic intervention was performed in over 400 patients with proteinuria (>500mg/24hr) and Type 1 diabetes mellitus [69]. The patients received the ACE inhibitor, captopril, or a "placebo". Blood pressure control in each group could be achieved with any therapies other than calcium channel blockers. The study was to last 5 years and the end points were time to doubling of serum creatinine, initiation of renal replacement therapy or death. The Collaborative Study Group reported their dramatic and efficacious findings of ACE inhibitor therapy in the *New England Journal of Medicine* in 1993 [69].

Subsequently, a 7 year follow up was reported in almost 100 patients with Type 2 diabetes given the ACE inhibitor, enalapil. The study showed all of the patients had microalbuminuria, a normal serum creatinine, and they were normotensive. In the placebo group, urine microalbumin doubled over the time period studied, but in the patients treated with ACE inhibitor, it did not. Patients in the EUCLID study (Type 1 diabetic nephropathy), the HOPE, BENEDICT, and ADVANCE studies (Type 2 diabetic nephropathy), numbering well over 12,000, all showed decreased microalbumin excretion with ACE inhibitors over the time period studied (see Ref 70 for original citations) [70-73].

The ACE inhibitors were developed in 1970 to be used in the therapy of hypertension. Their mechanism of action is specifically to inhibit the conversion of AngI to AngII, thereby interrupting the renin-angiotensin-aldosterone cascade in the kidney and adrenal cortex. Thus, these patients have low AngII levels and high AngI levels (they also have low aldosterone levels). At the time these drugs were synthesized AngII was well known to be a potent vasoconstrictor of vascular smooth muscle; the salt retaining properties of aldosterone were also well known. All forms of hypertension have either a volume or vasoconstrictor component (or both) and a class of drugs targeted to attack either component should be a very useful form of therapy. Thus, it was felt the ACE inhibitors would alter the vasoconstrictor component of hypertension. Forty years ago we did not know just how efficacious this class of drugs would be in the prevention of diabetic nephropathy, nor did we know of the many diverse actions this class of drugs seems to have. In the kidney, the ACE inhibitors appear to preserve renal function primarily by decreasing glomerular capillary pressure secondary to a marked fall in efferent arteriolar resistance.

In the early 1990s, a second class of drugs was introduced which also disrupted the renin-angiotensin-aldosterone axis, but by a different mechanism. These drugs are collectively known as "sartans" and are blockers of the AT1 receptor, hence the name ARBs, or angiotensin receptor blockers [73]. Patients who take these drugs have a high Ang II levels but it is unable to exert its action because the tissue receptors are blocked. In the kidney, these drugs lower glomerular capillary pressure by a mechanism similar to that described above for the ACE inhibitors. While they lower systemic blood pressure only modestly, their therapeutic window is very narrow. There are really only two doses one can use, the lower dose being at about the threshold of the dose-response curve, while the higher dose is at the plateau. This is rather unusual in the pharmacology of drug action and therefore, in our view, the drugs are of limited usefulness. Note that any other effect of AngII not mediated by the AT1 receptor (i.e., mediated by AT2 receptor, calcium, PKC, etc) will not be altered by ARB administration and indeed, could even be made worse because AngII levels rise significantly following the use of these drugs.

Now a number of studies clearly show that the ARBs are renoprotective and/or decreasing all cause mortality in diabetic nephropathy[74-79]. The combination of ACE inhibitors and ARB may be more beneficial [80-84], but there clearly are hazards [85].

As regards the third class of drugs, there is currently only one anti-renin agent on the market in the United States. Aliskiren (Rasilez®) is the first of a new class of antihypertensives that inhibits renin formation. The drug is orally active and patients receiving this drug should have low plasma renin activity, low AngII, and low aldosterone levels. It was thought this drug would be a breakthrough in blood pressure therapy and be renoprotective. Whether it provides long term protection in diabetic nephropathy is not yet known. Recent studies suggest that, at least in the short term, it does decrease albuminuria and that when combined with an ARB it is more efficacious [85-87].

One troubling finding of aliskiren is the observation that it stimulates *renal* renin secretion to a greater extent than either ACE inhibitors or ARBs especially when the drug is given at higher doses. We shall wait to see the role this class of drugs as regards the preservation of renal function both in diabetes mellitus and other proteinuric renal diseases.

The final group of drugs which affect the renin-angiotensin-aldosterone axis are the aldosterone antagonists. Here we have spironolactone, eplerenone and canrenone. These agents act by blocking the aldosterone mineralocorticoid receptors in various tissues, including the kidney. For years the drugs were given as a mild diuretic, primarily in salt-retaining states. In the last several decades it became apparent that these drugs were also useful in the treatment of heart failure because of their beneficial effects on cardiovascular remodeling [88, 89]. These effects are separate and distinct from the effects of ACE inhibitors possibly by decreasing cardiac and vascular smooth muscle fibrosis. Whether they are of value in decreasing the progression of diabetic renal disease is now being examined [90].

Hyporeninemic Hypoaldosteronism

In the late 1970s and early 1980s our laboratory at the University of Illinois College of Medicine in Chicago, identified patients who were admitted to hospital (either the University Hospital or the West Side VA) with hyperkalemia. We would scan the admitting lab work and if the patients had hyperkalemia, regardless of other diagnoses, we would further evaluate a number of aspects of renal function and endocrinology[91-94].

While there were many patients with hyperkalemia, a subset were those with diabetes mellitus and some degree of chronic renal insufficiency [88]. It now appears that fully two-thirds of patients with hyporeninemic hypoaldosteronism have diabetes mellitus, predominately Type 2.

Why this syndrome is seen in diabetes mellitus is not known but it has been suggested that prorenin is nonezymatically glycated, thereby rendering it inactive. Consequently, plasma and intrarenal renin release would be lowered. This would then decrease the conversion of AngI to AngII causing a fall in aldosterone release. These patients would develop hyperkalemia, a powerful and direct stimulus to aldosterone release. But there is no rise in aldosterone when these patients develop hyperkalemia. Why they don't respond is unknown. It's possible that either there is atrophy of the *zona glomerulosa* or that the vessels supplying the adrenal cortex and medulla are atherosclerotic such that the usual stimuli can no longer bind to their receptors and exert their actions.

Aldosterone is needed under normal conditions to allow the kidney to excrete adequate amounts of potassium when a subject is on a low sodium high potassium diet, i.e. the diet on which our species evolved. When on a high salt diet, non-aldosterone dependent potassium and acid excretion is sufficient to maintain homeostasis. Thus, aldosterone deficiency becomes clinically manifest under conditions of reduced distal sodium delivery. Thus, this disease requires both heart and renal disease to be expressed.

In general, the resulting hyperkalemia is not life threatening in most patients unless some intercurrent event such as heart failure develops. Treatment with the aldosterone analogue (Florinef®) is usually not required in patients with diabetes mellitus. The other feature of hyporeninemic hypoaldosteronism which may occur is Type IV distal renal tubular acidosis. This typically does require a small amount of bicarbonate therapy. Alternatively, the combination of increase salt intake with generous doses of loop diuretics can effectively treat the hyperkalemia and metabolic acidosis associated with this syndrome.

Integrating the pathophysiology of this interesting syndrome in our understanding of diabetic nephropathy is difficult. We eagerly await studies addressing this.

Summary

The pathogenesis of diabetic nephropathy is doubtless multifactorial. Hyperfiltration secondary to a rise in glomerular capillary pressure is key in increasing SN_{GFR} in early disease. It appears that physical factors, (i.e., stretch or sheer stress) lead to events at the cellular level which increase certain growth factors including epidermal growth factor, TGF-$\beta1$, AngII, and VEGF. All of these stimulate an increase in mesangial matrix either by stimulating collagenous or non-collagenous protein synthesis or both. This enlargement of the mesangium affects the glomerular podocytes and their negative charge on the glomerular basement membrane, thus allowing proteins to be excreted in the urine. The cascade for diabetic nephropathy is now set in motion. Identifying patients early so that regression of the renal abnormalities, not progression, is key [95].

References

[1] Bliss, M. (2005). Resurrections in Toronto: the emergence of insulin. *Hormone Research*, 64, 98s-102s.
[2] USRD. *2008 Annual Data Report: Atlas of Chronic Kidney Disease and End-Stage Renal Disease in the United States*. Bethesda, MD: US Renal Data System; 2008.
[3] Estacio, R. O., and Schrier, R. W. Pathogenesis and Treatment of Hypertension in the Diabetic Patient. In: Schrier RW, editor. *Diseases of the Kidney and Urinary Tract* (Eighth Edition). Philedelphia, PA: Lippincott Williams and Wilkins; 2007; 1351-1360.
[4] Khairallah, W., Merheb, M., Chaiban, J. and Badr, K. F. Hormones and the Kidney. In: Schrier RW, editor. *Diseases of the Kidney and Urinary Tract* (Eighth Edition). Philedelphia, PA: Lippincott Williams and Wilkins; 2007; 234-284.
[5] Nelson, RG. (2008). Kidney disease in childhood-onset diabetes. *Am J Kidney Disease*, 52, 407-411.
[6] Podymow, T; August, P. (2007). Hypertension in pregnancy. *Adv Chronic Kidney Dis*, 14, 178-190.
[7] Knauf, F; Aronson, PS. ESRD as a window in America's cost crisis in health care. *J Am Soc Nephrol*, 2009;20:2093-2097.
[8] Parving, H-H; Mauer, M; Ritz, E. Diabetic nephropathy. 8th ed. Philadelphia: Saunders, 2008.
[9] Kimmelsteil, P; Wilson, C. (1936). Intercapillary lesions in glomeruli of kidney. *Am J Pathology*, 12, 83-97.
[10] Perkins, BA; Krolewski, AS. (2009). Early nephropathy in type 1 diabetes: the importance of early renal function decline. *Curr Opin Nephrol Hypertens*, 18, 233-240.
[11] Brenner, BM; Troy, JL; Daugharty, TM. (1971). The dynamics of glomerular ultrafiltration in the rat. *J Clin Invest*, 50, 1776-1780.
[12] Deen, WM; Robertson, CR; Brenner, BM. (1972). A model of glomerular ultrafiltration in the rat. *Am J Physiol*, 223, 1178-1183.
[13] Brenner, BM; Troy, JL; Daugharty, et al. (1972). Dynamics of glomerular ultrafiltration in the rat. II. Plasma-flow dependence of GFR. *Am J Physiol*, 223, 1184-1190.
[14] Robertson, CR; Deen, WM; Troy, JL; et al. (1972). Dynamics of glomerular ultrafiltration in the rat. III. Hemodynamics and autoregulation. *Am J Physiol*, 223, 1191-1200.
[15] Deen, WM; Troy, JL; Robertson, CR; et al. (1973). Dynamics of glomerular ultrafiltration in the rat. IV. Determination of the ultrafiltration coefficient. *J Clin Invest*, 52, 1500-1508.
[16] Daugharty, TM; Ueki, IF, Mercer, PF; et al. (1974). Dynamics of glomerular ultrafiltration in the rat. V. Response to ischemic injury. *J Clin Invest*, 53, 105-116.
[17] Maddox, DA; Deen, WM; Brenner, BM. (1974). Dynamics of glomerular ultrafiltration. VI. Studies in the primate. *Kidney Int*, 5, 271-278.
[18] Deen, WM; Maddox, DA; Robertson, CR; et al. (1974). Dynamics of glomerular ultrafiltration. VII. Response to reduced renal mass. *Am J Physiol*, 227, 556-562.

[19] Myers, BD; Deen, WM; Robertson, CR; et al. (1975). Dynamics of glomerular ultrafiltration in the rat. VIII. Effects of hematocrit. *Circ Res,* 36, 425-435.
[20] Baylis, C; Ichikawa, I; Willis, WT, et al. (1977). Dynamics of glomerular ultrafiltration. IX. Effects of plasma protein concentration. *Am J Physiol,* 232, F58-F71.
[21] Briggs, JP; Kriz, W, Schnermann, JB. Overview of renal function and structure. In: Greenberg A, editor. *Primer on Kidney Diseases.* San Diego, California: Academic Press; 1998; 3-20.
[22] Hostetter, TH; Troy, JL; Brenner, BM. (1981). Glomerular hemodynamics in experimental diabetes mellitus. *Kidney Int,* 19, 410-415.
[23] Hostetter, TH; Rennke, HG, Brenner. (1982). The case for intrarenal hypertension in the initiation and progression of diabetic and other glomerulopathies. *Am J Med,* 72, 375-380.
[24] Zatz, R; Meyer, TW; Rennke, HG; et al. (1985). Predominance of hemodynamic rather than metabolic factors in the pathogenesis of diabetic glomerulopathy. *Proc Natl Acad Sci USA,* 82, 5963-5967.
[25] Zatz, R; Dunn, BR; Meyer, TW; et al. (1986). Prevention of diabetic glomerulopathy by pharmacological amelioration of glomerular capillary hypertension. *J Clin Invest,* 77, 1925-1930.
[26] Meyers, BD; Deen, WM; Brenner, BM. (1975). Effects of norepinephrine and angiotensin II on the determinants of glomerular ultrafiltration and proximal tubule fluid reabsorption in the rat. *Circ Res,* 37, 101-110.
[27] Baylis, C; Brenner, BM. (1978). The physiologic determinants of glomerular ultrafiltration. *Rev Physiol Biochem Pharmacol,* 80, 1-46.
[28] Arendshorst, W. J., and Navar, L. G. Renal Circulation and Glomerular Hemodynamics. In: Schrier RW, editor. *Diseases of the Kidney and Urinary Tract* (Eighth Edition). Philedelphia, PA: Lippincott Williams and Wilkins; 2007; 54-95.
[29] Ichikawa, I; Maddox, DA; Cogan, MG; et al. (1978). Dynamics of glomerular ultrafiltration in euvolemic Munich-Wistar rats. *Renal Physiol,* 1, 121-131.
[30] Morrin, PA; Bricker, NS, Kime, SW Jr; et al. (1962). Observations on the acidifying capacity of the experimentally diseased kidney in the dog. *J Clin Invest.* 41, 1297-1302.
[31] Bricker, NS; Morrin, PA; Kime, SW Jr. (1960). The pathologic physiology of chronic Bright's disease. An exposition of the "intact nephron hypothesis." *Am J Med* 28, 77-98.
[32] Seyer-Hansen, K. (1976). Renal hypertrophy in streptozotocin-diabetic rats. *Clin Sci Mol Med,* 51, 551-555.
[33] Jensen, PK; Christiansen, JS; Steven, K; et al. (1981). Renal function in streptozotocin-diabetic rats. *Diabetologia,* 21, 409-414.
[34] Imaeda, A; Kaneko, T; Aoki, T; et al. (2002). DNA damage and the effect of antioxidants in streptozotocin-treated mice. *Food Chem Toxicol,* 40, 979-987.
[35] Palm, F; Ortsater, H; Hansell, P; et al. (2004). Differentiating between effects of streptozotocin per se and subsequent hyperglycemia on renal function and metabolism in the streptozotocin-diabetic rat model. *Diabetes Metab Res Rev,* 20, 452-459.
[36] Breyer, MD, Bottinger, E; Brosius, FC; et al. (2005). Diabetic nephropathy: of mice and men. *Adv Chronic Kidney Dis,* 12, 128-145.
[37] Levine, DZ; Iacovitti, M; Robertson, SJ; et al. (2006). Modulation of single-nephron GFR in the db/db mouse model of type 2 diabetes mellitus. *Am J Physiol Regul Integr Comp Physiol,* 290, R975-R981.
[38] Levine, DZ; Iacovitti, M; Robertson, SJ; et al. (2008). Modulation of single-nephron GFR in the db/db mouse model of type 2 diabetes mellitus. II. Effects of renal mass reduction. *Am J Physiol Regul Integr Comp Physiol,* 294, R1840-R1846.

[39] Schnermann, J. (1999). Micropuncture analysis of tubuloglomerular feedback regulation in transgenic mice. *J Am Soc Nephrol*, 10, 2614-2619.
[40] O'Bryan, GT; Hostetter, TH. (1997). The renal hemodynamic basis for diabetic nephropathy. *Semin Nephrol*, 17, 93-100.
[41] Hostetter, TH. (2001). Hypertrophy and hyperfunction of the diabetic kidney. *J Clin Invest*, 107, 161-162.
[42] Remuzzi, G; Benigni, A; Remuzzi, A. (2006). Mechanisms of progression and regression of renal lesions of chronic nephropathies and diabetes. *J Clin Invest*, 116, 288-296.
[43] Wesson, DE. (2006). Moving closer to an understanding of the hyperfiltration of type 2 diabetes mellitus. *AM J Physiol Regul Integr Comp Physiol*, 290, R973-R974.
[44] Brenner, BM. (2007). Remission of renal disease: recounting the challenge, acquiring the goal. *J Clin Invest*, 110, 1753-1758.
[45] Cortes, P; Riser, B; Narins, RG. (1996). Glomerular hypertension and progressive renal disease: the interplay of mesangial cell stretch, cytokine formation and extracellular matrix synthesis. *Contrib Nephrol*, 118, 229-233.
[46] Riser, BL; Cortes, P; Zhao, X; et al. (1992). Intraglomerular pressure and mesangial stretching stimulate extracellular matrix formation in the rat. *J Clin Invest*, 90, 1933-1943.
[47] Homma, T; Akai, Y; Burns, KD; et al. (1992). Activation of S6 kinase by repeated cycles of stretching and relaxation in rat glomerular mesangial cells. Evidence for involvement of protein kinase C. *J Biol Chem*, 267, 23129-23135.
[48] Flyvbjerb, A. (2000). Putative pathophysiological role of growth factors and cytokines in experimental diabetic kidney disease. *Diabetologia*, 43, 1205-1223.
[49] Yasuda, T; Kondo, S; Homma, T; et al. (1996). Regulation of extracellular matrix by mechanical stretch in rat glomerular mesangial cells. *J Clin Invest*, 98, 1991-2000.
[50] Gruden, G; Thomas, S; Burt, D; et al. (1997). Mechanical stretch induces vascular permeability factor in human mesangial cells: mechanisms of signal transduction. *Proc Natl Acad Sci USA*, 94, 12112-12116.
[51] Cooper, ME; Vranes, D; Yousseff, S; et al. (1999). Increased renal expression of vascular endothelial growth factor (VEGF) and its receptor VEGFR-2 in experimental diabetes. *Diabetes*, 48, 2229-2239.
[52] De Vriese, AS; Tilton, RG; Elger, M; et al. (2001). Antibodies against vascular endothelial growth factor improve early renal dysfunction in experimental diabetes. *J Am Soc Nephrol*, 12, 993-1000.
[53] Ferrara, N; Davis-Smyth, T. (1997). The biology of vascular endothelial growth factor. *Endocr Rev*, 18, 4-25.
[54] Miner, JH. (1999). Renal basement membrane components. *Kidney Int*, 56, 2016-2024.
[55] Schena, FP; Gesualdo, L. (2005). Pathogenetic mechanisms of diabetic nephropathy. *J Am Soc Nephrol*, 16, S30-S33.
[56] Dronavalli, S; Duka, I; Bakris, GL. (2008). The pathogenesis of diabetic nephropathy. *Nat Clin Pract Endocrinol and Metab*, 4, 444-452.
[57] Pavkov, ME; Bennet, PH; Knowler, WC; et al. (2006). Effect of youth-onset type 2 diabetes on incidence of end-stage renal disease and mortality in young and middle-aged Pima Indians. *JAMA*, 296, 421-426.
[58] Lee, HB; Cha, MK; Song, KI; et al. (1997). Pathogenic role of advanced glycosylation end products in diabetic nephropathy. *Kidney Int Suppl*, 60, S60-S65.
[59] Anderson, S; Meyer, TW; Rennke, HG; et al. (1985). Control of glomerular hypertension limits glomerular injury in rats with reduced renal mass. *J Clin Invest*, 76, 612-619.

[60] Ikoma, M; Kawamura, T; Kakinuma, Y; et al. (1991). Cause of variable therapeutic efficiency of angiotensin converting enzyme inhibitor in glomerular lesions. *Kidney Int*, 40, 195-202.
[61] Fioretto, P; Steffes, MW; Sutherland, DE; Goetz, FC; Mauer, M. (1998). Reversal of lesions of diabetic nephropathy after pancreas transplantation. *N Engl J Med*, 339, 69-75.
[62] Simpson, SA; Tait, JF; Wettstein, A; et al. (1954). Constitution of aldosterone, a new mineralocorticoid. *Experientia*, 10, 132-133.
[63] Williams, JS; Williams, GH. (2003). 50th anniversary of aldosterone. *J Clin Endocrinol Metab*, 88, 2364-2372.
[64] Epstein, M. (2006). Aldosterone blockade: an emerging strategy for abrogating progressive renal disease. *Am J Med*, 119, 912-919.
[65] Sowers, JR; Whaley-Connell, A; Epstein, M. (2009). Narrative Review: The emerging clinical implications of the role of aldosterone in the metabolic syndrome and resistant hypertension. *Ann Intern Med*, 150, 776-783.
[66] The Diabetes Control and Complications Trial Research Group. (1993). The effect of intensive treatment of diabetes on the development and progression of long-term complications in insulin-dependent diabetes mellitus. *N Engl J Med*, 329, 977-986.
[67] UK Prospective Diabetes Study (UKPDS) Group. Intensive blood-glucose control with sulphonylureas or insulin compared with conventional treatment and risk of complications in patients with type 2 diabetes (UKPSA 33). *Lancet*, 1998;352:837-853.
[68] Marsenic, O. (2009). Glucose control by the kidney: an emerging target in diabetes. *Am J Kidney Disease*, 53, 875-883.
[69] Lewis, EJ; Hunsicker, LG; Bain, RP; et al. (1993). The effect of angiotensin-converting-enzyme inhibition on diabetic nephropathy. *N Engl J Med*, 329, 1456-1462.
[70] The EUCLID Study Group. (1997). Randomised placebo-controlled trial of lisinopril in normotensive patients with insulin-dependent diabetes and normoalbuminuria or microalbuminuria. *Lancet*, 349, 1787-1792.
[71] Mann, JF; Gerstein, HC; Yi, QL; et al; HOPE Investigators. (2003). Progression of renal insufficiency in type 2 diabetes with and without microalbuminuria: results of the Heart Outcomes and Prevention Evaluation (HOPE) randomized study. *Am J Kidney Disease*, 42, 936-942.
[72] Ruggenenti, P; Fassi, A; Ilieva, AP; et al; Bergamo Nephrologic Diabetes Complications Trial (BENEDICT) Investigators. (2004). Preventing microalbuminuria in type 2 diabetes. *N Engl J Med*, 351, 1941-1951.
[73] Sarafidis, PA; Bakris, GL. (2008). Renin-angiotensin blockade and kidney disease. *Lancet*, 372, 511-512.
[74] Parving, HH; Lehnert, H; Brochner-Mortensen, J; Gomis, R; Andersen, S; Arner, P; Irbesartan in Patients with Type 2 Diabetes and Microalbuminuria Study Group. (2001). The effect of irbesartan on the development of diabetic nephropathy in patients with type 2 diabetes. *N Engl J Med*, 345, 870-878.
[75] Brenner, BM; Cooper, ME; deZeeuw, D; et al; RENAAL Study Investigators. (2001). Effects of losartan on renal and cardiovascular outcomes in patients with type 2 diabetes and nephropathy. *N Engl J Med*, 345, 861-869.
[76] Mann, JF; Schmieder, RE; McQueen, M; et al. (2008). Renal outcomes with telmisartan, ramipril, or both, in people at high vascular risk (the ONTARGET study): a multicentre, randomized, double-blind, controlled trial. *Lancet*, 372, 547-553.
[77] Bilous, R; Chaturvedi, N; Sjolie, AK; Fuller, J; Klein, R; Orchard, T; Porta, M; Parving, H-H. (2009). Effect of candesartan on microalbuminuria and albumin excretion rate in diabetes. *Ann Intern Med*, 151, 11-20.

[78] Mann, JFE; Schmieder, RE; Dyall, L; et al. (2009). Effect of telmisartan on renal outcomes. *Ann Intern Med,* 151, 1-10.

[79] Rossing, K; Schjoedt, KJ; Jensen, BR; Boomsma, F; Parving, HH. (2005). Enhanced renoprotective effects of ultrahigh doses of irbesartan in patients with type 2 diabetes and microalbuminuria. *Kidney Int,* 68, L1190-L1198.

[80] Mogensen, CE; Neldam, S; Tikkanen, I; et al. (2000). Randomised controlled trial of dual blockade of renin-angiotensin system in patients with hypertension, microalbuminuria, and non-insulin dependent diabetes: the Candesartan and Lisinopril Miroalbuminuria (CALM) study. *BMJ,* 321, 1440-1444.

[81] Jacobsen, P; Andersen S; Rossing, K; Jensen, BR, Parving, HH. (2003). Dual blockade of the renin-angiotensin system versus maximal recommended dose of ACE inhibition in Diabetic Nephropathy. *Kidney Int,* 63, 1874-1880.

[82] Azizi, M; Wuerzner, G. (2007). Rationale for combining blockers of the renin-angiotensin system. *Semin Nephrol,* 27, 544-554.

[83] Sengual, AM; Altuntas, Y; Kurklu, A; Aydin, L. (2006). Beneficial effect of lisinopril plus telmisartan in patients with type 2 diabetes, microalbuminuria and hypertension. *Diabete Res Clin Pract,* 71, 210-219.

[84] Toto, R; Palmer, BF. (2008). Rationale for combination angiotensin receptor blocker and angiotensin-converting enzyme inhibitor treatment and end-organ protection in patients with chronic kidney disease. *Am J Nephrol,* 28, 372-380.

[85] Parving, HH; Persson, F; Lewis, JB; et al. (2008). Aliskiren combined with losartan in type 2 diabetes and nephropathy. *N Engl J Med,* 358, 2433-2446.

[86] Aliskiren trial in type 2 diabetes using cardiovascular and renal disease endpoints (ALTITUDE); ClinicalTrials.gov. Accessed October 16, 2008.

[87] Delea, TE; Sofrygin, O; Palmer, JL, et al. (2009). Cost-effectiveness of aliskiren in type 2 diabetes, hypertension, and albuminuria. *J Am Soc Nephrol,* 20, 2205-2213.

[88] Cooper, SA; Whaley-Connell, A; Habibi, J; et al. (2007). Renin-angiotensin-aldosterone system and oxidative stress in cardiovascular insulin resistance. *Am J Physiol Heart Circ Physiol,* 293, :H2009-H2023.

[89] Wei, Y; Whaley-Connell, AT; Habibi, J; et al. (2009). Mineralocorticoid receptor antagonism attenuates vascular apoptosis and injury via rescuing protein kinase B activation. *Hypertension,* 53, 158-165.

[90] Epstein, M; Williams, GH; Weinberger, M; et al. (2006). Selective blockade with eplerenone reduces albuminuria in patients with Type 2 diabetes. *Clin J Am Soc Nephrol,* 1, 940-951.

[91] Batlle, DC; Arruda, JAL; Kurtzman, NA. (1981). Hyperkalemia distal renal tubular acidosis associated with obstructive uropathy. *N Engl J Med,* 304, 373-380.

[92] Batlle, D; Roseman, MK; Sehy, JT; et al. (1981). Clinical and pathophysiologic spectrum of acquired distal renal tubular acidosis. *Kidney Int* 20: 389-396.

[93] Eiam-Ong, S; Kurtzman, NA. Renal tubular acidosis. In: Massry SG, Glassock RJ, editors. *Textbook of Nephrology* (Third edition). Boston, Massachusetts: Williams and Wilkins, 1995; 457-469.

[94] Batlle, D; Moorthi, WS; Kurtzman, N. (2006). Distal Renal Tubular Acidosis and the Potassium Enigma. *Semin Nephrol,* 26, 471-478.

[95] Fogo, AB. Progression versus regression of chronic kidney disease. (2006). *Nephrol Dial Transplant,* 21, 281-284.

In: Advances in Pathogenesis of Diabetic Nephropathy
Editor: Sharma S. Prabhakar

ISBN: 978-1-61122-134-3
© 2012 Nova Science Publishers, Inc.

Chapter IV

Experimental Approaches to Investigate Pathogenesis of Diabetic Nephropathy

Sharma S. Prabhakar[1]

Abstract

Nephropathy complicating diabetes is an important complication of both type I and type II diabetes and is the most frequent etiology of end stage renal failure. The currently used preventive and treatment options are far from being effective since majority of patients with overt diabetic nephropathy (DN) eventually progress at variable rates to end stage needing renal replacement. Although hyperglycemia and hypertension (both systemic and glomerular) play an important role in the pathogenesis, several factors have been incriminated recently and DN remains a vigorously investigated area in terms of etio-pathogenesis and hence interventions. While clinical investigations have helped us in understanding the pathophysiology and clinical prevention, most of our current knowledge of the pathogenesis has evolved from experimental investigations. Experimental studies to investigate pathogenesis of DN have mainly been of two approaches- in vitro experimentation using cell culture and tissue culture models and whole animal studies using models of diabetic models of type I and type II. Recent advances in knock out models and transgenic techniques have enabled investigators to refine the animal models to replicate human DN in them which lends to better understanding of pathogenesis and hence interventions targeting DN, both preventive and therapeutic. This review focuses on recent experimental advances that utilized both these approaches which contributed to our current understanding of pathogenesis of DN.

---

[1] Address for correspondence: Sharma S Prabhakar MD MBA FACP FASN, Professor and Chief, Division of Nephrology and Hypertension, Vice-Chairman, Department of Medicine Texas Tech University Health Sciences Center, Lubbock, TX 79430, T (806)743-3155 ext 252, F (806)743-3148.

Introduction

Diabetic nephropathy has swiftly increased in prevalence to lead the causes of end stage renal falure in most parts of the world. While the causes for such a steady increase remain multiple and debatable, the reasons why only about 30% of all diabetics develop nephropathy also remains an enigma. The genetics might play a role in such predisposition while factors in diabetic milieu are still quite instrumental in development as well as progression of diabetic nephropathy. Several chapters in this book are dedicated to a detailed discussion of such independent and individual pathogenic factors. Since significant gaps exist in our understanding of the pathogenesis, the current management options are effective in slowing the progression but cannot prevent or cure the condition. This has necessitated a vigorous search for new pathogenic pathways, signaling proteins and growth factors which have opened doors for new therapeutic targets [1]. Most studies to understand the pathogenesis of diabetic nephropathy were performed using in vitro studies in which conditions simulating diabetes are created in a cell culture or isolated kidney preparation. While such studies are in general useful to understand the impact of such individual factors on individual cells or tissues, there are several shortcomings of such in vitro observations. One of the major causes for the lack of understanding of the pathogenesis is the lack of a suitable animal model. In the past few decades several rodent and other animal models have been described with diabetes that go on to develop vascular complications including nephropathy. The development of genetic manipulation techniques such as knock out and transgenic approaches to animal experimentation has led to a rapid expansion of the knowledge base related to diabetic nephropathy. A detailed discussion of such cell culture and in vitro techniques and a broad overview of the animal models of diabetic nephropathy is the focus of this chapter.

In-Vitro Techniques

Cell-Culture Studies: Generally speaking, cell culture studies offer a pure and unique way of testing a hypothesis in a very controlled microenvironment. However the observations derived from such studies may not always be relevant to the whole animal especially in a disease state because of the complex interplay of several organ systems. Notwithstanding the shortcomings, cell culture experiments have been widely used to advance the knowledge of pathogenesis of various clinical disorders including diabetic nephropathy. Many renal cells have been studied both in primary cultures and established cell lines. The following paragraphs provide an overview of the commonly examined cell lines and some of the major contributions from such studies.

1. *Mesangial cells*: Mesangial cells play a vital role in the development and progression of diabetic nephropathy. Mesangial cell proliferation and mesangial matrix deposition in glomeruli are early ultrastructural changes in the diabetic kidney. Many investigators have evaluated the effects of various factors in diabetic milieu on the responses of mesangial cells (both murine and human) as they may play a direct role in the pathophysiological alterations of diabetic nephropathy. Mesangial expansion and hypercellularity is regulated by nitric oxide production amongst many other

factors. Besides mesangial cells are a rich source of inducible nitric oxide synthase. Experiments from our laboratory reported the inhibitory effects of high ambient glucose concentration on the mesangial nitric oxide synthesis. We further described that the mechanism underlying such an inhibition involved the stability rather than synthesis of tetrahydrobiopterin, a cofactor for NOS [2]. Several other studies using murine and human mesangial cells [3] have contributed significantly to our current understanding of the pathophysiology of diabetic nephropathy.

2. Renal microvascular endothelial cells: Because diabetic nephropathy is a microvascular complication of diabetes and endothelial dysfunction is an early feature of diabetic complications, there has been a significant interest in examining the renal microvascular endothelial cells to gain further insight into the pathogenesis of diabetic nephropathy. The recent availability of glomerular endothelial cells from both murine and human sources have lent a major support to investigation in this front. Since alterations in endothelial NOS are recognized as major contributors to diabetic nephropathy and since eNOS knock-out mice (vide infra) develop most features of human diabetic nephropathy, the initial focus of such investigation was to determine the effects of ambient glucose levels on nitric oxide production in glomerular endothelial cells [4]. More recent studies [5] have examined the role of several other factors such as angiotensin, prostaglandins, lipids and oxidative stress and their interplay in contributing to the endothelial dysfunction of diabetic nephropathy.

3. Podocytes: Podocyte loss in the kidney and podocyte excretion in the urine are features of early diabetic nephropathy The role of podocyte biology and alternations thereof have become the focus of investigation in the past decade in many glomerulopathies including diabetic nephropathy. A detailed discussion of podocyte abnormalities in diabetic nephropathy is presented elsewhere in a separate chapter devoted exclusively to this topic. Increased expression of GLUT-1 leads to glomerulopathy that resembles diabetic nephropathy. While most of the GLUT-1 expression is believed to due to mesangial cell effects, Zhang et al. [6] have examined the role of GLUT-1 expression in podocytes on mesangial matrix production. Two podocyte specific GLUT-1 transgenic mouse lines were studied. Interestingly, the authors found decreased mesangial expansion in diabetic transgenic mice. They concluded that increased podocyte GLUT-1 expression in diabetic mice did not contribute to early diabetic nephropathy. A recent review [7] illustrates how cell culture studies are being pursued to examine the role of inflammation in diabetic nephropathy particularly in cells other than macrophages such as podocytes.

4. Renal Epithelial cells: Renal epithelial cells especially proximal tubular cells have been extensively used to study the effects of mediators in the context of diabetes. Several investigators have invoked high glucose induced oxidative stress as a mediator of proximal tubule cell apoptosis. Recently Braznecianu et al. [8] has studied the mechanisms of reactive oxygen species (ROS) mediated apoptosis that leads to tubular atrophy in diabetic nephropathy. Using a human proximal tubule cell (HK2) line, the authors demonstrated that ROS induced by proteinuria resulted in tubular cell apoptosis and atrophy. In an editorial comment that followed this publication, Sanchez-Nino et al. [9] was pointed out that the discrepancy between such in vitro observations and mechanisms of human diabetic nephropathy preclude

extrapolating these concepts to human diabetic nephropathy. Ortiz-Munoz et al. [10] in a recent publication demonstrated the significance of inhibition of JAK-STAT signaling pathway by downstream target genes by suppressors of cytokine signaling pathways or SOCS (especially SOCS1 and SOCS3) These are activated in diabetic nephropathy particularly in proximal tubular cells and some glomerular cells and inhibit the JAK-STAT pathway. Brosius et al. [11] commented on this observation as a potential therapeutic target in diabetic kidney disease given the ongoing success of inhibitors of JAK2 pathway in meloproliferative disorders. Other investigators have shown the utility of studying tubular epithelial cells in identifying profibrotic processes such as epithelial-mesenchymal transition (EMT). Understanding the mechanisms underlying EMT and similar processes help develop therapeutic strategies to limit fibrosis in diabetic nephropathy [12]

Isolated Renal Tissue:

Isolated glomeruli and arterioles from diabetic animals have been studied to understand the pathophysiology of diabetic nephropathy. For instance the localization of ACE2 and its role in diabetic nephropathy was studied using this approach [13]. Functional abnormalities in isolated arteries from two different rat models of diabetes viz. STZ diabetic rats (type I diabetes) and Goto-kakizaki (GK) rat- a model of type II diabetes were the focus of a recent study. [14] In our laboratory, we have also utilized isolated renal tissue to examine renal nitric oxide generation in hyperglycemic rats specifically in response to angiotensin infusion to address the relative cortical versus medullary generation of NO (15)

Human renal biopsy tissue has also been utilized for purposes beyond histopathology. For example, Jiang et al. [16] demonstrated the role of Nrf2, a primary transcription factor that regulates cellular redox homeostasis provides a protective role in diabetic nephropathy. This observation was confirmed using Nrf2 knockout diabetic mice as well by the same investigators.

Proteomics:

Proteomics have found broad applications in kidney disease research and more specifically in diabetic nephropathy [17]. Proteomic methods helped to develop new insights into tubular and glomerular pathology and continue to uncover additional mechanisms of diabetic nephropathy [18].

Whole Animal Studies

While the information derived from cell culture and other in vitro techniques is valuable and has a unique place in understanding the pathogenesis of diabetic nephropathy, there are distinct concerns about the usefulness of this information in the context of interaction of these individual variables in the diabetic milieu and the whole animal or organism. Thus the ideal approach to understanding the pathogenesis is to study the natural history in humans or whole animals [19] and examine the contribution of various potential pathogenic factors and variables in the development and progression of diabetic nephropathy. For many decades in the past, animal models of diabetes were developed and were studied to understand the role of hemodynamics [20] hyperfiltration [21]and metabolic consequences of chronic diabetic state [22]. Over the years such animal studies also helped us understand the role of new pathogenic factors such as endothelin [23] as well as genes that predispose to renal injury as a consequence of diabetes [24, 25]. However a number of animal models of diabetes used up until recently to study renal disease had serious concerns such a lack of severe hypertension or progression of renal failure that precluded from being used as representative of human diabetic nephropathy. The past decades has witnessed a significant progress in the development of such models driven by mainly by the research needs and by support from NIH initiated Animal Models of Diabetic Complications Consortium (AMDCC).

Human Diabetic Nephropathy

To recapitulate, human diabetic nephropathy is heralded by increased urinary albumin excretion progressing to nephrotic state, development of hypertension and advancing renal failure. Histologically the disease is characterized by thickening of the glomerular basement membrane, mesangial expansion, arteriolar hyalinosis, tubulointerstial inflammation and fibrosis and ultimately glomerular sclerosis. A significant number of patients demonstrate mesangial nodules – typically focal or Kimmelsteil Wilson lesions, although it is less common in nephropathy from type II diabetes, where diffuse mesangial sclerosis is more common. Nephropathy in diabetes sometimes may be due a nondiabetic glomerular disease. Occasionally, a non-diabetic glomerulopathy may supervene over an established diabetic nephropathy and complicate the picture.

Animal Models of Diabetic Nephropathy

Over the past many decades several animal models of diabetic nephropathy were developed including murine (rats and mice), swine, baboon etc. However, the rat and mice models are the most commonly used animals for experimentation. Furthermore, there are animal models of type I diabetes and those with type II diabetes. But what propelled our knowledge in this field is the development of specific knockout and transgenic models involving particularly the mice [26]. Two Americans and a Briton won the 2007 Nobel Prize in medicine for developing the immensely powerful *"knockout" technology*, which allows scientists to create *animal models of human disease in mice.* the Nobelists are Martin Evans of Cardiff University, Wales; Mario R. Capecchi of the University of Utah; and Oliver Smithies of the University of North Carolina at Chapel Hill.

Problems with the Animal Models of Diabetic Nephropathy

The absence of progression, the lack of development of severe hypertension and inconsistent occurrence of hyperfiltration precluded the usage of the animal models hitherto used as representative of human diabetic nephropathy. The general problems with the use of animal models to simulate human diabetic nephropathy also include the lack of progression of albuminuria in most models. In addition, the use of different technologies to measure albumin excretion rates, and different units used in reporting further complicates the matter. AMDCC has recommended using Anti-mouse ELISA kits and reporting as µg/mg of creat. Using these criteria, db/db mouse and KK-ay mouse have the highest albumin excretion rates. Additionally from a histopathological perspective, thickening of the glomerular basement membrane and mesangial expansion is seen in most but not all mice models. Arteriolar hyalinosis is often absent due to lack of severe hypertension in most models. Diffuse glomerulosclerosis is seen often but not consistently in the mice models.

Transgenic Mice:

A transgenic animal is one that carries a foreign gene that has been deliberately inserted into its genome. Transgenic mice have provided the tools for exploring many biological questions including pathogenesis of diabetic nephropathy [27]. Two methods of producing transgenic mice are generally in use.

- -Transforming embryonic stem cells (ES cells) growing in tissue culture with the desired DNA;
- -injecting the desired gene into the pronucleus of a fertilized mouse egg

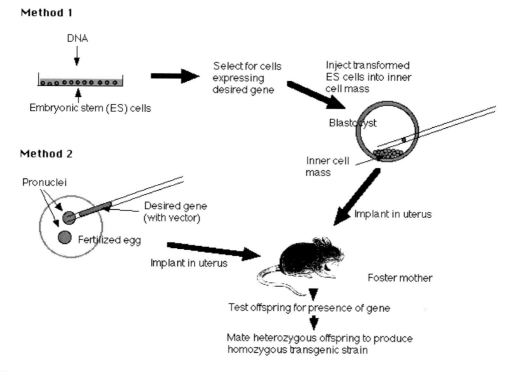

Figure. 1. Creation of a transgenic animal model.

Knockout Technology:

A *knockout mouse* is a genetically engineered mouse in which one or more genes have been turned off through a gene knockout. Knockout mice are important animal models for studying the role of genes which have been sequenced, but have unknown functions. Gene knockout technology in rats is much harder to accomplish, hence the paucity of such models but the last few years have witnessed a growth of rat knockouts of various genes yielding valuable research resources. However in general, the lack of adult mice limits studies to embryonic development and often makes it more difficult to determine a gene's function in relation to human health.

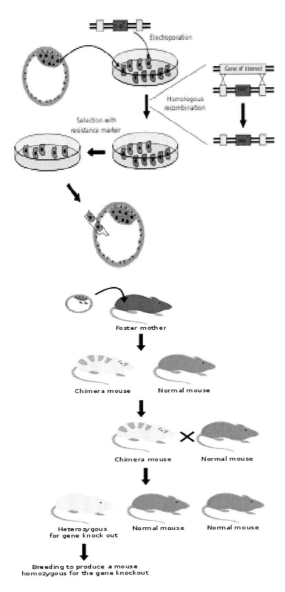

Figure 2. Creation of Knock out Model.

General Strains of Mice Used:

Amongst the mice models, C57BL/6 is the most commonly used strain and is the source of first mouse genome. This model demonstrates easily inducible obesity, diabetes and atherosclerosis. However it is resistant to renal injury. The db/db mice in this strain produces mild hyperglycemia and albuminuria.

The other common strain is C57LBKS: (16% genome from DBA/2 strain) db/db mice in this strain develop more florid changes of DN and with severe hyperglycemia and albuminuria. These mice also develop heart disease.

Specific Mouse Models of DN

As mentioned elsewhere in this chapter, there has been a lot of focus in the last few years on the mouse models of diabetic nephropathy more than any other animal species partly because of the better feasibility of developing transgenic and knockout models in mice than in other animals. But the complexity still remains in selecting the optimal model to examine the pathogenesis of diabetic nephropathy [28].

a) *Streptozotocin models* : Streptozotocin (STZ) has been used for decades to produce an insulin deficient state since STZ is toxic to pancreatic β islet cells thus producing a model of type I diabetes. C57BL is the most commonly used strain for this purpose since it yields a highly reproducible model with albuminuria and severe oxidative stress. The effects of STZ are greatly dependent on the dose. Thus toxicity of STZ is always a concern- higher doses resulting in toxic effects in many tissues including kidney. Besides it has mutagenic and biohazardous effects.. Lower doses yield diabetes in less than 50% animals and also yield lesser glomerular hypertrophy and mesangial expansion besides lower degrees of albuminuria. At such lower doses, podocyte loss often seen as a standard feature in diabetic nephropathy is not seen.

b) *Db/db mice:* This very commonly used mice model of type II diabetes is generated from the strains C57BLKS and C57BL [LeptR^{db}/LeptR^{db}] by manipulation of leprin receptor gene. Db gene encodes a mutation of leptin receptor . The resultant model develops hyperinsulinemia and hyperglycemia besides generalized glomerulomegaly, proteinuria, mesangial expansion, arteriolar hyalinosis. However there are also many limitations of this commonly used model . firstly the proteinuria is non-progressive and there is no GBM thickening. In addition they do not display interstitial or nodular sclerosis or even tubular atrophy. To complicate further they show immune complexes in glomeruli. [29].

c) *Ob/Ob mice:* In this mouse model, the mutation is in leptin (not receptor) and the animals exhibit more obesity than the other diabetic mouse models. However the renal structural and functional changes are mild.

d) *New Zealand Obese (NZO) mice:* These mice have polygenic inherited diabetes and obesity. Histologically they exhibit glomerulomegaly, mild GBM thickening and glomerulosclerosis . But evidence of autoimmune "lupus like nephropathy" with eosinophilic glomerular deposits in the kidney complicates the renal disease. It is suspected these features may represent a form of subacute arteritis that occurs in NZO mice.

e) *KK mice:* These are quite commonly used inbred Japanese mice with mild insulin resistance but the renal lesions resemble human DN. Insertion of Agouti allele into KK mice (KK-Ay) increases insulin resistance and leads to severe albuminuria, glomerulosclerosis. But yet, they do not exhibit significant renal failure. A specific variant of this mice, KK/Ta mice develop renal lesons that mimic human disease very closely [30].

f) *DBA/2J:* These mice develop diabetic albuminuria but no atherosclerosis. ardiac calcification is a problem in terms of pathogenesis and survival. The genetic mouse models of diabetic nephropathy described above along with other mice models are broadly reviewed in a recent report by Allen et al. [31]

Specific Monogenic Mutations in Mice

a) Apolipoprotein E: In mice with targeted disruption of APO E2 gene, elevated triglycerides and and cholesterol and atherosclerosis is observed. Interestingly APOE2- knockout in STZ C5BL6 mice develop severe diabetic nephropathy. So these models represent diabetic nephropathy in the background of severe hyperlipidemia and atherosclerosis

b) eNOS: Polymorphisms of eNOS (↓eNOS) has been demonstrated to be associated with advanced DN in experimental and human diabetic nephropathy. Renal disease in eNOS knockout diabetic mice is currently under active study. These animals however develop endothelial dysfunction [32] and severe HTN. Nakagawa et al. [33] has further defined the pathophysiological significance of eNOS knockout models in explaining the uncoupling VEGF and resulting in advanced diabetic nephropathy. Using these eNOS knockout mice Kosugi et al. [34] demonstrated that they develop advanced diabetic nephropathy and that they have less renal protection from renn angiotensin blockade compared to aldosterone receptor blockade.

c) GLUT1: Normoglycemic GLUT1 over-expressing transgenic mice develop glomerular gluco-toxicity which leads to albuminuria and mesangial expansion.

d) In addition, knockout technology was used in mice to examine and establish the critical role of osteopontin, a pro-fibrotic adhesion molecule. [35,36]. Recently Meier et al. [37] described how mice models with knock out of specific isoforms of protein kinase C help in evaluating the therapeutic potential of such an approach.

Rat Models of DN

Although many more mice models have been described, there are quite a few rat models developed to examine nephropathy in diabetes. Indeed, the knock out technology is now being extended to develop rat models to simulate human disease. Some of the commonly used rat models are described below.

a) *STZ rat*: These are the models for type I diabetes: renal disease significant only in spontaneously hypertensive rat (SHR) strains. In this model, the UAER or urine albumin excretion rate increases three fold. The STZ model can be established in genetically modified rodents for investigating the role of molecular mechanisms and genetic susceptibility in the development of diabetic nephropathy [38]. Several important observations came out of studies in STZ rat models. For example the role of AGEs in the development of nephropathy and other vascular complications of diabetes was evaluated using this model [39]. Furthermore renal effects of curcumin through inhibiting p300 and NFκB [40] and the ameliorative potential of angiotensin 1-7/Mas receptor axis [41] were described in STZ rat models. Using STZ diabetic Munich Wistar rats, Teles et al. [42] demonstrated that angiotensin receptor blockade not only prevent the progression but caused partial regression of glomerular lesions in diabetic nephropathy.

b) *Zucker Diabetic Fat rat:* -These are obese and diabetic (type II) rats and develop proteinuria, and renal failure. However the model is limited by development of hydronephrosis and only mild hypertension. Also to be noted is the fact that several of obese rodent models of type II diabetes are also obese and have been studied to examine the mechanisms of obesity related chronic kidney disease [43]. This model was also used extensively to study the role of PPAR-γ agonists in diabetic nephropathy as reviewed by Boulanger et al. [44]. A closely related species Zucker Obese rat was studied [45] to demonstrate that elevated intrarenal angiotensin II causes proteinuria by decrease in nephrin and glomerulosclerosis via TGF-β1 mediated matrix components.

c) *G-K rat:* These rats model for type II diabetes but no obesity, hypertension or hyperlipidemia. The renal disease is characterized by mild proteinuria, GBM thickening. No overt proteinuria or nephrosis or renal failure. Renal lesions mimic changes of aging in kidney [46].

d) *T2DN/Mcwi strain* Crossbreed of GK rats with FHH/EurMcwi *(Fawn hooded hypertensive non-diabetic rat).* These rats develop proteinuria at 6 m –18 m progressive (but less impressive than FHH) and mesangial expansion, GBM thickening, focal and finally diffuse GS, often with nodules (18m). However the problems include mild arteriolar hyalinosis, mild hypertiglyceridemia, no hypertension and no obesity. Renal failure by Scr measured by Jaffe reaction. [47].

Other Animal Models

A. *Pig:* Chinese minipigs fed on high carbohydrate and high lipid diet develop insulin resistance (using HOMA-IR index), hyperglycemia, dyslipidemia, albuminuria and glomerulosclerosis . However they do not develop renal failure. *(48)*. Swine models of diabetic nephropathy also have been used to evaluate the success of composite islet-kidney transplantation which may have a potential in patients with type I diabetes [49].

B. *Baboon*: This is a non-human primate STZ-model of DN. After 5 yrs of diabetes, they developed GBM thickening, mesangial expansion, which progressed to proteinuria by 10th year. Again, they do not exhibit renal failure *(50)*. The effects of calorie reduction and weight control on diabetic nephropathy was also demonstrated in non-human primates besides the rodent models of diabetic nephropathy [51]

AMDCC (Http://Www.Amdcc.Org)

Driven by the need to develop suitable if not ideal animal model to study the pathogenesis and treatment of diabetic nephropathy, the NIH came up with an initiative in 2001 and created the Animal Models for Diabetic Complications Consortium (AMDCC) to develop and test animal models with particular emphasis on the mouse models for diabetic nephropathy[52]. Mice were chosen because the knock-out models were easily developed in them and mice offer more flexibility for studying mammalian diseases than other species. Since its inception, this Consortium developed valuable information on the validation criteria for early and advanced diabetic nephropathy, current best models and negative models and future directions [53]. Such validation should significantly facilitate the understanding of the pathogenesis underlying the genetic mechanisms that contribute to the development of diabetic nephropathy as well as identifying potential therapeutic targets [54, 55]. Indeed animal models are now widely being used to evaluate traditional [56, 57] and nontraditional therapeutic agents [58] as well as to understand the mechanism of action of some the established therapies in diabetic nephropathy [59].

Criteria for an Optimal Animal Model of DN

A. >50% decline in GFR over life time of the animal
B. >100-fold increase in UAER compared to controls of the same strain, age and gender
C. Renal Histology: GBM thickening (>25% increase by EM morphometry), >50% increase in volume, Mesangial sclerosis, arterilolar hyalinosis, tubulointerstial fibrosis.

ZSF Rats- Basic Characters

In our laboratory, we characterized recently nephropathy in ZSF rats, a model of type II diabetes and obesity (60). Obese ZDFxSHHF-fa/facp model was developed by crossing lean female Zucker Diabetic Fatty (ZDF./fa) and lean male Spontaneously Hypertensive Heart Failure (SHHF/Mcc-facp, ./fa) rats. These rats are phenotypically normal until 8 weeks and then develop progressive obesity, hyperglycemia and hypertension after 8 weeks. Other features are nephropathy, heart failure and hyperlipidemia. The characteristics at 20th week are listed in the table below.

Phenotypic Features of ZSF Rats

As can be realized, they are very lipemic and hypertensive obese and hyperglycemic and thus provide an excellent model for metabolic syndrome. Hydronephrosis that is commonly seen with ZDF rats is rarely seen. The proteinuria and renal failure are progressive and result in end stage renal failure by 40 weeks of age by which time most glomeruli exhibit sclerosis. Ultrastructually the glomeruli demonstrate thickened basement membrane , mesangial expansion, arteriolar hyalinosis and sclerosis. These features are demonstrated in the figures shown below.

Table 1. Characteristics of ZSF1 rats at 8 weeks and 20 weeks.

	ZSF_1 (8 wks)	ZSF_1 (20 wks)
Body wt (g)	365±35	695±47*
Systolic BP (mm/Hg)	132±19	176±23*
Diastolic BP (mm/Hg)	88±8	103±11*
Plasma glucose (mg/dL)	126±12	196±22*
Serum creatinine (mg/dl)	0.77±0.19	1.47±0.25*‡
Creatinine Clearance (L/kg/day)	5.72±0.19	1.87±0.43‡
Proteinuria (mg/kg/day)	139±39	534±54* (80% albumin)
Urinary 8-OHdG (ng/day/kg)	746±110	5322±336‡
Total Cholesterol (mg/dL)	276±87	525±121*
Triglycerides (mg/dL)	369±62	1956±254‡
Tubular casts (0-4)	0	3+*
Tubular dilation/ atrophy(0-4)	0	4+*
Glomerular sclerosis(0-4)	0	1+
Arteriolar sclerosis(0-4)	0	4+*

N=12 in each group, * $P<0.01$ vs. 8 wks ZSF1-8 wk rats, ‡ $P<0.001$ vs. ZSF1 -8 wk rats

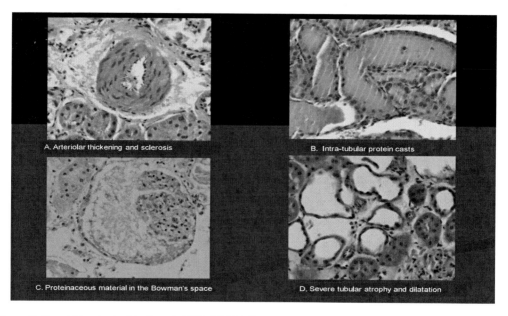

Figure 3. Renal histological lesions in ZSF (20 WKS) rats.

Experimental Approaches to Investigate Pathogenesis of Diabetic Nephropathy 61

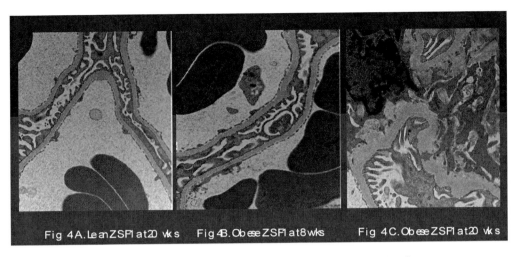

Figure 4 Electron microscopy of ZSF-1 rat kidneysGlomerular Basement Membrane.

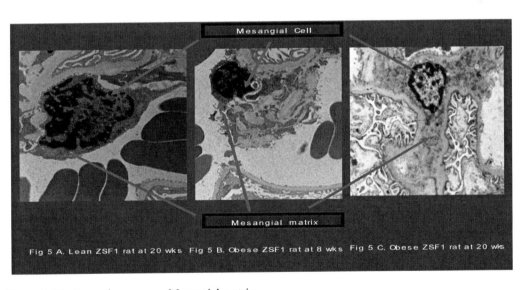

Figure 5. Electron microscopy – Mesangial matrix.

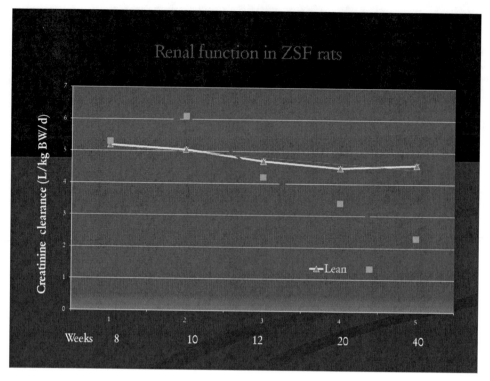

Figure 6. Renal function in ZSF rats – GFR.

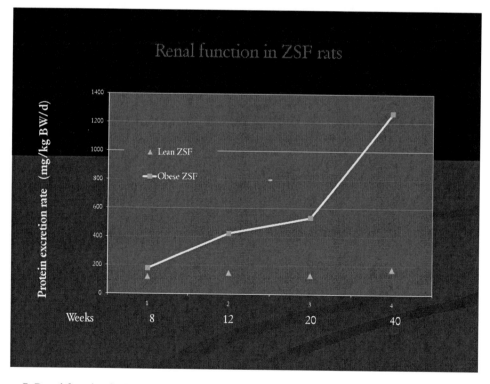

Figure 7. Renal function in ZSF rats – proteinuria.

Differences in DN in ZSF rat and humans

However there are some limitations to the ZSF rat as an ideal rodent model of diabetic nephropathy. These include

A. Rather rapid onset of nephropathy after development of sustained severe hyperglycemia
B. Lack of obvious glomerulopathy in the early phases
C. Lack of nodular sclerosis
D. Severe hyperlipidemia

We recently started investigating the functional genomics of diabetic nephropathy. At first we performed a meta-analysis of the publicly available and published studies and then compared the commonly misexpressed genes with those in obese diabetic ZSF rats. We found a significant correlation as reflected in the figure below.

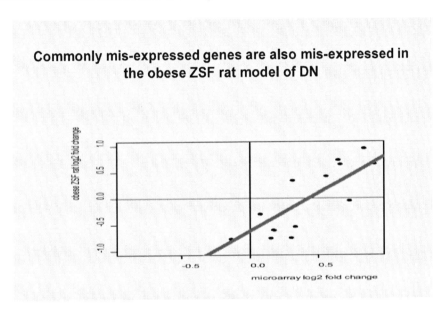

Figure 8. Functional genomics in diabetic nephropathy.

Plotted on the y-axis is the log fold change from the obese ZSF rats compared with lean rats at 16 weeks of age (established DN), while on the x-axis is the average log fold change calculated from the three different microarray experiments. The red line represents the best-fit line for the data

Summary

While diabetes is increasing in epidemic proportions and nephropathy from diabetes has become the most common cause of end stage renal failure, the pathogenesis of diabetic nephropathy remains incompletely understood. There has been an explosive growth of investigation in the past few decades to examine the pathogenesis of this condition from several approaches. Cell culture studies involving various cells derived from the kidney of both human and murine origin remain a major methodology to study the pathogenesis. Some of the significant clues to understanding the development of diabetic nephropathy were derived from such in vitro studies. Others have used isolated renal tissues and vasculature to further our understanding in this field. But the most significant advance in investigating diabetic nephropathy has been development of newer and better animal models that simulate human disease. The transgenic and knockout technologies have inspired formation of animal disease consortia that have been instrumental recent surge in the knowledge of pathogenesis of diabetic nephropathy (61). A sustained effort in utilizing all these and newer technologies is crucial to better defining the pathogenic basis and developing newer therapeutic strategies for this devastating condition.

References

[1] Flyvbjerg A. Inhibition and reversibility of renal changes: lessons from diabetic kidneydisease. *Acta Paediatr. Suppl.* 2006 Apr;95(451):83-92.

[2] Prabhakar SS. Tetrahydrobiopterin reverses high glucose mediated nitric oxide inhibition cultured murine mesangial cells. *Am. J. Physiol.* (Renal Physiology) 2001,281,p F0179-F0188.

[3] Prabhakar SS Inhibition of inducible nitric oxide synthase in mesangial cells by reduced extracellular pH is associated with uncpoupling of NADPH oxidation. *Kidney Intl.* 2002, 61 (5) 2015-2024.

[4] Hoshiyama M, Li B, Yao J, Harada T, Morioka T, Oite T. Effect of high glucose on nitric oxide production and endothelial nitric oxide synthase protein expression in human glomerular endothelial cells. *Nephron .Exp. Nephrol.* 95: e62–e68, 2003.

[5] Jaimes EA, Hua P, Tian RX, Raij L. Human glomerular endothelium: interplay among glucose, free fatty acids, angiotensin II, and oxidative stress. *Am. J. Physiol. Renal. Physiol.* 2010 Jan;298(1):F125-32. Epub 2009 Oct 28.

[6] Zhang H, Schin M, Saha J, Burke K, Holzman LB, Filipiak W, Saunders T, Xiang M,Heilig CW, Brosius FC 3rd. Podocyte-specific overexpression of GLUT1 surprisingly reduces mesangial matrix expansion in diabetic nephropathy in mice. *Am. J. Physiol. Renal Physiol.* 2010 Jul;299(1):F91-8. Epub 2010 Apr 7.

[7] Fornoni A, Ijaz A, Tejada T, Lenz O. Role of inflammation in diabetic nephropathy. *Curr. Diabetes Rev.* 2008 Feb;4(1):10-7.

[8] Sanchez- Marie-Luise Brezniceanu*, Cara J. Lau*, Nicolas Godin*, Isabelle Chénier*, Alain Duclos*, Jean Éthier*, Janos G. Filep, Julie R. Ingelfinger, Shao-Ling Zhang* and John S.D. Chan* Reactive Oxygen Species Promote Caspase-12 Expression and Tubular Apoptosis in Diabetic Nephropathy *J. Am. Soc .Nephrol.* 21: 943-954, 2010.

[9] Niño MD, Sanz AB, Ortiz A. Caspase-12 and diabetic nephropathy: from mice to men? *J. Am. Soc. Nephrol.* 2010 Jun;21(6):886-8. Epub 2010 May 6.

[10] Guadalupe Ortiz-Muñoz, Virginia Lopez-Parra, Oscar Lopez-Franco, Paula Fernandez-Vizarra, Beñat Mallavia, Claudio Flores, Ana Sanz, Julia Blanco, Sergio Mezzano, Alberto Ortiz, Jesus Egido, and Carmen Gomez-Guerrero Suppressors of Cytokine Signaling Abrogate Diabetic Nephropathy *J. Am. Soc. Nephrol.* 2010 21: 763-772.

[11] Brosius FC 3rd, Banes-Berceli A. A new pair of SOCS for diabetic nephropathy. *J. Am.*

Soc. Nephrol. 2010 May;21(5):723-4. Epub 2010 Apr 22.

[12] Simonson MS. Phenotypic transitions and fibrosis in diabetic nephropathy. *Kidney Int.* 2007 May;71(9):846-54. Epub 2007 Mar 7.

[13] Batlle D, Soler MJ, Wysocki J. New aspects of the renin-angiotensin system: angiotensin-converting enzyme 2 - a potential target for treatment of hypertension and diabetic nephropathy. *Curr. Opin. Nephrol. Hypertens.* 2008 May;17(3):250-7.

[14] Brøndum E, Nilsson H, Aalkjaer C. Functional abnormalities in isolated arteries from Goto-Kakizaki and streptozotocin-treated diabetic rat models. *Horm. Metab. Res.* 2005 Apr;37 Suppl 1:56-60.

[15] McMahon KW, Iznaola O and Prabhakar SS. "Angiotensin- nitric oxide interactions". In "Advances in angiotensin research" pages 35-68, Nova-Science Publishers, New York, 2008

[16] Jiang T, Huang Z, Lin Y, Zhang Z, Fang D, Zhang DD. The protective role of Nrf2 in streptozotocin-induced diabetic nephropathy. *Diabetes.* 2010 Apr;59(4):850-60. *Epub* 2010 Jan 26.

[17] Merchant ML, Klein JB. Proteomics and diabetic nephropathy. *Semin. Nephrol.* 2007 Nov;27(6):627-36.

[18] Thongboonkerd V, Barati MT, McLeish KR, Pierce WM, Epstein PN, Klein JB. Proteomics and diabetic nephropathy. *Contrib. Nephrol.* 2004;141:142-54.

[19] Shike T, Funabiki K, Tomino Y. Animal models. *Contrib. Nephrol.* 2001;(134):9-15.

[20] Cherney DZ, Scholey JW, Miller JA. Insights into the regulation of renal hemodynamic function in diabetic mellitus. *Curr. Diabetes Rev.* 2008 Nov;4(4):280-90.

[21] Levine DZ. Can rodent models of diabetic kidney disease clarify the significance of earlyhyperfiltration?: recognizing clinical and experimental uncertainties. *Clin. Sci.* (Lond). 2008 Jan;114(2):109-18.

[22] Schena FP, Gesualdo L. Pathogenetic mechanisms of diabetic nephropathy. *J. Am. Soc. Nephrol.* 2005 Mar;16 Suppl 1:S30-3.

[23] Meli S, Bruno CM. Endothelin and diabetic nephropathy: a new pathogenetic factor? *Panminerva Med.* 2001 Mar;43(1):45-8.

[24] Gohda T, Tanimoto M, Watanabe-Yamada K, Matsumoto M, Kaneko S, Hagiwara S, ShiinaK, Shike T, Funabiki K, Tomino Y. Genetic susceptibility to type 2 diabetic nephropathy in human and animal models. *Nephrology* (Carlton). 2005 Oct;10 Suppl:S22-5.

[25] Breyer MD. Stacking the deck for drug discovery in diabetic nephropathy: in search of an animal model. *J. Am. Soc. Nephrol.* 2008 Sep;19(9):1623-4. Epub 2008 Aug 6.

[26] Tesch GH, Nikolic-Paterson DJ. Recent insights into experimental mouse models of diabetic nephropathy. *Nephron Exp. Nephrol.* 2006;104(2):e57-62. Epub 2006 Jun 19.

[27] Wogensen L, Krag S, Chai Q, Ledet T. The use of transgenic animals in the study of diabetic kidney disease. *Horm. Metab. Res.* 2005 Apr;37 Suppl 1:17-25.

[28] Schlöndorff D. Choosing the right mouse model for diabetic nephropathy. Keyidn Int. 2010 May;77(9):749-50.

[29] Kumar Sharma, Peter McCue, and Stephen R. Dunn Diabetic kidney disease in the *db/db* mouse *Am J Physiol Renal Physiol* 284: F1138-F1144, 2003.

[30] Tomino Y, Tanimoto M, Shike T, Shiina K, Fan Q, Liao J, Gohda T, Makita Y,Funabiki K. Pathogenesis and treatment of type 2 diabetic nephropathy: lessons from the spontaneous KK/Ta mouse model. *Curr. Diabetes Rev.* 2005 Aug;1(3):281-6.

[31] Allen TJ, Cooper ME, Lan HY. Use of genetic mouse models in the study of diabetic nephropathy. *Curr. Diab. Rep.* 2004 Dec;4(6):435-40.

[32] Nakagawa T, Segal M, Croker B, Johnson RJ. A breakthrough in diabetic nephropathy: the role of endothelial dysfunction. *Nephrol. Dial. Transplant.* 2007 Oct;22(10):2775-7. Epub 2007 Jun 25.

[33] Nakagawa T. A new mouse model resembling human diabetic nephropathy: uncoupling of VEGF with eNOS as a novel pathogenic mechanism. *Clin. Nephrol.* 2009 Feb;71(2):103-9.

[34] Kosugi T, Heinig M, Nakayama T, Matsuo S, Nakagawa T. eNOS knockout mice with advanced diabetic nephropathy have less benefit from renin-angiotensin blockade than from aldosterone receptor antagonists. Am J Pathol. 2010 Feb;176(2):619-29. *Epub* 2009 Dec 30.

[35] Nicholas SB, Liu J, Kim J, Ren Y, Collins AR, Nguyen L, Hsueh WA. Critical role for osteopontin in diabetic nephropathy. Kidney Int. 2010 Apr;77(7):588-600. *Epub* 2010 Feb 3.

[36] Heuer JG, Breyer MD. Osteopontin in diabetic nephropathy: signpost or road? *Kidney Int.* 2010 Apr;77(7):565-6.

[37] Meier M, Menne J, Haller H. Targeting the protein kinase C family in the diabetic kidney: lessons from analysis of mutant mice. *Diabetologia.* 2009 May;52(5):765-75. Epub 2009 Feb 24.

[38] Tesch GH, Allen TJ. Rodent models of streptozotocin-induced diabetic nephropathy. *Nephrology* (Carlton). 2007 Jun;12(3):261-6.

[39] Karachalias N, Babaei-Jadidi R, Ahmed N, Thornalley PJ. Accumulation of fructosyl-lysine and advanced glycation end products in the kidney, retina and peripheral nerve of streptozotocin-induced diabetic rats. *Biochem. Soc. Trans.* 2003 Dec;31(Pt 6):1423-5.

[40] Chiu J, Khan ZA, Farhangkhoee H, Chakrabarti S. Curcumin prevents diabetes-associated abnormalities in the kidneys by inhibiting p300 and nuclear factor-kappaB. *Nutrition.* 2009 Sep;25(9):964-72. Epub 2009 Mar 5.

[41] Singh T, Singh K, Sharma PL. Ameliorative potential of angiotensin1-7/Mas receptor axis instreptozotocin-induced diabetic nephropathy in rats. *Methods Find Exp. Clin. Pharmacol.* 2010 Jan-Feb;32(1):19-25.

[42] Teles F, Machado FG, Ventura BH, Malheiros DM, Fujihara CK, Silva LF, Zatz R. Regression of glomerular injury by losartan in experimental diabetic nephropathy. *Kidney Int.* 2009 Jan;75(1):72-9. Epub 2008 Oct 22.

[43] Mak RH, Kuo HJ, Cheung WW. Animal models of obesity-associated chronic kidney disease. *Adv. Chronic. Kidney Dis.* 2006 Oct;13(4):374-85.

[44] Boulanger H, Mansouri R, Gautier JF, Glotz D. Are peroxisome proliferator-activated receptors new therapeutic targets in diabetic and non-diabetic nephropathies? *Nephrol. Dial. Transplant.* 2006 Oct;21(10):2696-702. Epub 2006 Jul 31.

[45] Sharma R, Sharma M, Reddy S, Savin VJ, Nagaria AM, Wiegmann TB. Chronically increased intrarenal angiotensin II causes nephropathy in an animal model of type 2 diabetes. *Front Biosci.* 2006 Jan 1;11:968-76.

[46] Janssen U, Vassiliadou A, Riley SG, Phillips AO, Floege J. The quest for a model of type II diabetes with nephropathy: the Goto Kakizaki rat. *J. Nephrol.* 2004 Nov-Dec;17(6):769-73.

[47] Nobrega MA, Fleming S, Roman RJ, Shiozawa M, Schlick N, Lazar J, Jacob HJ. Initial characterization of a rat model of diabetic nephropathy. *Diabetes.* 2004 Mar;53(3):735-42.
[48] Liu Y, Wang Z, Yin W, Li Q, Cai M, Zhang C, Xiao J, Hou H, Li H, Zu X. Severe insulin resistance and moderate glomerulosclerosis in a minipig model induced by high-fat/ high-sucrose/ high-cholesterol diet. *Exp. Anim.* 2007 Jan;56(1):11-20.
[49] Vallabhajosyula P, Griesemer A, Yamada K, Sachs DH. Vascularized composite islet-kidney transplantation in a miniature swine model. *Cell Biochem. Biophys.* 2007;48(2-3):201-7.
[50] Thomson SE , McLennan S, Kirwan PD, Heffernan SJ , Hennessy A, Yue DK and Twigg SM. Renal connective tissue growth factor correlates with glomerular basement membrane thickness and prospective albuminuria in a non-human primate model of diabetes: possible predictive marker for incipient diabetic nephropathy Journal of Diabetes and its Complications, Volume 22, Issue 4, July-August 2008, Pages 284-294
[51] Stern JS, Gades MD, Wheeldon CM, Borchers AT. Calorie restriction in obesity: prevention of kidney disease in rodents. *J. Nutr.* 2001 Mar;131(3):913S-917S.
[52] Breyer MD, Böttinger E, Brosius FC 3rd, Coffman TM, Harris RC, Heilig CW, Sharma K; AMDCC. Mouse models of diabetic nephropathy. *J. Am. Soc. Nephrol.* 2005 Jan;16(1):27-45. Epub 2004 Nov 24.
[53] Brosius FC 3rd, Alpers CE, Bottinger EP, Breyer MD, Coffman TM, Gurley SB, Harris RC, Kakoki M, Kretzler M, Leiter EH, Levi M, McIndoe RA, Sharma K, Smithies O,Susztak K, Takahashi N, Takahashi T; Animal Models of Diabetic ComplicationsConsortium. Mouse models of diabetic nephropathy. *J. Am. Soc. Nephrol.* 2009 Dec;20(12):2503-12. Epub 2009 Sep 3.
[54] Miyata T, van Ypersele de Strihou C. Translation of basic science into clinical medicine: novel targets for diabetic nephropathy. *Nephrol. Dial. Transplant.* 2009 May;24(5):1373-7. Epub 2009 Feb 11.
[55] Breyer MD, Qi Z, Tchekneva EE, Harris RC. Insight into the genetics of diabetic nephropathy through the study of mice. *Curr. Opin. Nephrol. Hypertens.* 2008 Jan;17(1):82-6.
[56] Thompson CS. Animal models of diabetes mellitus: relevance to vascular complications. *Curr. Pharm. Des.* 2008;14(4):309-24.
[57] Bruno S, Cattaneo D, Perico N, Remuzzi G. Emerging drugs for diabetic nephropathy. *Expert. Opin. Emerg. Drugs.* 2005 Nov;10(4):747-71.
[58] Zhang J, Xie X, Li C, Fu P. Systematic review of the renal protective effect of Astragalus membranaceus (root) on diabetic nephropathy in animal models. *J. Ethnopharmacol.* 2009 Nov 12;126(2):189-96. Epub 2009 Sep 6.
[59] Shou I, Fukui M, Tomino Y. Efficacy of ACE inhibitor (captopril) on glomerular antioxidant enzyme activity and hypertension in diabetic hypertensive rats. *Contrib. Nephrol.* 2001;(134):74-8.
[60] Prabhakar SS, Shi Shuping, Starnes Joel and Tran Ruc. Nephropathy in a Novel Rat Model of Type II Diabetes Is Associated With Oxidative Stress and Decreased Renal Nitric Oxide Production. *J. Am. Soc. Neph.,* 18, 2945-2952, 2007.
[61] Breyer MD, Böttinger E, Brosius FC, Coffman TM, Fogo A, Harris RC, Heilig CW, Sharma K. Diabetic nephropathy: of mice and men. *Adv. Chronic. Kidney Dis.* 2005 Apr;12(2):128-45.

Chapter V

Role of Hyperglycemia and its Metabolic Effects in the Pathogenesis of Diabetic Nephropathy

Philip Abraham and Howard Trachtman[*]
Department of Pediatrics, Division of Nephrology,
Schneider Children's Hospital of North Shore-LIJ Health System,
Long Island Campus for Albert Einstein College of Medicine, New Hyde Park, NY, US

Abstract

Hyperglycemia is the cardinal abnormality that enables the diagnosis of type 1 and type 2 diabetes to be made. Although it triggers many other mediators and signaling pathways that are involved in the acute and chronic kidney damage observed in diabetic nephropathy, there is much evidence that high glucose per se is instrumental in this process. In experimental models, high glucose leads to increases in function and structure within the kidney. It has distinctive effects on cell survival and function in each of the specific intra-renal cell types, namely mesangial, endothelial, tubular epithelial cells and podocytes. High glucose directly promotes renal fibrosis and apoptosis. High glucose impacts on the production and activation of many growth factors starting with transforming growth factor-β and including connective tissue growth factor, and midkine. Increased glucose concentrations promote inflammation mediated by chemokines and cytokines and also stimulates the synthesis of reactive oxygen species that potentiate renal injury. Protein kinase C is central in many of these processes and its expression is also directly modulated by high glucose levels. The clinical impact of hyperglycemia is the subject of a vast literature. In this chapter select aspects of the problem are discussed including the impact of short- and long-term control of hyperglycemia on the development of diabetic nephropathy, whether there are pediatric antecedents to diabetic kidney disease that can be attenuated by improved control, and the effect of exposure to high glucose in utero on morphogenesis. In summary, there is ample evidence that

---
[*] Correspondence address: Schneider Children's Hospital Division of Nephrology 269-01 76th Avenue, New Hyde Park, NY 11040, TEL. NO. 718-470-3423, FAX. NO. 718-470-0887, Email: trachtma@lij.edu.

hyperglycemia is an important feature of diabetic nephropathy and that therapeutic strategies to optimize glucose control are likely to have clinical benefit.

Introduction

Hyperglycemia is the central metabolic abnormality in diabetes mellitus and it serves as the basis for making the diagnosis in both type 1 and type 2 diabetes. The primary goal of all treatments for diabetes is to achieve normal serum glucose concentrations in an effort to restore short-term well being and prevent long-term complications. The kidney is a major target organ in diabetes and control of hyperglycemia is considered a major component of any program to prevent the development of diabetic nephropathy (DN). This chapter will focus on the direct effects of glucose on renal function, the impact of high glucose concentrations on specific cells within the kidney, and detail the signaling pathways by which an elevated glucose concentration induces kidney injury.

There have numerous outstanding reviews that seek to provide either an overview of diabetic nephropathy (Adler 2004) or that focus on distinct aspects of diabetic renal disease. The main area of interest of this chapter will be experimental models of diabetes with targeted information on specific clinical effects of hyperglycemia. It is clear that hyperglycemia is the jump off point for numerous secondary metabolic and molecular changes that are associated with the development of DN. Most of these mediators and signaling are covered in detail in separate chapters in this volume. In an attempt to minimize overlap and redundant presentation of material, this chapter will be limited as best as possible to studies that involve changes in renal structure and function that are linked directly to high glucose levels in vitro or in vivo. Moreover, primary emphasis will be confined to reports published in the last five years.

I. Preclinical Studies

A. General Structural and Functional Effects of Hyperglycemia

1. Hypertrophy

Cellular hypertrophy is a key feature that develops very early during the pathogenesis of DN. Hypertrophy involves all components of the kidney including the glomeruli. In db/db mice, which are deficient in the leptin receptor and which are widely used as model of type 2 diabetes, stereological and light microscopy methods demonstrate increased surface area and length of glomerular capillaries [Guo 2005].

Recent studies have indicated a number of novel mediators that are linked to this process. High glucose stimulates protein synthesis in association with increased phosphorylation of eukaryotic initiation factor 4E binding protein and decreased phosphorylation of eukaryotic elongation factor 2. These events are dependent on phosphatidylinositol 3-kinase, Akt, and mammalian target of rapamycin (mTOR). High glucose reduces the phosphorylation of AMP-activated protein kinase and inhibition of this step reduces high glucose-induced protein synthesis. Inhibition of mTOR signaling with rapamycin lessens renal hypertrophy in mice with STZ-diabetes [Sakaguchi 2006]. A kinase inactive AMPK further enhances the high glucose-induced protein synthesis. In rats with type I diabetes, AMPK phosphorylation is reduced and associated with increased mTOR activity. Increasing AMPK phosphorylation with metformin, reverses mTOR activation and inhibits renal hypertrophy without affecting hyperglycemia [Lee 2007]. Decreased Akt activity and its downstream effector, mTOR, have been confirmed in rats with STZ-diabetes. Tight glycemic control and insulin therapy modulated these two signaling molecules and impacted on subsequent renal hypertrophy [Zdychová 2008].

The tumor suppressor PTEN, a negative regulator of the phosphatidylinositol 3-kinase-Akt pathway, also contributes to this pathway. Exposure of mesangial cells to high glucose reduces PTEN expression and similar changes are noted in animals with STZ diabetes. Expression of PTEN inhibited high glucose-induced hypertrophy in cultured mesangial cells [Mahimainathan 2006]. Phosphoinositide 3 kinase (PI3K)/Akt kinase is increased after exposure to high glucose and inhibition of this enzyme attenuated cell cycle-dependent (G0/G1 phase) hypertrophy and p21 WAF1 gene transcription triggered by the diabetic conditions [Chuang 2007]. The p38 MAPK/MK-2 signaling pathway does not appear to be involved in diabetic renal hypertrophy because knockout of this enzyme did not protect against hyperfiltration or hypertrophy [Park J 2008].

The role of hyperglycemia *per se* in triggering renal hypertrophy was evaluated in STZ diabetic Fisher rats that were treated with phlorizin, a sodium-glucose co-transport inhibitor. This treatment prevented proteinuria, hyperfiltration, and kidney hypertrophy but not glomerular hypertrophy. The later change occurs early after the onset of diabetes in the absence of mesangial expansion and persists despite improved glycemic control [Malatiali 2008].

Oxidant stress directly contributes to the development of renal hypertrophy and also acts as a mediator of other upstream signals that initiate diabetic kidney injury. Administration of N-acetyl cysteine or taurine prevented glucose-induced hypertrophy of renal tubule epithelial cells in association with attenuated activation of MAPK, JAK2, STAT1 and STAT3 signaling cascades. Moreover, these antioxidants increased cyclin D1/cdk4 activation and suppressed p21 and P27 expression [Manna 2009]. In addition to production of ROS, increased production of advanced glycosylation end products (AGE) in response to hyperglycemia may be involved in the initiation of renal hypertrophy in DN. In podocytes exposed to bovine serum albumin-AGE there was induction of p27(Kip1) mRNA [Rüster 2008]. This led to cell cycle arrest and hypertrophy of the podocytes that could be reversed by silencing RNA to p27(Kip1).

2. Hyperfiltration

Hyperfiltration is a characteristic feature of DN that precedes overt evidence of renal dysfunction, namely albuminuria, decreased GFR, and hypertension. It is conceivable that alterations in renal sodium handling contribute to the increase in GFR because increased expression of the epithelial sodium channel (ENaC) has been documented at 40 week old Otsuka Long Evans Tokushima Fatty (OLETF) rats, a model of type 2 diabetes [Oh 2007]. Increased expression of ENaC has also been demonstrated in vitro in human cortical collecting duct cells exposed to high glucose [Hills 2006]. In addition to high glucose, AGE produced in response to hyperglycemia may stimulate ENaC expression. In mouse renal cortical collecting tubule cells, exposure to AGE stimulated in a time and dose-dependent manner increased ENaC mRNA and sodium uptake [Chang 2007]. However, there are no comparable studies in the early stages of disease to determine the role of increased sodium reabsorption in the development of hyperfiltration.

3. Cell Specific Effects

It is clear from renal genome-wide gene expression studies that hyperglycemia induces different patterns of transcription regulation in two distinct models of diabetes – Goto-Kakizaki insulin resistant rats and Wistar Kyoto rats with STZ diabetes [Hu 2009]. High glucose also alters gene expression patterns in specific cells such as the podocyte [Han S 2008]. These findings provide the impetus to address the impact of high glucose on the kidney as a whole and in specific renal cell types. The later work may involve in vitro studies of whole kidney tissue samples or pure cell populations. Investigations of specific cell types may rely upon well defined cell lines established from non-human sources or cells isolated from clinical material.

A. *Mesangial cell function:* Mesangial cells are pericyte-like cells that are interposed between adjacent capillary loops are regulate glomerular filtration surface and that synthesize extracellular matrix. The function of these cells is profoundly altered by hyperglycemia. However, different alterations of the extracellular matrix proteins can have disparate effects on mesangial cells. If mesangial cells are grown on glucose-modified type IV collagen, they display reduced proliferation and migration and increased type IV collagen synthesis. In contrast, if mesangial cells are plated with type IV collagen exposed to the carbonyl compound methylglyoxal, they demonstrate decreased adhesion and migration. This underscores the broad impact of high glucose on the ambient environment and function of mesangial cells [Pozzi 2009].

B. *Endothelial cells*: Vascular endothelial cells are also adversely affected by high glucose. In primary porcine aortic endothelial cells, exposure to glucose (30 mM) decreased cell glycoaminoglycan content while concomitant treatment with high glucose and insulin increased release of glycosaminoglycans into the media [Han J 2009]. In addition, high glucose reduced expression of endothelial cell-selective adhesion molecule (ESAM). This change was also noted in glomerular endothelial cells in mice with STZ diabetes. The alteration in ESAM expression may contribute to glomerular dysfunction because ESAM knockout mice have increased albuminuria [Hara 2009]. Activated protein C (APC) formation, which is regulated by thrombomodulin, is reduced in endothelial cells of diabetic mice. The reduced APC leads to glucose-induced apoptosis in endothelial cells and podocytes. Finally, recent studies have shown that high glucose levels trigger the accumulation of the G protein-coupled succinate receptor GPR91 in glomerular endothelial cells and that this molecule acts via intracellular calcium, nitric oxide (NO) and prostaglandins to stimulate release of renin [Toma 2008]. Taken together, this work provides further evidence of specific adverse effects of hyperglycemia on the endothelium [Isermann 2007]. Reduced availability of NO is a hallmark of diabetic vascular injury. Within endothelial cells, adverse effects of high glucose are manifested as reductions in endothelial nitric oxide synthase (eNOS) expression and activity. In eNOS knockout mice ($eNOS^{-/-}$) with STZ-induced diabetes, there is reduced GFR, increased albuminuria, and exaggerated glomerulosclerosis compared to wildtype controls [Zhao 2006}. The contribution of NO deficiency may be more profound in the tubular regions of the kidney because control of blood pressure in STZ-diabetic eNOS$^{-/-}$ mice reduces glomerular injury without modulating interstitial fibrosis [Kosugi 2009]. However, the glomerular microcirculation may still be more sensitive than on the large aortic vessel [Mohan 2008]. The decreased production of NO by endothelial cells exposed to high glucose is linked to oxidative stress, namely increased production of superoxide, and contributes to increased expression of cyclooxygenase-2 [Aljofan 2009]. Increased levels of free fatty acids, which are observed in patients with diabetes, have no adverse effect of the enzymatic activity of eNOS in endothelial cells exposed to high glucose [Jaimes 2009]. High glucose directly reduces the levels of endogenous S-nitrosylated proteins like eNOS in endothelial cells [Wadham 2007]. A recent study suggests that a novel mechanism by which high glucose inhibits eNOS activity is by promoting increased interaction between heat shock protein-90 and inhibitor kappaB kinase [Mohan 2009]. Angiotensin II plays a role because administration of an angiotensin receptor type 1 blocker to STZ-diabetic mice leads to recoupling of eNOS activity with reduced production of superoxide and increased NO synthesis in the aorta [Oak 2007]. Augmentation of eNOS activity using a transcription enhancer (AVE3085) improved vascular function in rats with STZ-diabetes [Riad 2008].

C. *Podocytes:* In podocytes exposed to high glucose, there is a concentration-dependent increase in pp38 MAPK and phosphorylated heat shock protein 25. In rats with STZ-diabetes, glomerular pp38MAPK and phosphorylated HSP25 are noted after 1 week. The levels decline by 1 month and are below control levels at 4 months. This suggests that increased pp38MAPK and HSP25 is an acute adaptation to hyperglycemia in podocytes [Dai 2006]. Differential gene expression profiles in podocytes exposed to high glucose demonstrate increased expression of heme oxygenase-1, VEGF, and thrombospondin and downregulation of angiotensin converting enzyme-2 and PPAR-γ [Han S 2008].The structural integrity and phenotype of podocytes is altered by high glucose. Growth of podocytes on AGE-modified extracellular matrix or exposure to high glucose leads to movement of α-actinin-4 from the peripheral cytoplasm to inner actin filament complexes. The combined exposure to both high glucose and AGE additively decreased the amount of α-actinin-4 in the cytoplasm and suppressed mRNA expression of the cytoskeletal protein. α-actinin-4 transcription was not modified by either factor alone [Ha 2006]. Thus, high glucose in combination with AGE may explain the cytoskeletal changes that have been observed in podocytes in DN.

D. *Tubular epithelial cells:* In animals with experimental diabetes, renal epithelial cells are characterized by increased accumulation of glycogen in the distal tubule within 1 month of onset of disease [Kang 2005].

4. Fibrosis

High glucose *in vitro and in vivo* leads to thickening of the basement membrane, the cardinal sign of extracellular matrix accumulation, in retinal and glomerular capillaries [Cherian 2009]. Tight control of glucose levels is paralleled by reduced thickness of both basement membranes and lower levels of fibronectin expression [Cherian 2009]. High glucose-induced accumulation of extracellular matrix in diabetic animals correlates with GLUT-1 expression in the kidney of diabetic rats. Similar findings were noted in isolated mesangial cells [Ricci 2006]. There is evidence that mechanical stress within the glomerulus may contribute to the stimulation of GLUT-1 expression in mesangial and initiate the increased accumulation of extracellular matrix in the diabetic kidney [Gnudi 2007].

Hyperglycemia also leads to increased renal expression of SGK1 in the kidney of animals with STZ diabetes [Feng 2005]. The altered SGK1 expression potentiates the effect of high glucose and increases fibronectin formation in response to the diabetic milieu. Peroxisome proliferator activated receptor alpha (PPAR-α) may also modulate fibrosis in DN because knockout of PPAR-α in STZ diabetic mice resulted in exacerbation of DN with increased albuminuria and glomerulosclerosis [Park C 2006]. Transglutaminase plays a key role in renal fibrosis and DN. In cultured proximal tubule cells, exposure to high glucose stimulated increased expression of tissue transglutaminase and augmented epsilon (gamma-glutamyl) lysine cross linking [Skill 2004]. Effective inhibition of transglutaminase activity in STZ diabetic rats for 8 months was beneficial, evidenced by lower levels of albuminuria and less glomerulosclerosis and tubulointerstitial fibrosis [Huang 2009]. Increased tissue transglutaminase causes an NF-κB dependent increase in active TGF-β [Telci JBC 2009]. Because of the effects of high glucose on both mediators, this interaction may potentiate the pro-fibrotic actions of hyperglycemia in the development of DN.

High glucose may directly promote fibrosis by increasing expression of tissue factor, a key molecule in renal fibrin formation [Sommeijer 2005]. There is also increased expression of megsin, a novel member of the serine proteinase inhibitor superfamily, in mesangial cells of animals with DN. This proteinase inhibitor is induced by high glucose in cultured mesangial cells. Megsin may inhibit the enzymatic activities of matrix metalloproteinases-2 and -9 leading to mesangial matrix expansion [Ohtomo 2008]. In addition to direct effects of high glucose on the synthesis and degradation of extracellular matrix proteins, hyperglycemia may promote secretion of proteins by renal cells. In mesangial cells exposed to high glucose medium, constitutive protein secretion involving the Golgi proteins munc 13-2 and rab 34, is enhanced. Secretion of fibronectin can be abolished in response to high glucose by siRNA to munc 13-2 [Goldenberg 2009]. The p38 MAPK pathway may be involved in high glucose-mediated fibrosis because a p38 inhibitor can reduce fibronectin mRNA and protein expression in mesangial cells in vitro and lower the amount of fibronectin in glomeruli removed from rats with STZ diabetes [Jung 2008].

5. Apoptosis:

Apoptosis occurs via an extrinsic pathway that activates caspase 8 or an intrinsic pathway that activates caspase 9. The two pathways converge on caspase 3, the enzyme that executes the programmed cell death. Hyperglycemia causes apoptosis of mesangial cells, podocytes, and renal tubular epithelial cells. Induction of p38 MAPK is a pivotal element in this response. In mesangial cells, the apoptosis-promoting effects of high glucose are on the intrinsic pathway with increased mitochondrial release of cytochrome c and activation of caspase 9 rather than caspase 8 [Mishra 2005]. In vitro studies with mesangial cells indicate that Akt phosphorylation precedes p38 MAPK activation. Overexpression of constitutively active Akt abrogates high glucose induced p38 MAPK phosphorylation and silencing of Akt induces p38 MAPK phosphorylation. This suggests that Akt modulates p38 MAPK induced apoptosis and decreased Akt activation in chronic DN, due to altered heat shock protein 25 and PTEN activity, and may exacerbate diabetic nephropathy. In diabetes, expression of TNF-related apoptosis-inducing ligand (TRAIL) is increased within the kidney and high glucose sensitizes cells to the apoptosis induced by TRAIL [Lorz C]. Insulin growth factor binding protein-3 (IGFBP-3) mediates apoptosis in mesangial cells treated with high ambient glucose, an effect that involves blockade of Akt phosphorylation at threonine 308 [Vasylyeva 2005]. The renin-angiotensin system may also play a role in renal apoptosis in DN. In STZ diabetic rats, there is increased expression of angiotensinogen. The resulting activation of the renin-angiotensin axis leads to increased caspase-3 activity and apoptosis. Treatment with an angiotensin receptor blocker or insulin but not hydralazine reversed these changes. This suggests that high glucose leads directly to increased apoptosis via the renin-angiotensin system, independent of systemic hypertension [Liu F 2007]. Finally, endoplasmic reticulum stress, triggered by unfolded protein response genes, may also contribute to renal cell apoptosis in diabetes. In patients with mild DN, there is increased expression of the transcription factor XBP1 and the endoplasmic reticulum chaperones HSPA5 and HYOU1. These findings were replicated in renal epithelial cells exposed to high glucose [Lindenmeyer 2008]. While this response may initially protect cells from endoplasmic stress, sustained hyperglycemia may eventually lead to apoptosis. In patients with DN, renal tubular epithelial cells display increased expression of the scavenger receptor CD36 and increased apoptosis. In contrast, paucity of CD36 in proximal tubular epithelial cells is paralleled by diminished apoptosis [Susztak[a] 2005].

High glucose also induces apoptosis in podocytes in models of type 1 Ins2 (Akita) mice and type 2 (db/db mice) diabetes. The onset of podocyte apoptosis was triggered by the p38 MAPK-induced generation of ROS and loss of podocytes coincided with the onset of albuminuria [Susztak[b] 2006].

There are several counter-regulatory mechanisms that may antagonize the proapoptotic stimuli triggered by diabetes. GTPase Ras proximate 1 (Rap1b), which increases the activity of B-Raf, an antiapoptotic protein, is upregulated in hyperglycemic states [Sun 2008]. In contrast, in proximal tubule cells exposed to high glucose, the levels of Bcl-2 and GTPase Ras proximate 1 (Rap1b) activity are decreased. Further work is needed to determine whether Rap1b reduces apoptosis in DN. Wnt/catenin signaling protects glomerular mesangial cells against high glucose-induced apoptosis. High glucose downregulates Wnt/catenin expression and nuclear translocation of catenin and increases caspase-3 activity and mesangial cell apoptosis [Lin 2006]. Strategies to promote Wnt/catenin signaling might be beneficial in the treatment of DN. Finally, connexin43 may attenuate mesangial cell senescence induced by diabetes. RNA interference with connexin43 expression resulted in enhanced mesangial cell senescence in response to high glucose [Zhang X 2006].

It is also important to recognize the tight interplay between apoptosis and necrosis in glucose-induced cell death. Most studies have demonstrated apoptosis triggered by high-glucose. However, in LLC-PK1 cells exposed to high glucose, there is an increase in cytosolic calcium, and activation of the cysteine protease calpain leading to necrosis. Inhibition of calpain prevented necrosis. In contrast, inhibition of PARP activity noted at 24 hours after exposure to high glucose did not reduce cell necrosis [Harwood 2007]. This finding underscores the complex control of the type of renal cell death that occurs in the diabetic milieu.

B. Signaling Effects of Hyperglycemia

1. Growth Factors: TGF-β/CTGF/BMP/FGF-2

TGF-β is a key mediator of DN by promoting the accumulation of extracellular matrix protein in the kidney. It does this by promoting synthesis and inhibiting degradation of these proteins. In addition, TGF-β may modulate renal inflammation and other processes involved in the development of DN. This pro-fibrotic cytokine can act via SMAD-dependent and independent pathways and is covered in greater detail in other chapters in this book. High glucose stimulation of TGF-β is mediated at least in part by the transcription factor, upstream stimulatory factor 2 (USF2), which binds to an 18 base pair sequence of the thrombospondin gene. Overexpression of USF2 in transgenic mice leads to more severe DN compared to wild type controls, manifested by increased albuminuria glomerular hypertrophy and increased glomerular accumulation of fibronectin [Liu S 2007]. The regulation of TGF-β expression by glucose is mediated by a number of other novel factors including angiogenesis inhibitors such as vasohibin-1 (VASH-1). Enhanced expression of VASH-1 in cultured murine mesangial cells suppresses the increase in TGF-β in response to high ambient glucose levels [Nasu 2009]. Recent studies suggest that specific microRNA molecules expressed in the kidney may mediate the effects of high glucose on TGF-β in diabetes [Kato 2009]. High glucose stimulates mRNA expression of connective tissue growth factor (CTGF) and production of extracellular matrix in human vascular smooth muscle cells [Liu X 2007]. This is important because CTGF appears to be an important downstream mediator of the deleterious actions of TGF-β in the development of DN. The impact of high glucose on CTGF expression has served as the impetus for ongoing clinical trials of an anti-CTGF antibody in the treatment of early DN.

BMP-7 is a member of the TGF superfamily of proteins and is also implicated in DN. In streptozocin (STZ)-diabetic rats, the reduced BMP-7 and BMP-7 type II receptor expression in the kidney, was reversed by treatment with insulin of phloridizin through correction of the hyperglycemia [Yeh 2009].

VEGF has also been implicated in the development of DN. Both high and low levels of this growth factor have been described in experimental models of DN and in clinical specimens. In immortalized proximal tubule cells, high glucose blunted the expression of VEGF mRNA and protein in response to hypoxic conditions (1% O_2 for 24 hours) [Katavetin 2006]. This change was paralleled by reduced involvement of the hypoxia inducible factor/hypoxia-response element.

Basic fibroblast growth facror-2 (bFGF-2), which plays a role in renal fibrosis, is upregulated within the renal interstitium of kidneys removed from patients with DN compared to controls. Fibroblasts grown in high glucose medium had increased bFGF-2 mRNA expression and higher proliferation rates that were reversed by addition of anti-bFGF-2 antibody. The effects of bFGF-2 may be mediated by PKC-β1 [Vasko 2009].

Less recognized growth factors have also been linked to DN. In mice with knockout of midkine, a growth factor involved in inflammation, the severity of STZ-induced DN was less based on reduced levels of collagen, diminished expression of monocyte chemoattractant protein-1 (MCP-1), and less infiltration of macrophages into the renal interstitium [Kosugi 2007]. Pigment epithelium-derived factor (PEDF), an inhibitor of angiogenesis, is decreased at the level of mRNA and protein in the diabetic kidney [Wang 2005]. High glucose inhibits

PEDF release in human mesangial cells. Because PEDF inhibits high-glucose induced activation of TGF-β, deficiency of this growth factor might be instrumental in promoting DN.

A variety of signaling molecules may transduce the cytokine effects triggered by high glucose including JUN and p38. Stat3 may also play a role because DN is less severe in modified Stat3 knockout mice with STZ diabetes [Lu 2009]

2. Cytokines/Chemokines

Chemokines, such as monocyte chemoattractract protein-1 (MCP-1), have been demonstrated to be both diagnostic and therapeutic targets in DN [Tesch 2008]. High glucose stimulates the expression of the chemokine macrophage inflammatory protein-3 alpha (MIP-3α) in cultured human proximal tubule epithelial cells [Qi[a] 2007]. Similarly MIP-3α expression is increased in dilated tubules of diabetic rats. The induction of MIP-3α by high glucose was attenuated by the administration of an anti-TGFβ antibody or an angiotensin converting enzyme inhibitor [Qi[a] 2007]. Alternatively the expression of another chemokine, MCP-1, also induced by high glucose, is suppressed by1,25(OH)$_2$-Vitamin D$_3$, acting via NF-κB [Zhang Z 2007].

Furthermore, the chemokine migration inhibitory factor (MIF) is expressed at higher levels in the kidney of animals with DN. Interestingly, CD74, the molecule that transduces the signal from MIF, is increased in glomeruli and tubules of renal tissue specimens obtained from Pima Indians with type 2 diabetes. Immunohistochemical studies localized the CD74 to the podocyte [Sanchez-Niño 2008]. High glucose induces CD74 in human proximal tubule cells and subsequent addition of MIF led to activation of MCP-1 [Sanchez-Niño 2008].

3. Reactive Oxygen Molecules (ROS)/Oxidant Stress

Systemic and kidney-specific oxidant stress has been detected in diabetes using various markers. The mitochondrion may be a key source of this pathway for organ damage. In a rat proximal tubule cell line, high glucose induced superoxide production and hyperpolarization in mitochondria. These adverse effects were completely prevented by overexpression of manganese superoxide [Munusamy 2009]. Advanced glycosylation end products (AGE) produced in response to high glucose stimulate the mitochondrial production of superoxide [Coughlan[a] 2009]. Reduction of AGE production by alagebrium, pharmacologic inhibition of AGE-receptor for AGE (RAGE) interaction, or RAGE deficiency abrogated the increase release of ROS [Coughlan[a] 2009; Coughlan[b] 2009]. Asataxanthin, a carotenoid, can reduce production of reactive oxygen species, activation of AP-1 and NF-κB, and expression of TGFβ-1by mesangial cells exposed to high glucose [Manabe 2008]. Similarly, urocortin, a 40 amino acid peptide related to corticotrophin-releasing factor that suppresses reactive oxygen species production in endothelial cells, lowered mitochondrial production of superoxide and diminished mesangial matrix expansion, in db/db mice, a model of type 2 diabetes [Li 2008]. The enzyme NADPH oxidase (NOX) is upregulated in STZ diabetes after 8 weeks and is another means of producing reactive oxygen molecules. Similarly, high glucose induces NOX in mesangial cells in vitro [Xu M 2009]. The oxidant stress that develops in mesangial cell exposed to high glucose is mediated by TGF-β which activates PKC isozymes and consequent production of reactive oxygen molecules by NOX [Xia 2008]. The ROS produced in response to high glucose transducer amplifies glucose signaling and contributes to renal fibrosis by stimulating epithelial-mesenchymal transformation and accumulation of extracellular matrix proteins [Ha 2006].

High glucose induces the expression of thioredoxin interacting protein and CDK7, a thiol related gene, in renal epithelial cells and mesangial cells respectively [Qi[b] 2007]. The expression of thioredoxin interacting protein, but not thioredoxin, is increased within proximal tubules in the cortex [Advani 2009]. While high glucose induced increased expression of thioredoxin interacting protein in NRK (proximal) and MDCK (distal) cell lines, thioredoxin expression was diminished in mesangial cells [Advani 2009]. The high glucose-induced expression of thioredoxin-interacting protein in proximal tubule cells *in vitro* and in rats with STZ diabetes is mediated by Kruppel-like factor 6 and PPAR-γ in a positive and negative manner, respectively [Qi 2009]. These are among the various antioxidant molecules that have been implicated in the modulation of oxidant stress with the renal parenchyma.

In db/db mice, there is increased expression of poly-ADP-ribose polymerase (PARP), an enzyme associated with oxidative stress. PARP activation leads to depletion of NAD+, slowing the rate of glycolysis, electron transport and ATP generation and leads to endothelial dysfunction [Pacher 2005]. Administration of two structurally unrelated PARP inhibitors ameliorated DN with lower albuminuria, less mesangial expansion, and diminished podocyte apoptosis and loss [Szabó 2006]. The last effect was mediated by prevention of PKC and NF-κB activation in podocytes [Pacher 2005].

Glucose-induced oxidant stress is linked to the activity of the renin-angiotensin axis, another important contributing element in the pathogenesis of DN. In mice that transgenically overexpress catalase in the proximal tubule epithelial cells, there is less ROS generation and reduced expression of angiotensinogen and cellular apoptosis in kidney tissue, compared with wild type controls. Proximal tubules isolated from the transgenic mice also displayed less stimulation of ROS production and angiotensin gene transcription in response to high glucose [Chuang 2007].

There are a variety of functional consequences of high glucose induced oxidant stress. For example, exposure of proximal tubule cells to high glucose inhibits Na+-glucose co-transport by a sequence of steps that involves increased production of hydrogen peroxidase, advanced glycosylation end products, mitochondrial dysfunction, and increased NOX activity [Han HJ 2005].

Antioxidants defense systems within the kidney are also disturbed by hyperglycemia. Ascorbate levels in renal tubular epithelial cells are diminished after exposed to high glucose secondary to competition between glucose and dehydroascorbate for cellular uptake by a shared transport mechanism [Chen L 2005]. In addition, renal expression of glucose-6-phosphate dehydrogenase (G6PD), a key enzyme in the production of the intracellular reductant NADPH, is reduced in the kidneys of diabetic rats versus normal controls. Insulin treatment and correction of hyperglycemia reversed these changes [Xu Y 2005].

4. PKC

Hyperglycemia directly activates PKC delta and PKC epsilon with activation of MAPK and NFKB in renal tissue. The changes in PKC-delta lead, in turn, to increased expression of endothelin converting enzyme-1 and release of endothelin-1 by human umbilical vein endothelial cells [Khamaisi 2009]. Administration of arjunolic acid can prevent these abnormal responses and reduce the severity of histopathological injury. High glucose–induced changes in PKC have profound impact on glomerular structure and function. Thus, in rats with STZ-diabetes, deletion of the PKCα gene prevents the hyperglycemia-induced reduction in nephron expression. It has been suggested that the PKC effect on nephron is mediated by WT-1, a known direct transcription factor on the nephron promoter. PKC-β1 also mediates the increased expression of the GLUT-2 glucose transporter in the proximal tubule brush border membrane that is triggered by high serum glucose levels [Goestemeyer 2007]. In addition, PKC-β1 leads to Akt activation in response to high glucose which in turn leads to increased TGF-β release and extracellular matrix accumulation. Addition of ruboxistaurin, a PKC-β inhibitor, prevented this sequence of steps [Wu 2009].

PKC is also involved in the increased production of reactive oxygen species in diabetes. In cultured rat mesangial cells, exposure to high glucose leads to increased expression of PKC-zeta which leads to increased release of oxidant molecules. There appeared to be a positive feedback loop because the oxidant stress further enhanced ROS generation [Kwan 2005]. Increased PKC-delta expression induced by high glucose may stimulate collagen accumulation in mesangial via a pathway that is dependent on plasminogen activator inhibitor-1 (PAI-1) and independent of TGF-β [Baccora 2007]. Based on experiments with cultured mesangial cells the pathway for interaction of glucose, AGE, ROS, and PKC in the pathogenesis of DN, the sequence appears to be high glucose→AGE→PKC phosphorylation→NOX activation→ROS production [Thallas-Bonke 2007].

A Phase II randomized clinical trial involving 123 patients with type 2 diabetes demonstrated that administration of ruboxistaurin, the PKC inhibitor, 32 mg per day for 1 year, resulted in a decrease in albuminuria without any decline in GFR [Tuttle 2005]. These findings indicate that PKC inhibitors may be a promising new approach to the treatment of DN.

5. Renin- Angiotensin II

It is well established that high glucose leads to activation of the renin-angiotensin, a major factor in the development of DN [Ziyadeh 2008]. The glucose-induced stimulation of angiotensin II interacts with many other signaling mechanisms e\within the kidney and systemically. Blockade of angiotensin with candesartan reverses the increase in renal sympathetic nerve activity in hypertensive rats with STZ-diabetes [Takimoto 2008]. If endothelial cells are exposed to high glucose, the increased activity of angiotensin II inhibits the activation of PPAR-γ, an effect that can be blocked by silencing of the angiotensin II receptor, type 1. Moreover, prevention of the high glucose-angiotensin II-PPAR-γ interaction blocks the increased expression of proinflammatory adhesion molecules by endothelial cells [Min 2009]. Similarly, treatment with the angiotensin converting enzyme inhibitor, enalapril, corrects the reduced response to bradykinin in mesenteric arterioles isolated from rats with STZ-diabetes [Rastelli 2008]. Administration of 1,25(OH)2-vitamin D3 may reverse the detrimental effects of angiotensin II that are triggered by high glucose *in vitro* and hyperglycemia *in vivo*. Combined treatment of rats with STZ-diabetes with an angiotensin receptor blocker and the vitamin D analogue, paricalcitol, results in greater amelioration of kidney injury compared to either agent alone and that the improvement is associated with greater suppression of renin activity [Zhang 2008]. The effect of vitamin D on high-glucose mediated renin release involves suppression of angiotensinogen expression by blockade of the NF-κB pathway [Deb 2009]. Finally, treatment of diabetic rats with the aldosterone antagonist, spironolactone, inhibits the renin-angiotensin axis and reduces the renal expression of type I/IV collagen and TGF-β [Taira 2008].

6. Prostaglandins

Inhibition of COX2 with celecoxib reduces GFR in patients with type 1 diabetes who have hyperfiltration but increased GFR in patients with a normal level of kidney function [Cherney[a] 2008].

The interactions between the various actions of hyperglycemia in the development of DN are summarized in Figure 1.

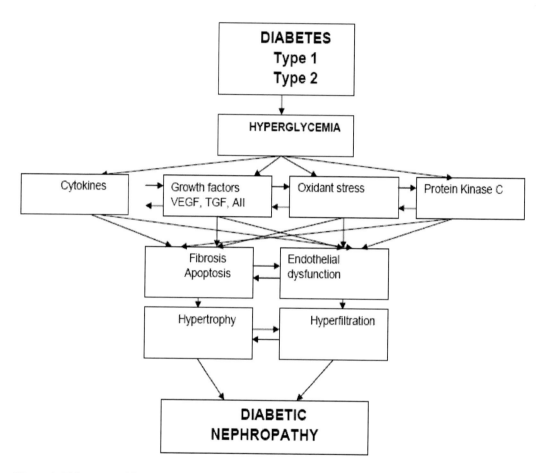

Figure 1. This cartoon illustrates some of the interactions between the various abnormalities triggered by hyperglycemia that contribute to the development of diabetic nephropathy.

II. Clinical Studies

A. Glucose Control

The impact of glycemic control on the morbidity and mortality of diabetes has been the subject of many investigations over many years. A recent editorial in JAMA [Kahn 2009] reviews older studies like the DCCT and UKPDS that demonstrate the beneficial effect of tight glycemic control on the development of DN. It also updates the status of newer trials such as the ACCORD, VADT, and ADVANCE trials which provided less clear-cut outcomes. In type 2 diabetes intensive blood glucose control targeting a HbA1c level below 6.5% was associated with a 10% reduction in the combined outcome of major macrovascular and microvascular complications [ADVANCE Collaborative Group 2008]. The improvement was driven primarily by a 21% relative reduction in DN, underscoring the role of hyperglycemia in the pathogenesis of diabetic kidney disease. While there is some controversy about whether cardiovascular outcomes are improved by tight control, long-term follow-up of the DCCT and UKPDS2 cohorts suggest that there are prolonged benefits of tight control even years after the period of intensive treatment of hyperglycemia, the so-called legacy effect. The clinical benefits of tight control of serum glucose concentration may be contingent on the age of the patient. When life expectancy is shorter than 5 years, intensive therapy of hyperglycemia produced little benefit [Pignone 2009]. This analysis would not be relevant to pediatric patients and young adults with type1 or type 2 diabetes.

The clinical task of achieving good glycemic control in young patients with diabetes is a monumental one. In the SEARCH for diabetes in Youth study involving 3947 patients with type 1 and 552 patients with type 2 diabetes at 6 centers in the United States, poor control (HbA1c$\geq$9.5%) was found in 17 and 27% of those with type 1 and 2 diabetes, respectively [Petiti 2009]. A recent study links the higher burden of type 2 diabetes in Latino Americans compared to non-Hispanic whites based on poor diseases control and higher HbA1c levels [Cabellero 2007]. Incorporation of HbA1c levels improves the accuracy of formula estimations of GFR, confirming the importance of hyperglycemia in increasing GFR [Yokoyama 2009].

In children with type 1 diabetes and normoalbuminuria, GFR is within the normal limits but the renal plasma flow is lower than in healthy controls, leading to an increased filtration fraction [Raes 2007]. There are gender differences in the renal responses to hyperglycemia. During clamped euglycemia, male adolescents with type 1 diabetes with normoalbuminuria had higher renal and plasma blood flow compared to females. Moreover, during hyperglycemia female adolescents had a reduction in renal blood flow while males had no significant alteration in renal hemodynamics. Following angiotensin converting enzyme inhibition, arterial blood pressure declined in both genders but only females had a reduction in GFR and filtration fraction [Cherney[b] 2005]. Interestingly, HbA1c levels do not correlate with any measure of activation of the renin-angiotensin axis [Stevanovic 2007]

Renal glucose uptake is markedly increased in patients with uncontrolled diabetes and short-term control of hyperglycemia with an insulin infusion for 2 hours reversed this abnormality [Meyer 2005]. This suggests that one of the benefits of improved metabolic control to prevent DN is to normalize glucose uptake as a trigger to renal injury. The increased renal uptake of glucose during hyperglycemia may involve upregulation of the GLUT1 transporter [Brosius 2005]. Polymorphisms in the GLUT1 gene may predispose to increased glucose flux that triggers the polyol pathway and PKC activation [Brosius 2005]. These changes may trigger accumulation of extracellular matrix proteins and culminate in renal fibrosis. Improved glucose control and avoidance of wide swings in serum glucose concentration may be protective against DN by limiting the production of ROS, assessed by urinary excretion of 8-isoPGF2 [Monnier 2006]. Short-term (4 weeks) treatment with an angiotensin receptor blocker improves endothelial dysfunction and reduces the release of proinflammatory cytokines by leukocytes in healthy volunteers exposed to high glucose [Willemsen 2007]. Similar studies need to be performed in patients with diabetes.

One interesting question is whether changes in serum glucose concentration within a range that is below levels that meet standard definitions of diabetes have an effect on kidney function. In a large sample of adults with CKD stage 3 or greater, serum levels of L-carboxymethyl-lysine (CML), a dominant AGE that reflects the serum glucose concentration correlated with the GFR. Even after excluding patients with diabetes, serum CML concentration was associated with CKD [Semba[a] 2009]. Similarly, in a group of older community dwelling women enrolled in the Women's Health and Aging Study, serum levels of CML and the soluble receptor for AGE (sRAGE) were associated with decreased GFR [Semba[b] 2009]. Finally, in a group of ambulatory patients without diabetes, serum AGE levels correlated with GFR. Moreover, high AGE levels were associated with suppression of endothelial nitric oxide synthase activity and endothelial dysfunction [Linden 2008]. It is well established that serum levels of AGE and advanced oxidation protein products are elevated in patients with type 2 diabetes and that the concentrations are correlated with the amount of albuminuria [Piwowar 2008]. Taken together, these findings in non-diabetic patients would suggest that adverse effects of high glucose levels on endothelial function and GFR are even more likely to occur in patients with clinically established diabetes and would support intensive efforts to achieve euglycemia.

B. Nephropathy

The search for early markers of DN in relationship to glucose control is an important area of clinical investigation. Even a transient elevation in serum glucose level for 2 hours in healthy volunteers leads to increased urinary excretion of TGF-β and F2-isoprostanes, a marker of oxidant stress [McGowan 2005]. Serum levels of TGF-β are increased in patients with type 2 diabetes and microalbuminuria; moreover, the serum TGF-β levels correlated with glycemic control, i.e., HbA1c levels and blood pressure [Ibrahim 2007]. This suggests that hyperglycemia triggers the activation of TGF-β leading to the initiation of progressive renal damage.

C. Pediatric Antecedents of DN

Diabetic nephropathy (DN) is an entity that occurs primarily in adult patients. Most surveys suggest that overt renal disease is rare in children and adolescents. In a large cohort study of 27,805 German children, age 9.9 years at baseline and 6.3 at the last visit, less than 1% had microalbuminuria or impaired kidney function [Schwab 2006]. However, the incidence of type 1 and type 2 diabetes has been rising at 2.5-7.5% annually in studies done in several western countries. This raises the important question of whether improved metabolic control of serum glucose levels in pediatric patients can delay or prevent the occurrence of DN in adults Microalbuminuria is often considered the most reliable sign of incipient DN. While the abnormality can revert to normal and should not be viewed as evidence of irreversible kidney damage, it represents the most easily measured and accessible marker of DN. The prevalence of microalbuminuria in pediatric patients ranges from 5-20%. In the Oxford Regional Prospective Study of 514 children and adolescents followed for at least 4.5 years, microalbuminuria was detectable on at the initial visit in 12.8% of the patients and it was persistent in 4.8%. After 11 years of type 1 diabetes, the prevalence of microalbuminuria was 40% but was persistent in only 18%. Interestingly, the cumulative prevalence of microalbuminuria was not impacted by the age at diagnosis of diabetes, i.e., <5, 5-10, or >10 years [Amin 2008]. In contrast, girls had a higher prevalence of new onset microalbuminuria compared to boys. Most importantly, the cumulative prevalence of microalbuminuria was directly related to the HbA1c level, i.e., <8.5%, 8.5-10, 10-12, and >12%. This suggests that improved glycemic control in children with type 1 diabetes can at least delay the incipient stages of DN.

Puberty may be a crucial phase in development that unmasks or accelerates the development of DN. If STZ diabetes was induced in experimental animals during puberty versus adulthood, only the later stage was marked by increased expression of CTGF [Langer 2008]. In adolescents (n=29) with type 1 diabetes, markers of oxidative stress such as serum levels of malondialdehyde and carbonyls were increased, and levels of antioxidants were reduced compared to healthy controls in direct relationship to glycosylated hemoglobin levels [Hernández-Marco 2009]. Similar findings were noted in a study of 100 children with type 1 diabetes age 2-17 years [Seckin 2006]. These findings indicate that early control of diabetes may inhibit key pathways that are implicated in the development of diabetic nephropathy. Figure 2 summarizes a proposed approach to prevent DN in pediatric patients with diabetes.

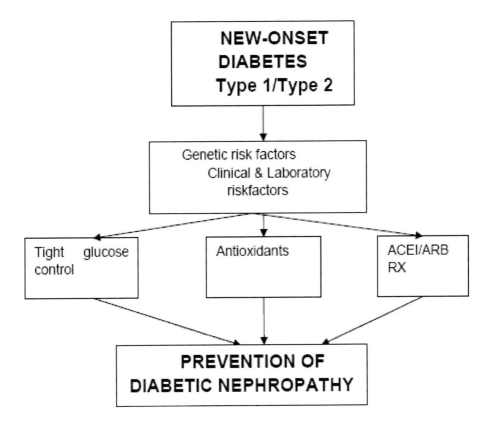

Figure 2. This figure summarizes a proposed approach to the treatment of pediatric patients with new-onset diabetes designed t prevent the development of diabetic nephropathy.

D. Congenital Malformations Induced by Hyperglycemia

Hyperglycemia during fetal development is associated with a wide spectrum of congenital anomalies including cardiovascular, central nervous system, skeletal and genitourinary systems [Kanwar[a] 2005]. In general, the retardation of renal morphogenesis caused by high glucose levels in utero reflects increased apoptosis and decreased organ size. Oxidant stress may contribute to this process. Exposure of embryonic metanephrons to graded levels of high glucose between days 13 to 17 of gestation results in a disruption of ureteric bud iterations and a reduced number of nascent nephrons. These changes occur in parallel with increased apoptosis and reduced renal specific oxidoreductase activity [Kanwar[b] 2005].

The pathway by which increased ROS production in the fetus leads to congenital malformations has been studied using mouse embryonic mesenchymal epithelial cells and *ex vivo* kidney explants. When these tissues are exposed to high glucose, there is increased ROS production mediated by the NF-κB pathway followed by increased PAX-2 gene expression [Chen 2006]. The finding is important because PAX-2 is essential for normal nephrogenesis. The high glucose effect on ureteric bud branching that occurs via increased ROS production also involves Akt signaling [Zhang[b] 2007]. It should be noted that there are studies that suggest that PAX-2 prevents hyperglycemia-induced apoptosis in mouse embryonic mesenchymal cells and that N-myc provides a positive autocrine feedback on PAX-2 gene expression [Zhang[a] 2007]. Finally, in the heart, reduced eNOS and increased VEGF expression are associated with apoptosis of myoblasts and cardiac abnormalities [Kumar 2008]. The role of these signaling molecules within the kidney requires further study.

Conclusion

High glucose in vitro and hyperglycemia in vivo are the defining abnormality in the definition of diabetes. This metabolic change is the starting point in virtually all experimental and clinical studies of diabetes. High glucose stimulates increased growth of the kidney and promotes enhancement of the glomerular filtration rate. In the long-term, it affects every cell in the kidney and provokes alterations in the expression of growth factors and oxidant stress. These changes lead to renal fibrosis and loss of cells via apoptosis. The importance of hyperglycemia is underscore by its association with a range of congenital malformations in the fetus exposed to high ambient glucose levels. There is ample evidence about the pivotal role of high glucose in the pathogenesis of DN to justify clinical efforts to improve the control of glycemia. Improved experimental models of DN and novel in vitro systems would help clarify the mechanism of action of high glucose in diabetic kidney disease and the design of safe and effective strategies to achieve normoglycemia in children and adults with type 1 and type 2 diabetes.

References

Adler S. Diabetic nephropathy: Linking histology, cell biology and genetics. *Kidney Int,* 2004 66: 2095-2106.

ADVANCE Collaborative Group, Patel A, MacMahon S, et al. Intensive Blood Glucose Control and Vascular Outcomes in Patients with Type 2 Diabetes. *N Engl J Med.,* 2008 358: 2560-72.

Advani A, Gilbert R, Thai K, Gow R M, Langham R G, Kelly D J et al. Expression, Localization, and Function of the Thioredoxin System in Diabetic Nephropathy. *J Am Soc Nephrol*, 2009 20: 730-741.

Aljofan M, Ding H. high glucose increases expression of cyclooxygenase-2, increases oxidative stress and decreases the generation of nitric oxide in mouse microvessel endothelial cells. *J Cell Physiol* 2009 [EPub ahead of print]

Amin R, Widmer B, Prevost AT, et al. Risk of microalbuminuria and progression to macroalbuminuria in a cohort with childhood onset type 1 diabetes: prospective observational study. *BMJ,* 2008 336:697-701.

Baccora M, Cortes P, Hassett C, Taube D, Yee J. Effects of long-term elevated glucose on collagen formation by mesangial cells. *Kidney Int,* 2007 72: 1216-1225.

Brosius F, Heilig C. Glucose transporters in diabetic nephropathy. *Pediatric Nephrology*, 2005 20: 447-451.

Cabellero AE, Tenzer P. Building cultural competency for improved diabetes care: Latino Americans and diabetes. *J Fam Pract.,* 2007 56: S7-13.

Chang CT, Wu MS, Tian YC, et al. Enhancement of epithelial sodium channel expression in renal cortical collecting ducts cells by advanced glycation end products. *Nephrol Dial Transplant,* 2007, 22:722-31.

Chen L, Jia RH, Qiu CJ, Ding G. Hyperglycemia inhibits the uptake of dehydroascorbate in tubular epithelial cell. *Am J Nephrol.,* 2005 25: 459-65.

Chen Y, Liu F, Tran S, Zhu Y, Hebert M, Ingelfinger J, Zhang S. Reactive oxygen species and nuclear factor-kappa B pathway mediate high glucose-induced Pax-2 gene expression in mouse embryonic mesenchymal epithelial cells and kidney explants. *Kidney Int,* 2006 70: 1607-1615.

Cherian S, Roy S, Pinheiro A, Roy S. Tight glycemic control regulates fibronectin expression and basement membrane thickening in retinal and glomerular capillaries of diabetic rats. *Invest Ophthalmol Vis Sci.,* 2009 50: 943-9.

Cherney DZ, Miller JA, Scholey JW, et al. The effect of cyclooxygenase-2 inhibition on renal hemodynamic function in humans with type 1 diabetes. *Diabetes.,* 2008 57: 688-95.

Cherney DZ, Sochett EB, Miller JA. Gender differences in renal responses to hyperglycemia and angiotensin-converting enzyme inhibition in diabetes. *Kidney Int.,* 2005 68: 1722-8.

Chuang T, Guh J, Chiou S, et al. Phosphoinositide 3-kinase is required for high glucose-induced hypertrophy and p21WAF1 expression in LLC-PK1 cells. *Kidney Int,* 2007 71: 867-874.

Coughlan MT, Thorburn DR, Penfold SA, et al. RAGE-Induced Cytosolic ROS Promote Mitochondrial Superoxide Generation in Diabetes. *J Am Soc Nephrol*, 2009 20:742-752.

Coughlan MT, Thorburn DR, Penfold SA, et al. RAGE-induced cytosolic ROS promote mitochondrial superoxide generation in diabetes. *J Am Soc Nephrol*, 2009 20:742-52.

Dai T, Natarajan R, Nast CC, et al. Glucose and diabetes: Effects on podocyte and glomerular p38MAPK, heat shock protein 25, and actin cytoskeleton. *Kidney Int,* 2006 69:806-814.

Deb DK, Chen Y, Zhang Z, Zhang Y, Szeto FL, Wong KE, Kong J, Li YC. 1,25-dihydroxyvitamin D3 suppresses high glucose-induced angiotensinogen expression in kidney cells by blocking NF-{kappa}B pathway. *Am J Physiol,* 2009;296:F1212-8.

Feng Y, Wang Q, Wang Y, Yard B, Lang F. SGK1-mediated fibronectin formation in diabetic nephropathy. *Cell Physiol Biochem,* 2005 16: 237-44.

Goestemeyer AK, Marks J, Srai SK, Debnam ES, Unwin RJ. GLUT2 protein at the rat proximal tubule brush border membrane kinase C (PKC)-beta-1 and plasma glucose concentration. *Diabetologia,* 2007 50: 2209-17.

Goldenberg NM, Silverman M. Rab34 and its effector munc13-2 constitute a new pathway modulating protein secretion in the cellular response to hyperglycemia. *Am J Physiol Cell Physiol.* 2009 297: 1053-8.

Gnudi L, Thomas SM, Viberti G. Mechanical forces in diabetic kidney disease: A trigger for impaired glucose metabolism. *J Am soc Nephrol* 2007;18:2226-2232.

Guo M, Ricardo SD, Deane JA, Shi M, Cullen-McEwen L, Bertram JF. A stereological study of the renal glomerular vasculature in the db/db mouse model of diabetic nephropathy. *J Anat,* 2005 207: 813-21.

Ha TS. High glucose and advanced glycosylated end-products affect the expression of alpha-actinin-4 in glomerular epithelial cells. *Nephrology (Carlton),* 2006 11:435-41.

Han HJ, Lee YJ, Park SH, Lee JH, Taub M. High glucose-induced oxidative stress inhibits Na+/glucose cotransporter activity in renal proximal tubule cells. *Am J Physiol Renal Physiol.,* 2005 288: 988-96.

Han J, Zhang F, Xie J, Linhardt RJ, Hiebert LM. Changes in cultured endothelial cell glycosaminoglycans under hyperglycemic conditions and the effect of insulin and heparin. *Cardiovasc Diabetol,* 2009. PMID: 19695080 (EPub ahead of print) http://www.ncbi.nlm.nih.gov/pubmed/19695080?ordinalpos=17anditool=EntrezSystem2.PEntrez.Pubmed.Pubmed_ResultsPanel.Pubmed_DefaultReportPanel.Pubmed_RVDocSum

Han S, Sanghwa Y, Jung D, et al. Gene expression patterns in glucose-stimulated podocytes. *Biochem Biophys Res Commun,* 2008 370:514-518.

Hara T, Ishida T, Cangara HM, Hirata K. Endothelial cell-selective adhesion molecule regulates albuminuria in diabetic nephropathy. *Microvasc Res,* 2009 77: 348-55.

Harwood S M, Allen D A, Raftery M J, Yaqoob M M. High glucose initiates calpain-induced necrosis before apoptosis in LLC-PK1 cells. *Kidney Int,* 2007 71: 655-663.

Hernández-Marco R, Codoñer-Franch P, Pons Morales S, Del Castillo Villaescusa C, Boix García L, Valls Bellés V. Oxidant/antioxidant status and hyperfiltration in young patients with type 1 diabetes mellitus. *Pediatr Nephrol,* 2009 24: 121-7.

Hills CE, Bland R, Bennett J, Ronco PM, Squires PE. High glucose up-regulates ENaC and SGK1 expression in HCD-cells. *Cell Physiol Biochem,* 2006 18: 337-46.

Hu Y, Kaisaki PJ, Argoud K, et al. Functional annotations of diabetes nephropathy susceptibility loci through analysis of genome-wide renal gene expression in rat models of diabetes mellitus. *BMC Med Genomics,* Jul 2009 2:41. http://www.ncbi.nlm.nih.gov/pubmed/19586551?ordinalpos=25anditool=EntrezSystem2.PEntrez.Pubmed.Pubmed_ResultsPanel.Pubmed_DefaultReportPanel.Pubmed_RVDocSum

Huang L, Haylor J, Hau Z, et al. Transglutaminase inhibition ameliorates experimental diabetic nephropathy. *Kidney Int,* 2009 76:383-394.

Ibrahim S, Rashed L. Estimation of transforming growth factor-beta 1 as a marker of renal injury in type II diabetes mellitus. *Saudi Med J.,* 2007 28: 519-23.

Isermann B, Vinnikov IA, Madhusudhan T, et al. *Nat Med,* 2007 13: 1349-58.

Jaimes EA, Hua P, Tian RX, Raij L. Human glomerular endothelium: Interplay among glucose, free fatty acids, angiotensin II and oxidative stress in hyperglycemia. *Am J Physiol* 2009 [EPub ahead of print].

Jung DS, Li JJ, Kwak SJ, et al. FR167653 inhibits fibronectin expression and apoptosis in diabetic glomeruli and in high-glucose-stimulated mesangial cells. *Am J Physiol Renal Physiol.,* 2008 295: 595-604.

Kahn, S. Glucose Control in Type 2 Diabetes: Still Worthwhile and Worth Pursuing. *JAMA,* 2009 301(15), 1590-1592.

Kang J, Dai XS, Yu TB, Wen B, Yang ZW. Glycogen accumulation in renal tubules, a key morphological change in the diabetic rat kidney. *Acta Diabetol.,* 2005 42: 110-6.

[a]Kanwar Y, Nayak B, Lin S, et al. Hyperglycemia: its imminent effects on mammalian nephrogenesis. *Pediatric Nephrology,* 2005 20: 858-868.

Kanwar Y, Akagi S, Nayak B, et al. Renal-specific oxidoreductase biphasic expression under high glucose ambience during fetal versus neonatal development. *Kidney Int.,* 2005 68:1670-83

Katavetin P, Miyata T, Inagi R, et al. High glucose blunts vascular endothelial growth factor response to hypoxia via the oxidative stress-regulated hypoxia-inducible factor/hypoxia-responsible element pathway. *J Am Soc Nephrol.,* 2006 17: 1405-13.

Kato M, Arce L, and Natarajan R. MicroRNAs and Their Role in Progressive Kidney Diseases. *Clin J Am Soc Nephrol,* 2009 4:1255-1266.

Khamaisi M, Dahan R, Hamed S, Abassi Z, Heyman SN, Raz I. Role of protein kinase C in the expression of endothelin converting enzyme-1. *Endocrinology,* 2009 150: 440-9.

Kosugi T, Yuzawa Y, Sato W, et al. Midkine is involved in tubulointerstitial inflammation associated with diabetic nephropathy. *Lab Invest.* 2007 87: 903-13.

Kosugi T, Heninig M, Nakayama T, Connor T, Yuzawa Y, Li Q, Hauswirth WW, Grant MB, Crocker BP, Campbell-Thompson M, Zhang L, Atkinson MA, Nakagawa T. lowering blood pressure blocks mesangiolysis and mesangial nodules, but not tubulointerstitial injury, in diabetic eNOS knockout mice. *Am J Pathol.* 2009 174:1221-1229

Kumar SD, Yong SK, Dheen ST, Bay BH, Tay SS. Cardiac malformations are associated with altered expression of vascular endothelial growth factor and endothelial nitric oxide synthase genes in embryos of diabetic mice. *Exp Biol Med* 2008;233:1421-32.

Kwan J, Wang H, Munk S, Xia L, Goldberg HJ, Whiteside CI. In high glucose protein kinase C-zeta activation is required for mesangial cell generation of reactive oxygen species. *Kidney Int,* 2005 68: 2526-41.

Langer W, Devish K, Carmines P and Lane P. Prepubertal onset of diabetes prevents expression of renal cortical connective tissue growth factor. *Pediatric Nephrology,* 2008 23: 275-283.

Lee MJ, Feliers D, Mariappan MM, et al. A role for AMP-activated protein kinase in diabetes-induced renal hypertrophy. *Am J Physiol Renal Physiol.,* 2007 292: 617-27.

Li X, Hu J, Zhang R, et al. Urocortin ameliorates diabetic nephropathy in obese db/db mice. *Br J Pharmacol.,* 2008 154: 1025-34.

Lin, C, Wang J, Huang Y, et al. Wnt/-Catenin Signaling Modulates Survival of High Glucose–Stressed Mesangial Cells. *J Am Soc Nephrol,* 2006 17: 2812-20.

Linden E, Cai W, He JC, et al. Endothelial dysfunction in patients with chronic kidney disease results from advanced glycation end products (AGE)-mediated inhibition of endothelial nitric oxide synthase through RAGE activation. *Clin J Am Soc Nephrol*, 2008 May 3:691-8.

Lindenmeyer Maja, Rastaldi M, Ikehata M, Neusser M A, Kretzler M, Cohen C D, and Schlöndorff D. Proteinuria and Hyperglycemia Induce Endoplasmic Reticulum Stress. *J Am Soc Nephrol*, 2008 19: 2225-2236.

Liu F, Brezniceanu M, Wei C, et al. Overexpression of Angiotensinogen Increases Tubular Apoptosis in Diabetes. *J Am Soc Nephrol*, 2007 19: 269-280.

Liu S, Shi L, Wang S. Overexpression of upstream stimulatory factor 2 accelerates diabetic kidney injury. *Am J Physiol Renal Physiol*, 2007 293: 1727-35.

Liu X, Luo F, Pan K, Wu W, and Chen H. High glucose upregulates connective tissue growth factor expression in human vascular smooth muscle cells. *BMC Cell Biology*, 2007 8:1. http://www/biomedcentral.com/1471-2121/8/1

Lorz C, Benito A, Ucero AC, Santamaría B, Ortiz A. Trail and kidney disease. *Front Biosci.* 2009 1: 3740-9.

Lu TC, Wang ZH, Feng X, Chuang PY, Fang W, Shen Y, Levy DE, Xiong H, Chen N, He JC. Knockdown of Stat 3 activity *in vivo* prevents diabetic nephropathy. Kid Int 76:63-71.

Mahimainathan L, Das F, Venkatesan B, Choudhury GG. Mesangial cell hypertrophy by high glucose is mediated by downregulation of the tumor suppressor PTEN. *Diabetes*, 2006 55: 2115-25.

Malatiali S, Francis I, Barac-Nieto M. Phlorizin prevents glomerular hyperfiltration but not hypertrophy in diabetic rats. *Exp Diabetes Res.* 2008 (EPub ahead of print) http://www.ncbi.nlm.nih.gov/pubmed/18769499?ordinalpos=100anditool=EntrezSystem 2.PEntrez.Pubmed.Pubmed_ResultsPanel.Pubmed_DefaultReportPanel.Pubmed_RVDoc Sum

Manabe E, Handa O, Naito Y, Mizushima K, Akagiri S, Adachi S. Astaxanthin protects mesangial cells from hyperglycemia-induced oxidative signaling. *J Cell Biochem*, 2008 103: 1925-37.

Manna P, Sinha M, Sil PC. Prophylactic role of arjunolic acid in response to streptozotocin mediated diabetic renal injury: activation of polyol pathway and oxidative stress responsive signaling cascades. *Chem Biol Interact*, 2009 181: 297-308.

McGowan T, Dunn S, Falkner B, and Sharma K. Stimulation of Urinary TGF-ß and Isoprostanes in Response to Hyperglycemia in Humans. *Clin J Am Soc Nephrol*, 2005 1: 263-268.

Meyer C, Tolias A, Platanisiotis D, Stumvoll M, Vlachos L, Mitrakou A. Increased renal glucose metabolism in Type 1 diabetes mellitus. *Diabet Med.*, 2005 22: 453-9.

Min Q, Bai YT, Jia G, Wu J, Xiang JZ. High glucose enhances angiotensin-II-mediated peroxisome proliferation-activated receptor-gamma inactivation in human coronary artery endothelial cells. Exp Mol Pathol 2009 [EPub ahead of print].

Mishra R, Emancipator SN, Kern T, Simonson MS. High glucose evokes an intrinsic proapoptotic signaling pathway in mesangial cells. *Kidney Int.*, 2005 67: 82-93.

Mohan S, Reddick RL, Musi N, Horn DA, Yan B, Prihoda TJ, Natarajan M, Abboud-Werner SL. Diabetic eNOS knockout mice develop distinct macro- and microvascular complications. *Lab Invest* 2008;88:515-528.

Mohan S, Konopinski R, Yan B, Centonze VE, Natarajan M. High glucose-induced IKK-Hsp-90 interaction contributes to endothelial dysfunction. *Am J Physiol* 2009;296:C182-92.

Monnier L, Mas E, Ginet C, et al. Activation of Oxidative Stress by Acute Glucose Fluctuations Compared With Sustained Chronic Hyperglycemia in Patients With Type 2 Diabetes. *JAMA,* 2006 295: 1681-1687.

Munusamy S, MacMillan-Crow LA. Mitochondrial superoxide plays a crucial role in the development of mitochondrial dysfunction during high glucose exposure in rat renal proximal tubular cells. *Free Radic Biol Med.,* 2009 46:1149-57.

Nasu T, Maeshima Y, Kinomura M, et al. Vasohibin-1 a negative feedback regulator of angiogenesis, ameliorates renal alterations in a mouse model of diabetic nephropathy. *Diabetes.* 2009 58: 2365-75.

Oak JH, Cai H. Attenuation of angiotensin II signaling recouples eNOS and inhibits nonendothelial NOX activity in diabetic mice. *Diabetes* 2007;56:118-26.

Oh YK, Joo KW, Lee JW, et al. Altered renal sodium transporter expression in an animal model of type 2 diabetes mellitus. *J Korean Med Sci.,* 2007 22:1034-41.

Ohtomo S, Nangaku M, Izuhara Y, et al. The role of megsin, a serine protease inhibitor, in diabetic mesangial matrix accumulation. *Kidney Int.,* 2008 74: 768-74.

Pacher P, Szabó C. Role of poly(ADP-ribose) polymerase-1 activation in the pathogenesis of diabetic complications: endothelial dysfunction, as a common underlying theme. *Antioxid Redox Signal,* 2005 7:568-80.

Park CW, Kim HW, Ko SH, et al. Accelerated diabetic nephropathy in mice lacking the peroxisome proliferator-activated receptor alpha. *Diabetes,* 2006 55: 885-93.

Park JK, Ronkina N, Höft A, et al. Deletion of MK2 signaling in vivo inhibits small Hsp phosphorylation but not diabetic nephropathy. *Nephrol Dial Transplant.,* 2008 23: 1844-53.

Petiti DB, Klingensmith GJ, Bell RA, et al. Glycemic control in youth with diabetes: The SEARCH for Diabetes in Youth Study. *J Pediatr,* 2009 155:668-672.

Pignone, M. Decisions About Intensity of Glycemic Control Should Depend on Age and Functional Status. *Clinical Diabetes,* 2009 27:147-148.

Piwowar A, Knapik-Kordecka M, Szczecińska J, and Warwas M. Plasma glycooxidation protein products in type 2 diabetic patients with nephropathy. *Diabetes Metab Res Rev.,* 2008 Oct;24(7):549-53.

Pozzi A, Zent R, Chetyrkin S, et al. Modification of collagen IV by glucose or methylglyoxal alters distinct mesangial cell functions. *J Am Soc Nephrol.* 2009 20: 2119-25.

Qi W, Chen X, Zhang Y, et al. High glucose induces macrophage inflammatory protein-3 alpha in renal proximal tubule cells via a transforming growth factor-beta 1 dependent mechanism. *Nephrol Dial Transplant.,* 2007 22: 3147-53.

Qi W, Chen X, Gilbert RE, et al. High glucose-induced thioredoxin-interacting protein in renal proximal tubule cells is independent of transforming growth factor-beta1. *Am J Pathol.,* 2007 171: 744-54.

Qi W, Chen X, Holian J, Tan CYR, Kelly DJ, Pollock CA. Transcription factors Kruppel-like factor 6 and peroxisome proliferator-activated receptor-γ mediate high glucose-induced thioredoxin-interacting protein. Am J Pathol 2009;175:1858-67.

Raes A, Donckerwolcke R, Craen M, Hussein MC and Walle JV. Renal hemodynamic changes and renal functional reserve in children with type I diabetes mellitus. *Pediatric Nephrology,* 2007 22:1903-1909.

Rane MJ, Song Y, Jin S, et al. Interplay between Akt and p38 MAPK Pathways in the Regulation of Renal Tubular Cell Apoptosis Associated with Diabetic Nephropathy. *Am J Physiol Renal Physiol,* 2009. PMID: 19726550 (EPub ahead of print) http://www.ncbi.nlm.nih.gov/pubmed/19726550?ordinalpos=13anditool=EntrezSystem2.PEntrez.Pubmed.Pubmed_ResultsPanel.Pubmed_DefaultReportPanel.Pubmed_RVDocSum

Rastelli VM, Oliveira MA, dos Santos R, de Cassia Tostes Passaglia R, Nigro D, de Carvalho MH, Fortes ZB. Enalapril treatment corrects the reduced response to bradykinin in diabetes increasing the B2 protein expression. *Peptides,* 2008;29:404-11.

Riad A, Westermann D, Van Linthout S, Mohr Z, Uyulmaz S, Becher PM, Rutten H, Wohlfart P, Peters H, Schulteiss HP, Tschope C. Enhancement of endothelial nitric oxide synthase production reverses vascular dysfunction and inflammation in the hindlimbs of a rat model of diabetes. *Diabetologia* 2008;51:2325-32.

Ricci C, Iacobini C, Oddi G, et al. Role of TGF-beta/GLUT1 axis in susceptibility vs resistance to diabetic glomerulopathy in the Milan rat model. *Nephrol Dial Transplant,* 2006 21:1514-24.

Rüster C, Bondeva T, Franke S, Förster M, and Wolf G. Advanced glycation end-products induce cell cycle arrest and hypertrophy in podocytes. *Nephrol Dial Transplant,* 2008 23:2179-91.

Sakaguchi M, Isono M, Isshiki K, Sugimoto T, Koya D, Kashiwagi A. Inhibition of mTOR signaling with rapamycin attenuates renal hypertrophy in the early diabetic nice. *Biochem Biophys Res Commun* 2006;340:296-301.

Sanchez-Niño M A, Sanz A B, Ihalmo P, al. The MIF Receptor CD74 in Diabetic Podocyte Injury. *J Am Soc Nephrol,* 2008 20: 353-362.

Schwab KO, Doerfer J, Hecker W, Grulich-Henn J, Wiemann D, Kordonouri O, Beyer P, Holl RW (DPV Initiative of the German Working Group for Pediatric Diabetology). *Diabetes Care* 2006;29:218-225

Seckin D, Ilhan N, Ilhan N, Ertugrul S. Glycaemic control, markers of endothelial cell act9ivation and oxidative stress in children with type 1 diabetes mellitus. *Diabetes Res Clin Pract* 2006;73:191-7.

Semba RD, Fink JC, Sun K, Windham BG, and Ferrucci L. Serum Carboxymethyl-Lysine, a Dominant Advanced Glycation End Product, Is Associated with Chronic Kidney Disease: The Baltimore Longitudinal Study of Aging. *J Ren Nutr,* 2009.

Semba RD, Ferrucci L, Fink JC, et al. Advanced glycation end products and their circulating receptors and level of kidney function in older community-dwelling women. 2009 53:51-8.

Skill NJ, Johnson TS, Coutts IG, et al. Inhibition of Transglutaminase Activity Reduces Extracellular Matrix Accumulation Induced by High Glucose Levels in Proximal Tubular Epithelial Cells. *J Biol Chem,* 2004 279: 47754 –762.

Sommeijer DW, Florquin S, Hoedemaker I, Timmerman JJ, Reitsma PH, Ten Cate H. Renal tissue factor expression is increased in streptozotocin-induced diabetic mice. *Nephron Exp Nephrol.,* 2005 101: 86-94.

Stevanovic RD, Fisher ND, Lansang CM, Freeman KD, Hollenberg NK. Short- and long-term glycaemic control and the state of the renin system in type 1 diabetes mellitus. *J Renin Angiotensin Aldosterone Syst,* 2007;8:85-92.

Sun L, Xie P, Wada J, et al. Rap1b GTPase Ameliorates Glucose-Induced Mitochondrial Dysfunction. *J Am Soc Nephrol,* 2008 19: 2293-2301.

Susztak K, Ciccone E, McCue P, Sharma K and Böttinger E P. Multiple Metabolic Hits Converge on CD36 as Novel Mediator of Tubular Epithelial Apoptosis in Diabetic Nephropathy. PLoS Med 2(2): e45. doi: 10.1371/ journal. pmed. 0020045 http://www.plosmedicine.org/article/info:doi/10.1371/journal.pmed.0020045

Susztak K, Raff AC, Schiffer M, Böttinger EP. Glucose-induced reactive oxygen species cause apoptosis of podocytes and podocyte depletion at the onset of diabetic nephropathy. *Diabetes,* 2006 55: 225-33.

Szabó C, Biser A, Benko R, Böttinger E, Suszták K. Poly(ADP-ribose) polymerase inhibitors ameliorate nephropathy of type 2 diabetic Lepr db/db mice. *Diabetes,* 2006 55: 3004-12.

Tiara M, Toba H, Murakami M, Iga I, Serizawa R, Murata S, Kobara M, Nakata T. Spironolactone exhibits renoprotective effects and inhibits renin-angiotensin-aldosterone system in diabetic rats. *Eur J Pharmacol,* 2008;589:264-71.

Takimoto C, Kumagai H, Osaka M, Sakata K, Onami T, Kamayachi T, Iigaya K, Hayashi K, Saruta T, Itoh H. Candesartan and insulin reduce renal sympathetic nerve activity in hypertensive type 1 diabetic rats. *Hypertens Res,* 2008;31:1941-51.

Telci D, Collighan RJ, Basaga H, Griffin M. Increased TGF expression can result in induction of transforming growth factor β1, causing increased synthesis and deposition of matrix proteins, which can be regulated by nitric oxide. J Biol chem. 2009;284:29547-29558

Tesch GH. MCP-1/CCL2: a new diagnostic marker and therapeutic target for progressive renal injury in diabetic nephropathy. *Am J Physiol,* 2008 294:F697-F701

Thallas-Bonke V, Thorpe SR, Coughlan MT, et al. Inhibition of NADPH oxidase prevents advanced glycation end product-mediated damage in diabetic nephropathy through a protein kinase C-alpha-dependent pathway. *Diabetes,* 2008 57:460-9.

Toma I, Kang JJ, Sipos A, Varfgas S, Bansal E, Hanner F, Meer E, Peti-Peterdi J. Succinate receptor GPR91 provides a direct link between high glucose levels and renin release in murine and rabbit kidney. *J Clin Invest* 2008;118:2526-2534.

Tuttle K, Bakris G, Toto R, et al. The Effect of Ruboxistaurin on Nephropathy in Type 2 Diabetes. *Diabetes Care,* 2005 28: 2686-2690.

Vasko R, Koziolek M, Ikehata M, et al. Role of basic fibroblast growth factor (FGF-2) in diabetic nephropathy and mechanisms of its induction by hyperglycemia in human renal fibroblasts. *Am J Physiol Renal Physiol.* 2009 296: 1452-63.

Vasylyeva TL, Chen X, Ferry RJ Jr. Insulin-like growth factor binding protein-3 mediates cytokine-induced mesangial cell apoptosis. *Growth Horm IGF Res,* 2005 15: 207-14.

Wadham C, Parker A, Wang L, Xia P. High glucose attenuates protein S-nitrosylation in endothelial cells: role of oxidative stress. *Diabetes* 2007;56:2715-21

Wang JJ, Zhang SX, Lu K, Chen Y, Mott R, Sato S, Ma JX. Decreased expression of pigment epithelium-derived factor is involved in the pathogenesis of diabetic nephropathy. *Diabetes,* 2005 54: 243-50.

Willemsen JM, Westerink JW, Dallinga-Thie GM, van Zonneveld AJ, Gaillard CA, Rabelink TJ, de Koning EJ. Angiotensin II type 1 receptor blockade improves hyperglycemia-induced endothelial dysfunction and reduces proinflammatory cytokine release from leukocytes. *J Cardiovasc Pharmacol,* 2007;49:6-12.

Wu D, Peng F, Zhang B, et al. PKC-β1 Mediates Glucose-Induced Akt Activation and TGF-β1 Upregulation in Mesangial Cells. *J Am Soc Nephrol,* 2009 20: 554-566.

Xia L, Wang H, Munk S, et al. High glucose activates PKC-zeta and NADPH oxidase through autocrine TGF-beta1 signaling in mesangial cells. *Am J Physiol Renal Physiol,* 2008 295: 1705-14.

Xu M, Dai DZ, Dai Y. Normalizing NADPH oxidase contributes to attenuating diabetic nephropathy by the dual endothelin receptor antagonist CPU0213 in rats. *Am J Nephrol,* 2009 29: 252-6.

Xu Y, Osborne BW, Stanton RC. Diabetes causes inhibition of glucose-6-phosphate dehydrogenase via activation of PKA, which contributes to oxidative stress in rat kidney cortex. *Am J Physiol Renal Physiol.,* 2005 289: 1040-7.

Yeh CH, Chang CK, Cheng MF, Lin HJ, Cheng JT. Decrease of bone morphogenetic protein-7 (BMP-7) and its type II receptor (BMP-RII) in kidney of type 1-like diabetic rats. *Horm Metab Res,* 2009 41: 605-11.

Yokoyama H, Kanno S, Takahashi S, Yamada D, Itoh H, Saito K, Sone H, Haneda M. Determinants of decline in glomerular filtration rate in nonproteinuric subjects with or without diabetes and hypertension. *Clin J Am Soc Nephrol,* 2009 4:1432-1440.

Zdychová J, Veselá J, Kazdová L, Komers R. Renal activity of Akt kinase in experimental Type 1 diabetes. *Physiol Res.,* 2008 57: 709-15.

[a]Zhang S, Chen Y, Tran S, et al. Pax-2 and N-myc regulate epithelial cell proliferation and apoptosis in a positive autocrine feedback loop. *Pediatric Nephrology,* 2007 22: 813-824.

[b]Zhang S, Chen YW, Tran S, Chenier I, Hébert MK and Ingelfinger JR. Reactive Oxygen Species in the Presence of High Glucose Alter Ureteric Bud Morphogenesis. *J Am Soc Nephrol,* 2007 18: 2105-2115.

Zhang X, Chen X, Wu D, et al. Downregulation of Connexin 43 Expression by High Glucose Induces Senescence in Glomerular Mesangial Cells. *J Am Soc Nephrol,* 2006 17: 1532-1542.

Zhang Z, Yuan W, Sun L, Szeto F, Wong K, Li X, Kong J, Li Y. 1,25-Dihydroxyvitamin D_3 targeting of NF-ΚB suppresses high glucose-induced MCP-1 expression in mesangial cells. *Kidney Int,* 2007 72: 193-201.

Zhang Z, Zhang Y, Ning G, Deb DK, Kong J, Li YC. Combination therapy with AT1 blocker and vitamin D analog markedly ameliorates diabetic nephropathy: Blockade of compensatory renin increase. *Proc Natl Acad Sci USA,* 2008;105:15896-901.

Zhao HJ, Wang S, Cheng H, Zhang MZ, Takahashi T, Fogo AB, Breyer MD, Harris RC. Endothelial nitric oxide synthase deficiency produces accelerated nephropathy in diabetic mice. *J Am Soc Nephrol,* 200 17:2664-2669

Ziyadeh FN, Wolf G. Pathogenesis of the podocytopathy and proteinuria in diabetic nephropathy. *Cur Diabetes Rev,* 2008;4:39-45.

In: Advances in Pathogenesis of Diabetic Nephropathy
Editor: Sharma S. Prabhakar

ISBN: 978-1-61122-134-3
© 2012 Nova Science Publishers, Inc.

Chapter VI

Advanced Glycation End Products and Diabetic Nephropathy

*Jaime Uribarri**
The Mount Sinai School of Medicine
One Gustave Levy Place
New York, NY 10021, US

Introduction

The prevalence of diabetic nephropathy is increasing dramatically and it currently represents the first cause of end-stage renal disease requiring renal replacement therapy in the United States [1]. Although the genetic background is important in determining susceptibility to diabetic nephropathy, exposure to chronic hyperglycemia leading to the subsequent activation of multiple pathogenic pathways appears to be the main initiating factor [2]. Activation of protein kinase C (PKC) pathway, enhanced polyol pathway, increased oxidative stress, and overproduction of advanced glycation end products (AGEs) have all been proposed as potential cellular mechanisms by which hyperglycemia induces diabetic complications, including nephropathy [2]

The high levels of AGEs present in diabetes mellitus patients are thought to underlie many of the complications of this disease [3]. In this chapter we will review the evidence linking AGEs to the initiation and progression of diabetic nephropathy. We will discuss in detail the role of dietary AGEs. Finally, we will review new work aimed at reducing the body AGE load suggesting potential therapeutic interventions to prevent and/or slow down the progression of this common clinical condition.

---

* Phone: 212-241-1887, Fax: 212-369-9330, email: jaime.uribarri@mssm.edu.

What are Advanced Glycation End Products (AGEs)?

AGEs are a large group of heterogeneous compounds produced by the non-enzymatic reactions of sugars with free amino groups on proteins, peptides, or amino acids. This sequence of events is known as the Maillard, or browning, reaction first identified in 1912. We now know that AGEs may also form through many other pathways, including oxidation of sugars, lipids, and amino acids to create reactive aldehydes that covalently bind to proteins. The normal metabolism of glucose generates glycolytic intermediates, which also contribute to the pool of reactive aldehydes. Moreover, neutrophils and monocytes, upon inflammatory stimulation, produce myeloperoxidase and activate NADPH oxidase, which form AGEs by oxidizing amino acids. εN-carboxymethyl-lysine (CML), pentosidine, and methylglyoxal (MG) derivatives are among some of the better-characterized AGEs.

AGEs can produce tissue damage by either protein cross-linking that causes direct alteration in the structure and therefore function of proteins or though a variety of mechanisms including activation of receptors which activate pro-inflammatory and pro-oxidative cellular signaling pathways [4] (Figure 1). There are two types of cell surface AGE receptors, those that bind AGEs and initiate cell activation and those that bind, internalize, and degrade AGEs [4]. The best-studied receptor that binds and initiates OS is the receptor for AGE (RAGE). It recognizes AGEs as one of many ligands, is not endocytic, and is upregulated by OS. Binding of AGEs to RAGE initiates a cascade of intracellular signaling leading to activation of several inflammatory responses and pathological gene expression that eventually increases oxidative stress (OS) [5]. The most extensively evaluated of the endocytic AGE receptors is AGER1, which has marked antioxidant properties modulating AGE responses via RAGE and nuclear factor kappa-B [5], but also via the epidermal growth factor receptor, extracellular receptor kinase, and p66shc [6,7]. Unexpectedly, AGER1 appears suppressed or down regulated in the presence of chronically elevated AGE levels, as is typical of severe diabetic complications or chronic kidney disease [8,9], a time at which increased function of this receptor would have been anticipated. It is unclear whether this down-regulation is a primary process or results from the AGE overload state. Finally, a group of circulating proteins such as lysozyme and transferrin bind AGEs, effectively keeping them from causing damage to other molecules [10].

Evidence Linking AGEs and Diabetic Nephropathy

In Vitro Studies

Increased extracellular matrix is a pathological hallmark of diabetic nephropathy. In addition to collagen, a variety of non-collagenous glycoproteins such as fibronectin also accumulate in the kidney of diabetics. Extracellular matrix accumulation may be the result of increased synthesis of matrix components and/or decreased degradation. AGEs may play a role in the pathogenesis of diabetic nephropathy by modulating extracellular matrix turnover.

BIOLOGICAL EFFECTS OF AGEs

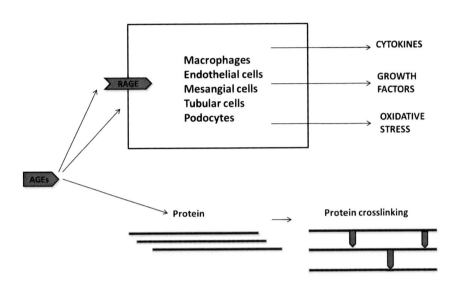

Figure 1. Biological effects of AGEs on different cell systems.

Direct cross-linking of slow-turnover proteins in the kidney extracellular matrix results in multiple abnormalities including altered matrix protein structure and function [11,12], aberrant cell–matrix interactions that change cellular adhesion, altered cell growth, and loss of the epithelial phenotype [13]; and inhibition of interactions required for self-assembly of type IV collagen and laminin [14].

In vitro, AGEs bind to renal mesangial cells through AGE receptors, which initiate overproduction of matrix proteins and diminish the expression of the major matrix metalloproteinase (MMP) responsible for degrading the non-collagenous matrix glycoprotein fibronectin [15,16]. AGEs also stimulate production of collagen IV and fibronectin in glomerular endothelial cells [17].

AGEs have been shown to play a role in tubular epithelial-myofibroblast transdifferentiation (TEMT) in diabetic nephropathy, but the intracellular signaling pathway remains unknown [18-21]. This effect is probably mediated by activation of the RAGE-ERK1/2 MAP kinase pathway to mediate the early TEMT process.

AGEs also have significant in vitro effect on podocytes, cells that play a major role in preventing protein passage through the glomerular capillary wall. Our group has shown that an AGE-RAGE interaction contributes to podocyte apoptosis by activation of the FOXO4 transcription factor [22]. The effect of increased podocyte apoptosis may explain the frequent decrease in the number of podocytes in kidney biopsies of patients with diabetic nephropathy. Other groups have demonstrated that the addition of AGEs to cultured human podocytes reduces expression of nephrin, a protein that is critical for normal function of podocytes in the glomerular filtration barrier [23], and of neuropilin (NRP1) [24].

Results of in vitro work with murine mesangial cells over expressing AGER1 are particularly interesting [7]. As expected, these cell prevented AGE-induced MAPK1, 2 phosphorylation and NF-κB activity and also increased AGE degradation. The authors demonstrated step by step that AGER1 negatively regulates AGE-mediated oxidant stress-dependent signaling via the EGFR and Shc/Grb2/Ras pathway [7]. Thus AGER1 could be a potentially useful molecule for developing therapeutic targets against vascular and kidney disorders related to diabetes [7].

Animal Studies

A direct role of AGEs in causing kidney damage is supported by several experimental observations. Short-term exogenous AGE administration to normal, nondiabetic mice led to increased glomerular expression of type IV collagen and laminin, indicators of mesangial matrix expansion and basement membrane thickening [25]. Furthermore, long-term treatment of normal rats with intravenous AGE-albumin induced albuminuria and morphologic changes of diabetic nephropathy, including glomerular hypertrophy, mesangial matrix expansion, and basement membrane thickening [26]. When the receptor for AGEs (RAGE) was over expressed in diabetic mice, features of kidney disease (albuminuria, elevated serum creatinine, kidney hypertrophy, mesangial expansion, and glomerulosclerosis) worsened [27]. Conversely, blockade of RAGE by a soluble truncated form of RAGE prevented structural and functional characteristics of nephropathy in db/db mice [28]. Finally, strategies to prevent AGE accumulation in the kidney of diabetic rats with AGE inhibitors such as aminoguanidine [29], benfotiamine [30], pyridoxamine [31, 32], OPB-9195 [33] and AGE breakers [34-36] have been shown to ameliorate diabetic nephropathy without influencing glycemic control.

The breakdown of preexisting AGEs with alagebrium, a putative AGE cross-link breaker, was associated with reduced renal fibrosis in experimental diabetes (35). A subsequent study by our group (36) confirmed these findings and further demonstrated that alagebrium was also beneficial when used as part of a delayed intervention protocol, suggesting that it may be useful in both preventing and retarding diabetic nephropathy. We also demonstrated that this compound significantly reduced serum, skin and kidney levels of AGEs, while increasing their urinary excretion [36].

The short-term (2 weeks) intraperitoneal administration of lysozyme in non-obese diabetic (NOD), db/db (+/+) mice, and non-diabetic, AGE-infused Sprague-Dawley rats reduced elevated basal serum AGE levels, increased urinary AGE excretion and improved albuminuria due to diabetes [37]. More recently, another group administered oral lysozyme, microencapsulated in orally administrable chitosan-coated alginate microspheres, to Wistar rats after diabetes induction with streptozotocin [38]. The lysozyme treatment significantly reduced the concentration of serum AGEs in the circulation and their deposition in the kidneys and prevented the development of microalbuminuria and morphological changes of diabetic nephropathy in the treated rats [38]. These results strongly suggest that lysozyme, by sequestering AGEs, may protect against diabetic renal damage.

Human Studies

The increase in circulating AGEs parallels the severity of renal functional impairment in diabetic nephropathy [39]. Biopsy samples from kidneys from diabetic subjects have demonstrated increased AGE deposition throughout the renal cortex [40,41]. CML, pyralline and pentosidine have been identified in renal tissue of diabetics with or without ESRD; AGE accumulation appeared to parallel the severity of diabetic nephropathy [40, 42]. Also, whereas low-level RAGE expression in normal control human subjects was restricted to podocytes, glomeruli of patients with diabetic nephropathy demonstrated diffuse up-regulation of RAGE expression in podocytes, colocalizing with synaptopodin expression [43]. A recent study in kidney biopsies from patients with diabetic nephropathy showed significant reduction of nephrin, an important regulator of the glomerular filter integrity. In the same study, cultured podocytes showed significant down-regulation in nephrin expression when glycated albumin was added [23].

Results from a phase 3 clinical trial using aminoguanidine in patients with diabetic nephropathy showed that the primary end point, time to doubling of serum creatinine, did not reach statistical significant [44]. Serum creatinine doubled in 26% [61/236] of the placebo-treated patients and in 20% [91/454] of those who received aminoguanidine (p = 0.099). Analyses of secondary end points including proteinuria and kidney function, however, were very positive. Therapy with aminoguanidine produced a statistically significant reduction in total urinary protein after 36 months compared with the placebo group (732 mg/24 h at the low dose and 329 mg/24 h at the high dose as compared with 35 mg/24 h in the placebo group; p = 0.001). Moreover, the estimated glomerular filtration rate decreased more slowly in the aminoguanidine-treated patients with a 36-month decrease from baseline of 6.26 ml/min as compared with 9.80 ml/min in the placebo-treated patients (p = 0.05) [44]. A report on two phase 2 studies on the use of pyridoxamine in patients with diabetic nephropathy shows that the drug is generally safe and well tolerated and significantly reduced the change from baseline in serum creatinine (p < 0.03), but with no reduction in albuminuria [45]. Although further clinical studies are warranted to more fully investigate the effects of these agents on diabetic nephropathy, these preliminary results support a significant role for AGEs in the pathogenesis of diabetic nephropathy.

Dietary AGEs

There are at least two sources of AGEs in diabetic as well as non-diabetic subjects: 1) those formed endogenously in the body and 2) those consumed with the standard diet or inhaled via tobacco smoking. The diet content of AGEs depends not only on the protein, lipid and carbohydrate content, but also and more importantly, on the temperature and conditions of cooking as clearly illustrated in table 1 [46]. Animal-derived foods cooked at high temperature, for prolonged time and under dry conditions have the highest AGE content [46].

The role of dietary AGEs (dAGEs) in human health and disease has been largely ignored in the past, mostly because of the assumption that these compounds are poorly absorbed. However, in recent years, is has become apparent that food is a major source of AGEs [46-49]. The oral administration of double-labeled single protein-AGEs, with or without specific AGE inhibitors, such as aminoguanidine in rats, or the enrichment of low-AGE experimental diets with specific AGEs in mice verified that dAGEs are absorbed [48, 49]. An estimated 10% of ingested AGEs are absorbed into the circulation, and two-thirds of those that are absorbed are retained in the body, thus contributing to the body AGE pool, indistinguishable from endogenously formed AGEs [48].

Table 1. AGE content in selected food items

REGULAR AGE DIET		LOW AGE DIET	
Food	AGE content (kilounits/100g)	Food	AGE content (kilounits/100g)
Chicken, broiled	5828	Chicken, boiled	1124
Beef, broiled	5963	Beef, stewed	2230
Salmon, broiled	4334	Salmon, boiled	1081
Lamb leg, broiled	2431	Lamb leg, boiled	1218
French fries	1522	Potato, boiled	17
Tuna, broiled	5113	Tuna, fresh	919
Egg, omelet, butter	507	Egg, omelet, corn oil	222

Data for this table has been obtained from reference 46

Common AGE compounds found in foods, such as εN-carboxymethyl-lysine (CML) or methylglyoxal (MG) derivatives have been shown to have similar in vitro pro-inflammatory and pro-oxidative actions as their endogenous counterparts [50]. In vivo links have been described between dietary AGEs and a variety of disease processes [51-55]. More importantly, a number of animal studies have shown that reduced consumption of dietary AGEs diminishes serum AGE levels and suppresses many disease processes, including insulin resistance in db/db (+/+) mice (50), atherosclerosis in apoE deficient mice [52,56] and diabetic nephropathy in NOD and db/db (+/+) mice [57].

These experimental findings have now been supported by studies in healthy subjects as well as in patients with diabetes or kidney disease, who responded to a low-AGE diet with marked reduction of circulating AGE levels [9,58,59]. More importantly, a low AGE diet for a period of only 4 weeks produced significant decrease of extracellular and intracellular markers of inflammation and oxidative stress, including TNF-α, VCAM-1, RAGE and p66 in a group of chronic kidney disease patients [9]. It is particularly noteworthy that peripheral mononuclear cell AGER1 mRNA, which was suppressed in CKD patients was restored after the low AGE diet, implicating oxidants rather than genetic causes in the loss of AGER1 in high OS conditions. Although peripheral mononuclear cells may not reflect other tissues with respect to AGER1, the data are in line with findings from aging mice fed a low AGE, linking increased tissue AGER1 to lower OS and extended lifespan [60].

All the above evidence supports a new paradigm in which the excessive consumption of AGEs and related oxidants secondary to a "Western lifestyle" represents an independent risk factor of inappropriate chronic oxidative stress during the healthy adult years, which over time facilitates the emergence of chronic diseases, such as diabetes and cardiovascular diseases [61].

The Effects of AGEs on Arteries

Elevated AGEs are also associated with macrovascular abnormalities, including atherosclerosis, which could indirectly contribute to renal disease in diabetic subjects by decreasing renal blood flow and by causing hypertension. AGEs have been shown to decrease both endothelial cell nitric oxide levels and activity by inhibiting endothelial nitric oxide synthase [62] and by quenching NO [63], thereby adversely affecting vascular endothelium and its protective functions, particularly vascular relaxation. Other actions on the endothelial cells include increased expression and release of VCAM-1 [64,65]. We recently showed that a single oral load of an AGE-rich beverage free of glucose or lipids to diabetic as well as to healthy subjects is associated with a significant rise of serum AGE levels in parallel with an acute impairment of endothelial function, as reflected both by a decrease in arterial vasodilation in response to ischemia and by an increase in circulating PAI-1 levels [66]. It is therefore reasonable to conclude that, during recurrent ingestion of high AGE foods, multiple insults to the vasculature can result in persistent endothelial dysfunction and, over time, in overt vascular disease.

AGEs also have direct influence on the structural integrity of the vessel wall affecting the physical properties of arteries, by decreasing their distensibility and elasticity in part induced by cross-linking of subendothelial matrix molecules, such as collagen, or by disruption of matrix–matrix and matrix–cell interactions. This interpretation is reinforced by the observation that AGE-breakers have been shown to improve arterial compliance is elderly subjects with predominantly systolic hypertension [67].

Dietary AGEs and the Pathogenesis of Diabetes

Up to this point, we have been discussing about the potential effect of AGEs in causing some of the complications of diabetes, namely diabetic nephropathy. Increasing evidence suggests that AGEs may actually play a role in the pathophysiology of insulin resistance, the most common underlying abnormality in the metabolic syndrome and in type 2 diabetes mellitus. At least three potential mechanisms could explain the effect of AGEs in inducing insulin resistance. The first mechanism is glycation of the insulin molecule [68], which alters the structure and significantly compromises biological activity of glycated insulin [69]. A second mechanism is the effect of AGEs inhibiting cytochrome c oxidase and ATP production, leading to the impairment of glucose-stimulated insulin secretion through iNOS-dependent nitric oxide production, as recently demonstrated [70]. A third mechanism is the effect of AGEs stimulating several intracellular signaling pathways leading to increased ROS production and thereby interference with insulin receptor downstream signaling [71]. In vitro incubation of skeletal muscle cells with AGEs impairs the metabolic function of insulin on these cells [72]. A high AGE diet induced insulin resistance in at least three animal models of diabetes, a situation prevented by a diet restricted in AGES [51,53,70]. In the clinical arena, we have described a direct correlation between serum AGE levels and HOMA, a marker of insulin resistance, in a large cross-section of healthy subjects [73]. Therefore, it seems that an excessive AGE intake may be an important factor in the increased incidence of type 2 diabetes mellitus in most modern societies.

Anti-AGE Therapies

On the basis on the above analyses, there are several possible approaches to decrease the body AGE load and therefore either prevent or slow down the progression of diabetic nephropathy. These strategies include decreasing the exogenous supply of AGEs by either restricting the AGE content of the diet or inhibiting the GI absorption of AGEs, decreasing endogenous AGE formation, reducing AGE effects on cells, breaking down AGE crosslinks or increasing urinary excretion of AGEs (Table 2). Lastly, combination therapy with drugs that act in part through different pathways such as blockers of the renin-angiotensin system could potentially have synergistic effects.

Table 2. Anti-AGE therapies

Mechanism of action	Therapy	Animal or human experience
Decreased exogenous AGE supply	Low AGE diet	-Proven effect decreasing circulating levels of AGEs
	Inhibition of GI absorption of AGEs	-Use of lysozyme in rats
-Current clinical trials with Kremezin
Decreased endogenous AGE formation	Control of hyperglycemia	-Proven to reduce AGE formation
	Use of medications	-Extensive animal experience with aminoguanidine, pyridoxamine and benfotiamine
-Clinical trials with Aminoguanidine and Pyridoxamine
Breakdown of existing tissue AGEs	Use of crosslink breakers	-Animal experience with alagebrium
-Clinical trials with alagebrium for arterial stiffness
Increased urinary excretion of AGEs	No specific therapy (some of above therapies increase urinary AGE excretion secondarily)	-No specific compound available
Reduced cellular effect of AGEs	Blockade of RAGE	-Animal experience with the use of the soluble form of RAGE
	Increased activity of AGER1	-Only of theoretical interest. No compound available.
	Use of antioxidants	-No specific trials for diabetic nephropathy reported
Blockade of the renin-angiotensin system	Several ACE inhibitors and angiotensin receptor blockers available	-Significant clinical experience with the use of these compounds for other clinical indications
Miscellaneous drugs	Hydralazine, thiazolidines, carnosine, etc.	-Significant clinical experience with the use of these compounds for other clinical indications

I) Low AGE Diet

Reduced intake of dAGEs can be achieved while consuming the usual amount of nutrients by simply changing the way of cooking the food from high heat dry application (roasting, barbecue) to low heat high humidity (stewing, etc) [46]. On the other hand, increasing the consumption of fish, legumes, vegetables, fruits, and whole grains and reducing intake of full fat dairy products, solid fats, fatty meats, and highly processed foods will also reduce dietary AGE intake. These guidelines are consistent with the dietary guidelines of the American Diabetes Association [74]. We have repeatedly shown that dietary AGE restriction is a feasible and safe strategy to decrease the body AGE burden in both healthy and sick populations [9,57,58].

II) Inhibition of Gastrointestinal Absorption of Dietary AGEs

Inhibition of gastrointestinal absorption of dietary AGEs may be a novel target for therapeutic intervention in diabetes and related diseases. AST-120 (Kremezin) is an oral adsorbent that attenuates the progression of chronic renal failure (CRF) [75]. It has recently been found that this compound binds CML in vitro and it decreases serum levels of AGEs in non-diabetic CRF patients [76]. These findings suggest that AST-120 could exert beneficial effects on CRF patients by adsorbing diet-derived AGEs and subsequently decreasing serum AGE levels raising a significant therapeutic potential for the treatment of patients with various AGE-related disorders as well. Currently, there are three ongoing clinical trials testing the effect of this compound in the progression of renal failure (www.clinicaltrials.gov) and results should be available in the future. The success of orally administered lysozyme in reducing serum AGEs and albuminuria in diabetic rats [38] raises the potential for using this compound in humans. Rice containing recombinant human lysozyme is currently available and has been successfully used to treat children with acute diarrhea [77].

III) Inhibition of Formation of New AGEs

A) Control of Hyperglycemia

Since hyperglycemia enhances AGE formation strict control of hyperglycemia should have a significant effect in reducing the body AGE pool [78]

B) Medications that Inhibit AGE Formation

Previous work with aminoguanidine, pyridoxamine and benfotiamine has already been discussed above. A review of the www.clinicaltrials.gov website reveals two ongoing clinical trials with these compounds:

1) A Double-Blind Clinical Trial of Benfotiamine Treatment in Diabetic Nephropathy. Sponsored by University Medical Center Groningen http://www.clinicaltrials.gov/ct2/show/NCT00565318?term=benfotiamineandrank=1
2) A Randomized, Double-Blind, Placebo-Controlled, Multi-Center, Phase 2b Study to Evaluate the Safety and Efficacy of Pyridorin (Pyridoxamine Dihydrochloride) in

Patients With Nephropathy Due to Type 2 Diabetes. Sponsored by NephroGenex, Inc.http://www.clinicaltrials.gov/ct2/show/NCT00734253?term=pyridoxamineandrank=3

IV) Breakdown of Existing AGEs

a) Alagebrium

Previous work with the use of AGE breakers such as alagebrium has been discussed above. A review of the www.clinicaltrials.gov website reveals one clinical trial with this compound that reportedly was terminated early because of financial constraints.

b) Increased AGER1 Activity

Increasing activity of AGER1 that destroys AGEs remains as a possibility in the future.

V) Increased Urinary Excretion of AGEs

At any particular time, circulating AGE levels reflect the balance between input of AGEs into the extracellular space from both exogenous and endogenous sources and output through tissue breakdown and more importantly, urinary excretion of AGEs. Tissue breakdown of AGEs is processed mostly through cellular endocytosis followed by intracellular degradation resulting in low molecular weight AGE peptides, which are then released to the extracellular space. AGE peptides filter across the glomerular basement membrane and undergo variable degree of reabsorption and catabolism in the proximal tubular cells, while the rest is excreted in the urine [79-81]. The development of compounds that affect renal tubular handling of AGEs and therefore their urinary excretion remains as a completely unexplored area.

VI) Reduce AGE Effects on Cells;

a) Modification of Cellular Receptors Of AGEs

Administration of the soluble form of RAGE (sRAGE) in an experimental model of diabetic nephropathy markedly diminished albuminuria and improved glomerulosclerosis [28] showing promise as a possible future therapy.

As mentioned above, mesangial cells over-expressing AGER1, the protector anti-oxidant AGE receptor, prevented the actions of AGEs. Increasing the expression of this receptor in the kidney could be an important mechanism against diabetic nephropathy, but this remains only speculative.

b) Use of Antioxidants

AGEs produce cellular injury by a cascade of receptor-dependent and independent events that lead to the intracellular generation of reactive oxygen species. Moreover, OS contributes to the generation of AGEs. Because of this reciprocal process through which AGEs and OS mutually enhance production of one another it makes sense that any drug with antioxidant action might have an anti-AGE effect. Experimentally, blockade of NADPH oxidase, a major source of cellular ROS, by apocynin decreased renal extracellular matrix accumulation of fibronectin and collagen IV in a model of diabetic nephropathy [82]. Several other antioxidant compounds have been used with variable success in animals [83-85]. Unexpectedly, however, no major therapeutic drugs have been developed in this area. A review of the www.clinicaltrials.gov website shows a completed study on the effect of N-Acetylcysteine for treatment of overt diabetic nephropathy from Shiraz University of Medical Sciences in Iran, but we found no reported results from the group in a pubMed search (December 2010).

VII) Blockade of the Renin-Angiotensin System

Activation of the renin-angiotensin system (RAS) elicits OS generation and subsequently stimulates growth factor and cytokine production by kidney cells as well, in a similar way as AGEs do [86]. Therefore, a cross talk between AGEs and the RAS has been proposed to participate in diabetic nephropathy [86]. This background suggests that combination therapy with inhibitors of the RAS and anti-AGE agents may be a good therapeutic option for diabetic nephropathy. Actually, a good number of ACE inhibitors and angiotensin receptor blockade of the renin-angiotensin system [87-89] have been shown to attenuate the accumulation of tissue AGEs. It remains to be seen whether this can be apply clinically since a recent study showed that irbesartan did not alter the increase in pentosidine and CML in serum of type 2 diabetic patients with progressive nephropathy [90].

VIII) Miscellaneous Drugs

Hydralazine, another antihypertensive agent whose effect does not involve the renin–angiotensin system, has AGE-inhibitory effects similar to those of low-dose olmesartan [91]. A number of antidiabetic agents including thiazolidines [92] and metformin [93] also reduce AGE formation. Carnosine is a dipeptide with both antiglycation and antioxidant action (94). It remains to be determined if it is the reduction in tissue AGE levels per se or inhibition of downstream signal pathways which is ultimately required for end organ protection.

References

[1] US Renal Data System, USRDS 2005 Annual Data Report. Atlas of End stage Renal Disease in the United States, National Institute of Health, National Institute of Diabetes and Digestive and Kidney Disease: Bethesda, MD 2005.

[2] Brownlee M. Biochemistry and molecular cell biology of diabetic complications. Nature. 2001;414:813-20.

[3] Ulrich P, Cerami A. Protein glycation, diabetes and aging. Recent Prog Horm Res. 2001; 56:1-21.

[4] Vlassara H, Uribarri J, Cai W, Striker G. Advanced glycation end product homeostasis: exogenous oxidants and innate defenses. Ann N Y Acad Sci. 2008;1126:46-52

[5] Yan SF, Du Yan S, Ramasamy R, Scmidt AM. Tempering the wrath of RAGE: An emerging therapeutic strategy against diabetic complications, neurodegeneration, and inflammation. Ann Med 2009; 25:1-15

[6] Cai W, He C, Zhu L, Vlassara H. Advanced glycation end product (AGE) receptor 1 suppresses cell oxidant stress and activation signaling via EGF receptor. PNAS USA 2006; 103: 13801-806

[7] Cai W, He JC, Zhu L, Chen X, Striker GE, and Vlassara H. AGE-receptor-1 counteracts cellular oxidant stress induced by AGEs via negative regulation of p66shc-dependent FKHRL1 phosphorylation. *AM. J. Physiol.* 2008; 294: 145-152

[8] He CJ, Koschinsky T, Buenting C, Vlassara H. Presence of diabetic complications in type 1 diabetic patients correlates with low expression of mononuclear cell AGE-receptor-1 and elevated serum AGE. *Mol. Med.* 2001 ;7:159-68.

[9] Vlassara H, Cai W, Goodman S, Pyzik R, Yong A, Zhu L, Neade T, Beeri M, Silverman JM, Ferrucci L, Tansman L, Striker GE, Uribarri J. Protection against loss of innate defenses in adulthood by low AGE intake; role of a new anti-inflammatory AGE-receptor-1. *J. Clin. End. Met.* 2009 ;94:4483-91.

[10] Liu H, Zheng F, Li Z, Uribarri J, Ren B, Hutter R, Tunstead JR, Badimon J, Striker GE, Vlassara H. Reduced acute vascular injury and atherosclerosis in hyperlipidemic mice transgenic for lysozyme. *Am. J. Pathol.* 2006 ;169:303-13

[11] Silbiger S, Crowley S, Shan Z, Brownlee M, Satriano J, Schlondorff D: Nonenzymatic glycation of mesangial matrix and prolonged exposure of mesangial matrix to elevated glucose reduces collagen synthesis and proteoglycan charge. *Kidney Int* 43:853 – 864,1993

[12] Mott JD, Khalifah RG, Nagase H, Shield CF 3rd, Hudson JK, Hudson BG: Nonenzymatic glycation of type IV collagen and matrix metalloproteinase susceptibility. *Kidney Int* 52:1302 –1312,1997

[13] Krishnamurti U, Rondeau E, Sraer JD, Michael AF, Tsilibary EC: Alterations in human glomerular epithelial cells interacting with nonenzymatically glycosylated matrix. *J. Biol. Chem.* ;272:27966 –27970,1997

[14] Charonis AS, Tsilbary EC: Structural and functional changes of laminin and type IV collagen after nonenzymatic glycation. *Diabetes* 41[Suppl 2] :S49 –S51,1992

[15] McLennan SV, Kelly DJ, Schache M, Waltham M, Dy V, Langham RG, Yue DK, Gilbert RE. Advanced glycation end products decrease mesangial cell MMP-7: a role in matrix accumulation in diabetic nephropathy? *Kidney Int* 72:481-488, 2007

[16] McLennan SV, Martell SK, Yue DK. McLennan SV, Martell SK, Yue DK. Effects of mesangium glycation on matrix metalloproteinase activities: possible role in diabetic nephropathy. *Diabetes.* 2002 ;51:2612-8

[17] Cohen MP, Lautenslager GT, Hud E, Shea E, Wang A, Chen S, Shearman CW.Inhibiting albumin glycation attenuates dysregulation of VEGFR-1 and collagen IV subchain production and the development of renal insufficiency. *Am. J. Physiol. Renal. Physiol.* 2007 ;292:F789-95

[18] Oldfield MD, Bach LA, Forbes JM, Nikolic-Paterson D, McRobert A, Thallas V, Atkins RC, Osicka T, Jerums G, Cooper ME: Advanced glycation end products cause epithelial-myofibroblast transdifferentiation via the receptor for advanced glycation end products (RAGE). *J. Clin. Invest.* 108:1853–1863, 2001

[19] Li JH, Wang W, Huang XR, Oldfield M, Schmidt AM, Cooper ME, Lan HY: Advanced glycation end products induce tubular epithelial-myofibroblast transition through the RAGE-ERK1/2 MAP kinase signaling pathway. *Am. J. Pathol.* 164 : 1389–1397, 2004

[20] Wang W, Huang XR, Li AG, Liu F, Li JH, Truong LD, Wang XJ, Lan HY. Signaling mechanism of TGF-beta1 in prevention of renal inflammation: role of Smad7. *J. Am. Soc. Nephrol.* 2005; 16:1371-1383

[21] Burns WC, Twigg SM, Forbes JM, Pete J, Tikellis C, Thallas-Bonke V, Thomas MC, Cooper ME and Kantharidis P. Connective Tissue Growth Factor Plays an Important Role in Advanced Glycation End Product–Induced Tubular Epithelial-to-Mesenchymal Transition: Implications for Diabetic Renal Disease *J. Am. Soc. Nephrol.* 17: 2484-2494, 2006

[22] Chuang PY, Yu Q, Fang W, Uribarri J, He J: Advanced glycation endproducts induce podocyte apoptosis by activation of the FOXO4 transcription factor. *Kidney Int* 72:965–976,2007

[23] Doubler S, Salvidio G, Lupia E, Ruotsalainen V, Verzola D, Deferrari G, camusi G. Nephrin expression is reduced in human diabetic nephropathy: evidence for a distinct roel for glycated albumin and angiotensin II. *Diabetes* 52:1023-1030, 2003

[24] Bondeva T, Ruster C, Franke S, Hammeerschmid E, Klagsbrun M, Cohen CD, Wolf G. Advanced glycation end-products suppress neuropilin-1 expression in podocytes. *Kidney Int* 2009; 75:605-616

[25] Yang CW, Vlassara H, Peten EP, He CJ, Striker GE, Striker LJ. Advanced glycation end products up-regulate gene expression found in diabetic glomerular disease. *PNAS* 91:9436-9440, 19994

[26] Vlassara H, Fuh H, Makita Z, Krungkrai S, Cerami A, Bucala R. Exogenous advanced glycosylation end products induce complex vascular dysfunction in normal animals: a model for diabetic and aging complications. *Proc. Natl. Acad Sci. U S A.* 1992 ;89:12043-7

[27] Yamamoto Y, Kato I, etc. Development and prevention of advanced diabetic nephropathy in RAGE-overexpressing mice. *J. Clin. Invest.* 108:261-168, 2001

[28] Wendt TM, Tanji N, Guo J, Kislinger TR, Qu W, Lu Y, Bucciarelli LG, Rong LL, Moser B, Markowitz GS, Stein G, Bierhaus A, Liliensiek B, Arnold B, Nawroth PP, Stern DM, D'Agati VD, Schmidt AM: RAGE drives the development of glomerulosclerosis and implicates podocyte activation in the pathogenesis of diabetic nephropathy. *Am. J. Pathol.* 162:1123 –1137,2003

[29] Soulis T, Cooper ME, Sastra S, Thallas V, Panagiotopoulos S, Bjerrum OJ, Jerums G: Relative contributions of advanced glycation and nitric oxide synthase inhibition to aminoguanidine-mediated renoprotection in diabetic rats. *Diabetologia* 40:1141 – 1151,1997

[30] Babaei-Jadidi R, Karachalias N, Ahmed N, Battah S, Thornalley PJ. Prevention of incipient diabetic nephropathy by high-dose thiamine and benfotiamine. *Diabetes* 2003; 52:2110-2120

[31] Tanimoto M, Gohda T, Kaneko S, Hagiwara S, Murakoshi M, Aoki T, Yamada K, Ito T, Matsumoto M, Horikoshi S, Tomino Y. Effect of pyridoxamine (K-163), an inhibitor of advanced glycation end products, on type 2 diabetic nephropathy in KK-A(y)/Ta mice. *Metabolism* 56:160-167, 2007

[32] Zheng F, Zeng YJ, Plati AR, Elliot SJ, Berho M, Potier M, Striker LJ, Striker GE. Combined AGE inhibition and ACEi decreases the progression of established diabetic nephropathy in B6 db/db mice. *Kidney Inter* 70:507, 2006

[33] Nakamura S, Makita Z, Ishikawa S, Yasumura K, Fujii W, Yanagisawa K, Kawata T, Koike T: Progression of nephropathy in spontaneous diabetic rats is prevented by OPB-9195, a novel inhibitor of advanced glycation. *Diabetes* 46:895–899,1997

[34] Joshi D, Gupta R, Dubey A, Shiwlaker A, Pathak P, Gupta RC, Chauthaiwale V, Dutt C. TRC4186, a novel AGE-breaker improves diabetic cardiomyopathy and nephropathy in Ob-ZSF1 model of type 2 diabetes. *J. Cardiovasc. Pharmacol.* 2009, June 17

[35] Forbes JM, Thallas V, Thomas MC, Founds HW, Burns WC, Jerums G, Cooper ME: The breakdown of preexisting advanced glycation end products is associated with reduced renal fibrosis in experimental diabetes. *FASEB J* 17:1762–1764,2003

[36] Peppa M, Brem H, Cai W, Zhang JG, Basgen J, Li Z, Vlassara H, Uribarri J. Prevention and reversal of diabetic nephropathy in db/db mice treated with alagebrium (ALT-711). *Am. J. Nephrol.* 2006; 26:430-6

[37] Zheng F, Cai W, Mitsuhashi T, Vlassara H.Lysozyme enhances renal excretion of advanced glycation endproducts in vivo and suppresses adverse age-mediated cellular effects in vitro: a potential AGE sequestration therapy for diabetic nephropathy? *Mol. Med.* 2001; 7:737-747

[38] Cocchietto M, Zorzin L, Toffoli B, Candido R, Fabris R, Stebel M, Sava G. Orally administered microencapsulated lysozyme downregulates serum AGE and reduces the severity of early-stage diabetic nephropathy. *Diabetes Metab.* 34:587,2008

[39] Makita Z, Radoff S, Rayfield EJ, Yang Z, Skolnik E, Delaney V, Friedman EA, Cerami A, Vlassara H.Advanced glycosylation end products in patients with diabetic nephropathy. *N. Engl. J. Med.* 1991 ;325:836-42

[40] Schleicher ED, Wagner E, Nerlich AG. Increased accumulation of the glycoxidation product N(epsilon)-(carboxymethyl)lysine in human tissues in diabetes and aging. *J. Clin. Invest.* 1997; 99:457-468

[41] Horie K, Miyata T, Maeda K et al. Immunohistochemical colocalization of glycoxidation products and lipid peroxidation products in diabetic glomerular lesions. Implications for oxidative stress in the pathogenesis of diabetic nephropathy. *J. Clin. Invest.* 1997; 100:2995-3004

[42] Sugiyama S, Miyata T, Horie K et al. Advanced glycation end-products in diabetic nephropathy. *Nephrol. Dial. Transplant.* 1996; 11(suppl 5):91-94

[43] Tanji N, Markowitz GS, Fu C et al. Expression of advanced glycatioen end products and their cellular receptor RAGE in diabetic nephropathy and nondiabetic renal disease. *J. Am. Soc. Nephrol* .200; 11:1656-1666

[44] Bolton WK, Cattran DC, Williams ME, Adler SG, Appel GB, Cartwright K, Foiles PG, Freedman BI, Raskin P, Ratner RE, Spinowitz BS, Whittier FC, Wuerth JP; ACTION I Investigator Group. Randomized trial of an inhibitor of formation of advanced glycation end products in diabetic nephropathy. *Am. J. Nephrol* .2004; 24:32-40

[45] Williams ME, Bolton WK, Khalifah RG, Degenhardt TP, Schotzinger RJ, McGill JB. Effects of pyridoxamine in combined phase 2 studies of patients with type 1 and type 2 diabetes and overt nephropathy. *Am. J. Nephrol.* 27:605, 2007

[46] Uribarri J, Woodruff S, Goodman S, Cai W, Chen X, Pyzik R, Yong A, Striker GE, Vlassara H. Advanced glycation end products in foods and a practical guide to their reduction in the diet. *J Am Diet Assoc* 2010 ; 110:911-16.

[47] Koschinsky T, He CJ, Mitsuhashi T, Bucala R, Liu C, Bueting C, Heitmann K, Vlassara H. Orally absorbed reactive advanced glycation end products (glycotoxins): an environmental risk factor in diabetic nephropathy. *Proc. Natl. Acad. Sci. USA.* 1997; 94: 6474–6479

[48] He C, Sabol J, Mitsuhashi T, Vlassara H. Dietary glycotoxins: inhibition of reactive products by aminoguanidine facilitates renal clearance and reduces tissue sequestration. *Diabetes* 1999; 48:1308-1315

[49] Cai W, He JC, Zhu L, Chen X, Zheng F, Striker GE, Vlasara H. Oral glycotoxins determine the effects of calorie restriction on oxidant stress, age-related diseases, and lifespan. *Am. J. Pathol* .2008; 173:327-36

[50] Cai W, Gao Q-d, Zhu L, Peppa M, He C, and Vlassara H. Oxidative stress-inducing carbonyl compounds from common foods: novel mediators of cellular dysfunction. *Mol. Med.* 2002; 8(7): 337-46

[51] Hofmann SM, Dong HJ, Li Z, Cai W, Altomonte J, Thung SN, Zeng F, Fisher EA, Vlassara H: Improved insulin sensitivity is associated with restricted intake of dietary glycoxidation products in the db/db mouse. *Diabetes 51*:2082 –2089,2002

[52] Lin RY, Choudhury RP, Cai W, Lu M, Fallon JT, Fisher EA, Vlassara H: Dietary glycotoxins promote diabetic atherosclerosis in apolipoprotein E-deficient mice. *Atherosclerosis* 168:213 –220,2003

[53] Sandu O, Song K, Cai W, Zheng F, Uribarri J, Vlassara H. Insulin resistance and type 2 diabetes in high-fat-fed mice are linked to high glycotoxin intake. *Diabetes* 2005; 54:2314-2319

[54] Peppa M, He C, Hattori M, McEvoy R, Zheng F, Vlassara H. Fetal or neonatal low-glycotoxin environment prevents autoimmune diabetes in NOD mice. Diabetes. 2003 ;52:1441-8.

[55] Peppa M, Brem H, Ehrlich P, Zhang JG, Cai W, Li Z, Croitoru A, Thung S, Vlassara H. Adverse effects of dietary glycotoxins on wound healing in genetically diabetic mice. *Diabetes.* 2003 ;52:2805-13.

[56] Lin RY, Reis ED, Dore AT, Lu M, Ghodsi N, Fallon JT, Fisher EA, Vlassara H. Lowering of dietary advanced glycation endproducts (AGE) reduces neointiminal formation after arterial injury in genetically hypercholesterolemic mice. *Atherosclerosis* 2002; 163: 303-11

[57] Zheng F, He C, Cai W, Hattori M, Steffes M, Vlassara H. Prevention of diabetic nephropathy in mice by a diet low in glycoxidation products. *Diab. Metab. Res. Rev.* 2002, 18: 224-37

[58] Vlassara H, Cai W, Crandall J, Goldberg T, Oberstein R, Dardaine V, Peppa M, Rayfield EJ: Inflammatory mediators are induced by dietary glycotoxins, a major risk factor for diabetic angiopathy. *Proc. Natl. Acad. Sci. U S A*99:15596 –155601,2002

[59] Uribarri J, Peppa M, Cai W, Goldberg T, Lu M, He C, Vlassara H: Restriction of dietary glycotoxins reduces excessive advanced glycation end products in renal failure patients. *J. Am. Soc. Nephrol.* 14:728 –731,2003

[60] Cai W, He JC, Zhu L, Chen X, Wallenstein S, Striker GE, Vlassara H. Reduced oxidant stress and extended lifespan in mice exposed to a low glycotoxin diet: association with increased AGER1 expression. *Am. J. Pathol.* 2007;170:1893-902.
[61] Vlassara H, Uribarri J. Glycoxidation and diabetic complications: modern lessons and a warning? *Rev. Endocr. Metab. Disord.* 2004;5:181-8
[62] Xu B, Chibber R, Ruggiero D, Kohner E, Ritter J, Ferro A. Impairment of vascular endothelial nitric oxide synthase activity by advanced glycation end products. *FASEB J.* 17:1289–1291, 2003
[63] Bucala R, Tracey KJ, Cerami A: Advanced glycosylation products quench nitric oxide and mediate defective endothelium-dependent vasodilatation in experimental diabetes. *J. Clin. Invest.* 87:432–438, 1991
[64] Cai W, He JC, Zhu L, et al.: High levels of dietary advanced glycation end products transform low-density lipoprotein into a potent redox-sensitive mitogen-activated protein kinase stimulant in diabetic patients. *Circulation* 110:285–291, 2004
[65] Basta G, Lazzerini G, Del Turco S, et al.: At least 2 distinct pathways generating reactive oxygen species mediate vascular cell adhesion molecule-1 induction by advanced glycation end products. *Arterioscler. Thromb. Vasc. Biol.* 25:1401–1407, 2005
[66] Uribarri J, Stirban A, Sander D, Cai W, Negrean M, Buenting CE, Koschinsky T, Vlassara H: Single oral challenge by advanced glycation end products acutely impairs endothelial function in diabetic and nondiabetic subjects. *Diabetes Care* 30:2579 – 2582,2007
[67] Kass DA, Shapiro EP, Kawaguchi M, Capriotti AR, Scuteri A, deGroof RC, Lakatta EG. Improved arterial compliance by a novel advanced glycation end-product crosslink breaker. *Circulation.* 2001;104:1464-70
[68] Guedes S, Vitorino R, Domingues MRM, Amado F and Domingues P. Mass Spectrometry Characterization of the Glycation Sites of Bovine Insulin by Tandem Mass Spectrometry *J. Am. Soc. Mass Spectrometry* 2009; 20:1319-26
[69] O'Harte FP, Boyd AC, McKillop AM, Abdel-Wahab YH, McNulty H, Barnett CR, Conlon JM, Højrup P, Flatt PR. Structure, antihyperglycemic activity and cellular actions of a novel diglycated human insulin.*Peptides.* 2000 Oct;21(10):1519-26
[70] Zhao Z, Zhao C, Zhang XH, Zheng F, Cai W, Vlassara H, Ma ZA. Advanced glycation end products inhibit glucose-stimulated insulin secretion through nitric oxide-dependent inhibition of cytochrome c oxidase and adenosine triphosphate synthesis. *Endocrinology.* 2009 Jun;150(6):2569-76
[71] Bashan N, Kovsan J, Kachko I, Ovadia H, Rudich A. Positive and negative regulation of insulin signaling by reactive oxygen and nitrogen species. *Physiol. Rev.* 2009;89:27-71
[72] Miele C, Riboulet A, Maitan MA, Oriente F, Romano Ch, Formisano P, Giudicelli J, Beguinot F, and Van Obberghen E. Human Glycated Albumin Affects Glucose Metabolism in L6 Skeletal Muscle Cells by Impairing Insulin-induced Insulin Receptor Substrate (IRS) Signaling through a Protein Kinase C-mediated Mechanism. *J. Biol. Chem.*, Vol. 278, Issue 48, 47376-47387, November 28, 2003
[73] Uribarri J, Cai W, Peppa M, Goodman S, Ferrucci L, Striker G, and Vlassara H. Circulating glycotoxins and dietary advanced glycation endproducts: two Links to

inflammatory response, oxidative stress, and aging. *J. Gerontol. A Biol. Sci. Med. Sci.* 2007; 62: 427-33

[74] American Diabetes Association position statement: Nutrition recommendations and interventions for Diabetes. *Diabetes Care* 2008; 31:S61-S78

[75] Shimizu H, Okada S, Shinsuke OI, Mori M.Kremezin (AST-120) Delays the Progression of Diabetic Nephropathy in Japanese Type 2 Diabetic Patients. *Diabetes Care 2005*; 28:2590

[76] Ueda S, Yamagishi S, Takeuchi M, Kohno K, Shibata R, Matsumoto Y, Kaneyuki U, Fujimura T, Hayashida A, Okuda S. Oral adsorbent AST-120 decreases serum levels of AGEs in patients with chronic renal failure.*Mol. Med.* 2006; 12:180-184

[77] Zavaleta N, Figueroa D, Rivera J, Sánchez J, Alfaro S, Lönnerdal B.Efficacy of rice-based oral rehydration solution containing recombinant human lactoferrin and lysozyme in Peruvian children with acute diarrhea. *J. Pediatr. Gastroenterol. Nutr.* 2007 ;44:258-64

[78] Monnier VM, Bautista O, Kenny D, Sell DR, Fogarty J, Dahms W, Cleary PA, Lachin J, Genuth S: Skin collagen glycation, glycoxidation, and crosslinking are lower in subjects with long-term intensive versus conventional therapy of type 1 diabetes: relevance of glycated collagen products versus HbA1c as markers of diabetic complications. DCCT Skin Collagen Ancillary Study Group. *Diabetes Control and Complications Trial Diabetes* 1999;48:870-880

[79] Gugliucci A, Bendayan M: Renal fate of circulating advanced glycated end products (AGE): Evidence for reabsorption and catabolism of AGE-peptides by renal proximal tubular cells. *Diabetologia* 39: 149–160, 1996

[80] Miyata T, Ueda Y, Horie K, Nangaku M, Tanaka S, van Ypersele de Strihou C, Kurokawa K: Renal catabolism of advanced glycation end products: The fate of pentosidine. *Kidney Int* 53: 416–422, 1998

[81] Saito A, Nagai R, Tanuma A, Hama H, Cho K, Takeda T, Yoshida Y, Toda T, Shimizu F, Horiuchi S, Gejyo F. Role of megalin in endocytosis of advanced glycation end products: implications for a novel protein binding to both megalin and advanced glycation end products. *J. Am. Soc. Nephrol.* 2003 May;14(5):1123-

[82] Thallas-Bonke V, Thorpe SR, Coughlan MT, Fukami K, Yap FY, Sourris KC, Penfold SA, Bach LA, Cooper ME, Forbes JM. Inhibition of NADPH oxidase prevents advanced glycation end product-mediated damage in diabetic nephropathy through a protein kinase C-alpha-dependent pathway. *Diabetes.* 2008 Feb;57(2):460-9

[83] S. Sharma, M. Anjaneyulu, S.K. Kulkarni and K. Chopra, Resveratrol, a polyphenolic phytoalexin, attenuates diabetic nephropathy in rats, *Pharmacology* 76 (2006), pp. 69–75

[84] S. Sharma, S.K. Kulkarni and K. Chopra, Curcumin, the active principle of turmeric (*Curcuma longa*), ameliorates diabetic nephropathy in rats, *Clin. Exp. Pharmacol. Physiol.* 33 (2006), pp. 940–945

[85] M. Anjaneyulu and K. Chopra, Quercetin, an anti-oxidant bioflavonoid, attenuates diabetic nephropathy in rats, *Clin Exp Pharmacol Physiol* 31 (2004), pp. 244–248

[86] Thomas MC, Tikellis C, Burns WM, Bialkowski K, Cao Z, Coughlan MT, Jandeleit-Dahm K, Cooper ME, Forbes JM. Interactions between renin angiotensin system and advanced glycation in the kidney. *J. Am. Soc. Nephrol.* 2005 ;16:2976-84

[87] Forbes JM, Cooper ME, Thallas V, Burns WC, Thomas MC, Brammar GC, Lee F, Grant SL, Burrell LA, Jerums G, Osicka TM: Reduction of the accumulation of advanced glycation end products by ACE inhibition in experimental diabetic nephropathy. *Diabetes* 2002; 51:3274-3282

[88] Miyata T, van Ypersele de Strihou C, Ueda Y, Ichimori K, Inagi R, Onogi H, Ishikawa N, Nangaku M, Kurokawa K: Angiotensin II receptor antagonists and angiotensin-converting enzyme inhibitors lower in vitro the formation of advanced glycation end products: biochemical mechanisms. *J. Am. Soc. Nephrol.* 2002; 13:2478-2487

[89] Liu XP, Pang YJ, Zhu WW, Zhao TT, Zheng M, Wang YB, Sun ZJ, Sun SJ. Benazepril, an angiotensin-converting enzyme inhibitor, alleviates renal injury in spontaneously hypertensive rats by inhibiting advanced glycation end-product-mediated pathways. *Clin. Exp. Pharmacol. Physiol.* 2009 ;36:287-96

[90] Busch M, Franke S, Wolf G, Rohde RD, Stein G; Collaborative Study Group.Serum levels of the advanced glycation end products Nepsilon-carboxymethyllysine and pentosidine are not influenced by treatment with the angiotensin receptor II type 1 blocker irbesartan in patients with type 2 diabetic nephropathy and hypertension. *Nephron. Clin. Pract.* 2008;108(4):c291-7

[91] Nangaku M, Miyata T, Sada T, Mizuno M, Inagi R, Ueda Y, Ishikawa N, Yuzawa H, Koike H, van Ypersele de Strihou C, Kurokawa K. Anti-hypertensive agents inhibit in vivo the formation of advanced glycation end products and improve renal damage in a type 2 diabetic nephropathy rat model. *J. Am. Soc. Nephrol.* 2003 ;14:1212-22

[92] Morcos M, Schlotterer A, Sayed AA, Kukudov G, Oikomonou D, Ibrahim Y, Pfisterer F, Schneider J, Bozorgmehr F, Rudofsky G Jr, Schwenger V, Kientsch-Engels R, Hamann A, Zeier M, Dugi K, Yard B, Humpert PM, van der Woude F, Nawroth PP, Bierhaus A. Rosiglitazone reduces angiotensin II and advanced glycation end product-dependent sustained nuclear factor-kappaB activation in cultured human proximal tubular epithelial cells. *Horm. Metab. Res.* 2008; 40:752-759

[93] Beisswenger P, Ruggiero-Lopez D: Metformin inhibition of glycation processes. Diabetes Metab 2003; 29:6S95-6S103

[94] Alhamdani MS, Al-Kassir AH, Abbas FK, Jaleel NA, Al-Taee MF: Antiglycation and antioxidant effect of carnosine against glucose degradation products in peritoneal mesothelial cells. *Nephron. Clin. Pract.* 2007; 107:c26-c34

In: Advances in Pathogenesis of Diabetic Nephropathy
Editor: Sharma S. Prabhakar

ISBN: 978-1-61122-134-3
© 2012 Nova Science Publishers, Inc.

Chapter VII

Growth Factors in the Pathogenesis of Diabetic Nephropathy

*Charbel C. Khoury[1] and Fuad N. Ziyadeh[2],**
[1]Feinberg School of Medicine, Northwestern University, Chicago, IL, US
[2]Faculty of Medicine, American University of Beirut, Beirut, Lebanon

Despite the growing toll of diabetic nephropathy on public health [1], the current armamentarium for treatment and prevention of the disease remains limited to the blocking of the renin-angiotensin-aldosterone system (RAAS) and the control of hyperglycemia. A number of large clinical trials attest to the effectiveness of such a treatment methodology [2, 3]. Yet recent evidence seems to show that a subset of patients continue to progress in their disease even with treatment [4, 5]. While the progression of nephropathy may be the result of incomplete patient adherence to therapeutic guidelines, this can also be viewed as a sign that the inhibition of the RAAS may not be equally efficient in all individuals. A number of additional therapies have been investigated over the past few years with no solid leads so far [6]. Growth factors have been associated with the development and progression of diabetic kidney disease (see Table 1). Understanding the role of these factors could generate future targets for therapy. In this chapter we will bring forth the current evidence and hypotheses on a number of these growth factors, focusing mainly on Transforming Growth Factor-beta (TGF-β) and the Vascular Endothelial Growth Factor (VEGF), the main players in the pathogenesis of the manifestations of diabetic nephropathy.

Overview of the TGF-β Family

In humans and other mammalians, the TGF-β superfamily is believed to include 33 known proteins [7].

---

[*] Address all correspondence to: Fuad N. Ziyadeh, M.D., Professor of Medicine and Biochemistry, Departments of Internal Medicine and Biochemistry, Faculty of Medicine, American University of Beirut, Bliss Street, Beirut, Lebanon, Phone: +961-1-350000, ext 5353, Fax: +961-1-370814, e-mail: fz05@aub.edu.lb; US Mail: 3 Dag Hammarskjold Plaza, 8th Floor, New York, NY, 10017, USA.

Table 1. Other Growth Factors in the Pathogenesis of Diabetic Nephropathy

Growth Factor	Role in pathogenesis	Type of Evidence	References
GH/IGF1	- Somatostatin analogs and Growth Hormone (GH) receptor antagonists decrease renal and glomerular growth, as well as urinary albumin excretion especially when initiated at the onset of diabetes	Experimental – Rodent type 1 DM	[337-344]
	- GHR/binding protein knockout mice are protected against diabetic glomerular changes	Experimental – Mice type 1 DM	[345]
	- No change in diabetic nephropathy markers upon inhibition with somatostatin analogue in type 2 diabetes model	Experimental type 2 DM – *db/db* mice	[346]
	- Possible correlation between serum or urinary GH, IGF-I, IGF binding protein levels and kidney function in type 1 diabetic patients	Human (results vary between studies)	[347-352]
	- Octreotide decreases glomerular hyperfiltration and kidney volume in type 1 diabetic patients	Human	[353]
	- IGF-I induces mesangial cell proliferation, migration, and matrix synthesis	Cell culture	[354-361]
	- GH may be protective to the podocytes. It results in actin reorganization, along with increased ROS production. IGF-1 specifically upregulates the angiogenic $VEGF_{xxx}$ in podocytes	Cell culture	[333, 362, 363]
	- IGF-I causes increased collagen synthesis in tubular cells, and has been found to augment CTGF (CCN2) activity	Cell culture	[236, 364, 365]
	- Endothelial cells respond to IGF-I with increased NO synthesis	Cell culture	[366]
PDGF	- upregulated Platelet-Derived Growth Factor (PDGF) in rodent diabetic models	Experimental	[367-370]
	- pharmacological administration to type 1 diabetic model results in transient mesangial proliferation but no long term effects on diabetic kidney disease	Experimental	[371]
	- non-specific inhibition results in amelioration of albuminuria, and glomerular and tubulointerstitial damage	Experimental	[368, 372]
	- upregulated in human diabetes	Human	[373-375]
	- induces mesangial cell proliferation and migration, may mediate TGF-β synthesis in diabetes	Cell culture	[376, 377]
HGF	- levels of Hepatocyte Growth Factor (HGF) are low in late stages of diabetic kidney disease, but may be increased early on	Experimental	[378]
	- improvement of glomerulopathy, albuminuria, tubulointerstitial fibrosis with exogenous administration of HGF (recombinant factor and gene therapy).	Experimental	[378-381]
	- variable renal levels in diabetic patients	Human	[382-384]

Growth Factor	Role in pathogenesis	Type of Evidence	References
	- HGF decreases TGF-β levels and effects in the kidney	Experimental and cell culture	[380, 385-387]
	-HGF decreases podocyte apoptosis	Cell culture	[388]
EPO	- administration of erythropoietin (EPO) reduced proteinuria, serum creatinine, glomerulosclerosis and tubulointerstitial fibrosis, and decreased TGF-β.	Experimental- STZ mice	[389]
	- SNP in the promoter of the EPO gene is associated with elevated EPO levels and is significantly associated with diabetic nephropathy	Human (combination of case–control association and functional studies)	[390]
	- Inefficient EPO or decreased levels may aggravate tubular hypoxia		[391]
Leptin	- administration of leptin induces proteinuria and increases glomerular matrix and TGF-β production	Experimental- rats	[392]
	- Leptin increases TGF-β synthesis and endothelial cell proliferation	Cell culture	[392]
	- Leptin stimulates glucose transport and the expression of TGF-βRII in mesangial cells	Cell culture	[393]

It encompasses, among others, the three isoforms of the TGF-β family (-1, -2, and -3), as well as the Bone Morphogenetic Proteins (BMP), the Growth and Differentiation Factors (GDF), the Activins, and the Inhibins [7]. These members share some similarities in their sequences, structure, and synthesis profiles. Their genes encode a prepropeptide with an amino-terminal signal peptide. Processing will result in a monomeric propeptide consisting of a prosegment (also referred to as Latency Associated Protein) and the monomeric polypeptide whose sequence is generally conserved across the TGF-β superfamily. These polypeptide molecules share a motif of three intramolecular disulphide bonds referred to as the "cysteine knot" [8]. While most of these cytokines are essentially secreted as disulfide-linked dimeric peptides, the number and the position of the cysteine amino acids differentiate between them [7,9].

To initiate its signaling pathways the TGF-β superfamily involves two sets of receptors: the Type I and the Type II receptors. Both are transmembrane proteins with an intracellular serine-threonine kinase domain, and differ mainly by the presence of a glycine-serine-rich (GS) region in the type I receptor. So far only seven type I and five type II receptors have been shown to associate with all the TGF-β superfamily, by creating different combinations of receptor-ligand interactions [7]. When the ligand engages the type II receptor, a heterotetrameric complex is formed, and the type II receptor phosphorylates the type I receptor at the GS region [10]. This induces a conformational change in the type I receptor and activates its kinase domain, thus leading to further downstream phosphorylation and signaling. The profibrotic and antiproliferative actions of TGF-β1 depend on the serine-threonine kinase activity [11, 12]. Nonetheless recent evidence indicates that the TGF-β receptor complex may also have a tyrosine kinase activity, the role of which remains to be clarified [13-15].

The characteristic pathway for the propagation of the TGF-β family signal involves a class of transducers referred to as the Smad proteins [16-18]. These can be divided into three subcategories. Typically, the receptor-activated (R-) Smads include Smad2 and Smad3 which are specific for the TGF-βs as well as activins, and Smad1, Smad5, and Smad8 for the BMPs. R-Smads are phosphorylated by the active type I receptors, and subsequently form complexes with the second group of Smads, the common mediator (co-) Smad or Smad4. These complexes usually interact with transcription modulators to coordinate -both positively and negatively- the transcription of many different genes including those involved the extracellular matrix (ECM) composition, regulation of the cell cycle, cell differentiation, among others. The third subcategory of Smad proteins, Smad6 and Smad7, are inhibitory in nature and participate in a negative feedback loop. These I-Smads cause dephosphorylation of the activated Type I receptor and compete for its binding; they also induce receptor down-regulation, interfere with the formation of the R-Smad/co-Smad complexes, and may repress gene transcription in the nucleus [7, 19]. Furthermore the I-Smads, and especially Smad7, could activate other routes of signaling, like MAP kinases and JNK, independently from the canonical R-Smad pathway [1]. In the podocytes Smad7 was shown to contribute to an apoptotic effect of TGF-β by inhibiting NF-κB signaling [20]. Currently, more and more experimental evidence is indicating that TGF-β may also signal through multiple non-Smad pathways including MAP kinase (MAPK) pathways, Rho-like GTPase signaling pathways, and phosphatidylinositol-3-kinase (PI3K)/AKT pathways [21]. The added intricacy of the signaling networks allows TGF-β to be central in a multitude and a variety of cellular processes.

TGF-β as a Mediator of Diabetic Nephropathy

The interest in TGF-β as a mediator of diabetic kidney disease stems from the panoply of data that implicate it in the regulation of cell proliferation and ECM production [22]. These cellular responses are reminiscent of the tubuloglomerular hypertrophy, basement membrane thickening, mesangial matrix expansion, and tubulointerstitial fibrosis observed in the kidney of diabetic patients. TGF-β's stimulating effects on ECM accumulation involve a double hit to the homeostatic balance maintaining the matrix. On the one hand, the cytokine regulates the composition of the ECM by inducing the expression of fibronectin, and matrix glycoproteins like osteonectin, osteopontin, tenascin, thrombospondin, biglycan, and decorin; it also regulates the expression of several collagen isotypes both directly and indirectly via its ability to induce the profibrotic cytokine Connective Tissue Growth Factor (CTGF) through both the Smad and MAP kinase pathways. On the other hand, TGF-β decreases ECM degradation by inhibiting the expression of enzymes that degrade the ECM such as interstitial collagenase and Plasminogen Activator as well as by stimulating Plasminogen Activator Inhibitor-1 (PAI-1) and Tissue Inhibitor of Metalloproteinases-3 (TIMP-3). Additionally, TGF-β induces or represses numerous members of the integrin family, the end effect being an increase in cell-matrix adhesion [1].

Three different isoforms of the TGF-β ligand have been described in mammalian tissues: TGF-β1, 2, and 3. While part of the TGF-β activity in the adult kidney may be contributed to by platelets, macrophages, and vascular smooth muscle cells, resident renal cells have been shown to produce their own. Accordingly the TGF-β1 isoform is found in both proximal and distal tubular epithelial cells, in interstitial cells, and more so in glomerular mesangial, endothelial, and epithelial cells [23-27]. Though TGF-β3 shares a comparable pattern in the kidney, its expression levels are lower in the glomerulus [27]. TGF-β2 protein seems to be mostly limited to the juxtaglomerular apparatus colocalizing with renin [28]. In the kidney TGF-β1 is the most highly expressed of the three isoforms and will be the focus of this review unless otherwise specified.

Other elements of the TGF-β system are present and active in the normal adult kidney. Indeed receptors for TGF-β have been identified in glomerular endothelial, mesangial, and epithelial cells [24, 29]. The TGF-β-linked Smads are also expressed in glomerular, tubular, and interstitial cells of the kidney, albeit with some cell-to-cell and Smad-to-Smad variation [30-35].

TGF-β in Experimental Diabetic Kidney Disease

Over the past decade or so, a multitude of research articles have implicated TGF-β in different models of diabetic kidney disease. In rodents with type 1 diabetes, urine and at times plasma levels of TGF-β are elevated [36-38]. However the kidneys of these diabetic animals specifically show increased expression and activation of the TGF-β1 pathway in parallel with the different stages of the renal disease [39-48]. Few days after the onset of glycosuria, both the mRNA and protein levels of TGF-β were increased in the kidney cortex of the non-obese diabetic (NOD) mouse and the diabetic Biobreeding (BB) rat. This coincided with the development of renal hypertrophy in the animals [39]. Similarly, in the streptozotocin (STZ)-diabetic rat and mouse models, the cortical and glomerular TGF-β mRNA increased within one to three days of the onset of the diabetic state [37, 40]. This early up-regulation of the TGF-β system is further emphasized by the finding of enhanced expression of TGF-β type II receptor (TGF-βRII) mRNA and protein in the early phases of STZ-induced diabetes [37, 47, 49].

When followed for 4 weeks or longer, NOD mice continued to show high levels of the cytokines [42]. Likewise, in STZ-diabetic rats, TGF-β mRNA and protein expression were further increased in the glomeruli and tubular interstitium. In parallel, there was an associated increase in ECM expression, suggesting that the cytokine may play a role in the subsequent manifestations of diabetic kidney disease, namely glomerusclerosis and tubulointerstitial fibrosis [41, 43-45]. The reduction of hyperglycemia with insulin treatment was shown to control the overexpression of TGF-β1 as well as reduce matrix deposition [40, 41, 43, 44]. Other models of type 1 diabetes also seem to point to an involvement of the TGF-β system. In the OVE26 mice, Calmodulin is transgenically over-expressed in the pancreatic β-cells, resulting in hypoinsulinemia, early onset of hyperglycemia, and progressive albuminuria [50]. Recent work on these animals has also shown a possible association between TGF-β and the tubulointerstitial fibrosis witnessed in the late proteinuric stages of the disease model [48].

As for type 2 diabetes, studies performed with *in situ* hybridization and immunohistochemistry on *db/db* mouse kidneys showed an upregulation of TGF-β1 in the glomeruli [51]. Concurrently, higher levels of TGF-βRII mRNA and protein were noted in both the glomerular and tubular compartments [51]. The result may be an increased sensitization of the kidney to both autocrine and paracrine TGF-β signals leading to extracellular matrix deposition and renal hypertrophy. Indeed the diabetic mice showed upregulation of the downstream signaling pathways in the glomeruli and tubules. Smad3 accumulated in the nuclei of glomerular and tubular cells as would be expected in a cell with active signaling [51]. Moreover southwestern histochemsitry indicated increased transcription of end genes, as significantly more nuclear protein binding to the Smad binding element (SBE) was seen in the diabetic glomerular and tubular cells. The response of TGF-β in type 2 diabetes was further proven in other models of the disease namely the obese Zucker [52] and OLETF rats [53].

Inhibition of TGF-β System: Answers and Questions

There is more to TGF-β in diabetic renal disease than a mere association. Indeed inhibiting the cytokine and its signaling with different strategies has shed some light into the depth and strength of this relationship. When STZ-diabetic mice received a short-term treatment with a pan-isoform TGF-β neutralizing antibody, the result was a marked decrease in glomerular hypertrophy as well as control of the upregulation of fibrotic signals represented by fibronectin, α1(IV) collagen, and TGF-β1 mRNA [37]. After this first analysis showing a potential causality, our group switched focus to the *db/db* mouse model and conducted a series of experiments to examine whether TGF-β inhibition can prevent and/or treat diabetic kidney disease. Long term (8 weeks) therapy with anti-TGF-β antibody was systemically administered to *db/db* mice shortly after the onset of the diabetic state. Accordingly we found a significant decrease in mesangial matrix expansion as well as renal Collagen IV and fibronectin expression [54]. More importantly, neutralization of this growth factor prevented the decrease in creatinine clearance which is seen in more advanced stages of the disease. However, no reduction in albuminuria was observed [54]. All in all, it is safe to say that TGF-β is involved in aspects of both the structural and functional deteriorations of the kidney in diabetes. Next to these preventive effects, anti-TGF-β antibody also showed a therapeutic potential. In a separate experiment, *db/db* mice were given the same treatment but this time after the establishment of diabetic kidney disease [55]. The glomerular basement membrane thickening and mesangial matrix expansion were consequently improved or reversed, approaching the normal measurements seen in the non-diabetic controls [55].

Interference with TGF-β signaling through Smad3 in diabetic mice confirmed an etiologic role for this component of TGF-β signaling in the manifestations of diabetic renal disease. The knockout (KO) of Smad3 in genetically engineered mice lacking exons 2 and 3 and then rendered diabetic by STZ showed prevention of renal hypertrophy, mesangial matrix expansion, fibronectin overexpression, glomerular basement membrane thickening, and increased plasma creatinine and blood urea nitrogen [56]. Interestingly, diabetic Smad3-KO mice also continued to exhibit marked albuminuria [56]. This dissociation of albuminuria from renal function and glomerulosclerosis may be explained by two hypotheses. Proteinuria, a pathogenic factor by itself, may mediate its downstream fibrotic effects on the tubulointerstitium through the TGF-β system [57]. Alternatively, the growth factor's widespread role in diabetic nephropathy may not extend to the pathophysiological drive behind albuminuria [57, 58]. In fact, the diabetic Smad3 KO mice failed to improve the decreased podocyte slit pore density, a histological change seen across a good number of proteinuric glomerular diseases [56].

A number of other articles have replicated the effects of the cytokine on diabetic renal pathology. Tampering with TGF-β by (a) using another panselective antibody (1D11) with or without add-on angiotensin converting enzyme (ACE) inhibitor [59, 60], (b) decreased expression of the TGF-β type II receptor (TGF-βRII) in TGF-βRII gene heterozygous mice [61], (c) administering pharmacological inhibitors such as SMP534 and GW788388 [62, 63], and (d) utilizing soluble TGF-β receptor like soluble Betaglycan and soluble TGF-βIIR [64, 65] all show marked improvement in glomerulosclerosis, ECM deposition, glomerular basement membrane thickening, or other histological and molecular parameters of diabetic renal disease. However, only the soluble Betaglycan study reports a significant effect on renal function [64]. The main controversy resides in the improvement in albuminuria noted in these articles as well as a different genetically engineered Smad3 KO mouse [59-66]. While differences in technical design can be identified among these studies, two main hypotheses for the TGF-β-albuminuria relationship stand out. In the study by Benigni's group using an anti-TGF-β antibody, the effectiveness of TGF-β inhibition was highly dependent on the timing of treatment. While capable of decreasing albuminuria when given early on in diabetes, anti-TGF-β antibody would do so in later stages of the disease only if combined with an ACE Inhibitor [60]. On the other hand, Russo's group using soluble TGF-βRII posits that diabetic albuminuria is in fact a result of a decrease in postglomerular albumin processing by the tubules, a process that is highly regulated via TGF-β [65]. In our opinion, whether or not this cytokine is central in the development of albuminuria remains to be clarified with additional studies and alternative methods of TGF-β inhibition. However, if indeed true, the "tubular vs glomerular" origin of albuminuria may explain why our experiments have repeatedly shown persistent albuminuria with general improvement of glomerular structure.

Human Diabetic Nephropathy and TGF-β

Studies in human patients corroborate the findings of animal research, implicating TGF-β in diabetic renal disease. Analysis of kidney biopsy from diabetic patients has revealed an upregulation of all three isoforms of TGF-β in the glomerular and tubulointerstitial compartments [43, 67, 68]. Similarly, when assayed by competitive RT-PCR, TGF-β1 mRNA had a marked elevation even in the early stages of diabetic nephropathy [69]. These results correlated with collagen IV deposition as well as one of the clinical markers of diabetes, mainly HBA1c [69].

To determine the renal production of TGF-β, Sharma et al. studied 14 type-2 diabetic and 11 non-diabetic patients undergoing an elective cardiac catheterization [70]. Both groups were relatively matched with respect to renal function, proteinuria, and hypertension. TGF-β levels were measured in the femoral artery, renal vein, and urine. The net mass balance (ng/min) across the kidney was calculated using the renal blood flow. The results demonstrated that while the kidneys of a non-diabetic subject extracts an average of 3500 ng/min of TGF-β protein from the circulation, the kidneys of a diabetic patient actually produces an average net amount of 800 ng/min. Furthermore, urinary TGF-β was increased up to four-fold in diabetic patients. The latter effect did not seem to be a consequence of enhanced glomerular permeability to circulating proteins, as both diabetic normo- and microalbuminuric patients showed a comparable increase in urinary TGF-β levels. Recently the same group conducted a second bedside experiment with 13 healthy volunteers [71]. After inducing acute hyperglycemia in the range of 200 to 250 mg/dl for a period of just 2 h, urinary levels of TGF-β increased seven-fold. The cytokine returned to normal values overnight. With the absence of any change in plasma levels of TGF-β throughout the hyperglycemic episode, the authors concluded that their results are most likely secondary to increased renal production. However the design of this study cannot exclude a delayed TGF-β response in the plasma coinciding with the time of urine collection. Taken together, these studies provide good evidence that the kidney is overproducing TGF-β in diabetes possibly very early on in the disease. Fluctuations in blood glucose are certainly common in diabetic patients. Consequently the TGF-β system may perhaps be increased in a pulsatile cumulative fashion at first due to rapidly induced signals, and then becomes constantly upregulated as more steady pathways become activated by the disease. Identification of these different pathophysiological processes, the contribution of different renal cells, and the activity of the secreted cytokine are all questions that remain to be addressed.

TGF-β also seems to be associated with the renal outcomes of the disease. When classified according to the level of mesangial expansion, type 2 diabetic patients with more severe histology had higher levels of urinary TGF-β [72]. On the other hand, in a nested case-control study from the EURODIAB Prospective Complications Study, urinary TGF-β measurements were found to be significantly elevated in type 1 diabetic patients with micro- or macro-albuminuria [73]. The strength of this correlation appeared to be partly dependent on glycemic control, the level of Amadori albumin, and blood pressure. The bivariate and multivariate analyses in this study allude to possible mechanistic pathways, whereby the increase in TGF-β is due partly to hypertension and hyperglycemia acting through increased Amadori-glycated albumin.

TGF-β as a Genetic Risk Factor for Diabetic Nephropathy

Development of renal disease shows familial clustering and ethnic variations in type 1 and type 2 diabetes [74, 75]. While genetic factors may very well influence diabetic nephropathy, the role of TGF-β system as susceptibility genes remains unclear. Studies have looked into DNA polymorphism in the TGF-β1, TGF-βR1, and TGF-βR2 loci, but a strong reproducible association is yet to be made [74-81]. The small sample sizes, as well as the environmental, demographic and ethnic factors that complicate such studies certainly play a role in the results. In so far, polymorphisms at position +869 (Thymine or Cytosine), which changes codon 10 (Leucine or Proline) of the TGF-β1 protein appears to be a plausible candidate. Despite one negative result [76], different groups have reported this polymorphism in type 1 and type 2 diabetes in Asian and European ethnic backgrounds [77-79].

Pathophysiological Mechanisms of TGF-β in Diabetic Kidney Disease

Upregulation of TGF-β in Diabetic Nephropathy: A Collaborative Effect

Classically diabetic nephropathy is viewed as a compilation of hemodynamic and metabolic changes. In fact, hyperglycemia and hemodynamic stress activate a number of metabolic pathways that seem to generally converge towards activation of the TGF-β system. Most kidney cell types in tissue culture show a direct effect of high ambient glucose on TGF-β expression. Mesangial cells [82, 83], glomerular endothelial cells [84], proximal tubular cells [85], and interstitial fibroblasts [86] upregulate the expression of the cytokine when grown in high glucose media; podocytes and mesangial cells show increased expression of its receptor, TGF-βR-II [49, 87]. Very early in the disease process, the glomerulus shows evidence of hyperfiltration and hyperperfusion [88]. It is believed that a defective autoregulation leads to a decrease in both afferent and efferent arteriolar resistances, mounting to an increase in glomerular plasma flow and the elevation of glomerular transcapillary hydrostatic pressure [89-91]. Apparently the resulting mechanical forces are capable of inducing a TGF-β signal. To mimic glomerular hypertension in culture, layers of mesangial and podocyte cells exposed to alternating stretch and relaxation cycles have shown increased synthesis of the growth factor and occasionally of ECM proteins [92-95]. Similarly TGF-β mRNA and protein levels are elevated in bovine aortic endothelial cells exposed to fluid shear stress in vitro [96]. In mesangial cells, the mechanical stimulus may in fact be transduced intracellularly by a protein kinase C (PKC) / p38 MAP kinase dependent pathway [97].

Moreover, many diverse factors like the prostanoids, nitric oxide (NO), atrial natriuretic peptide, growth hormone, glucagon, insulin, and angiotensin II (ANG II) have been suggested as agents causing the hemodynamic changes of diabetic nephropathy [98, 99]. Thromboxane A2 is a powerful vasoconstrictor that decreases renal blood flow, lowers single-nephron glomerular filtration rate, and was found to have a direct contractile effect on mesangial cells in vitro [100, 101]. Diabetic animal models have been shown to have increased renal Thromboxane expression [102] and an elevated urinary Thromboxane B2 (a metabolite of Thromboxane A2) shortly after the onset of the disease [103-107]. The prostanoid may accordingly be upregulated to counter the vasodilation of renal arteries [108]. Nonetheless proving its involvement in the hemodynamic presentation at hand has been inconclusive [105, 109-111], with some studies suggesting a decreased responsiveness of the kidney vasculature to Thromboxane A2 [112-114]. It appears, however, that the prostanoids may have a fibrogenic effect in mesangial cells that may be mediated by TGF-β [102, 115-118].

Angiotensin II (AngII) is another vasoactive humoral factor that has amassed large interest as a key mediator of diabetic nephropathy. Blockade of the RAAS is currently the predominant option available for the management of diabetic kidney disease [119, 120]. Although ACE inhibitors reduce systemic hypertension, normalize intraglomerular capillary pressure, and attenuate the increased glomerular capillary permeability [121-126], evidence points that their beneficial effects extend beyond the hemodynamic properties [127-129]. ANGII acts both independently and in synergy with high glucose to cause hypertrophy of proximal tubular cells and mesangial cells [130-133] and to stimulate ECM protein deposition

[130, 134-137]. Since various anti-TGF-beta regimens have been shown to abolish the nonhemodynamic effects of AngII, it appears that the hypertrophic and profibrotic effects of AngII are mediated, at least in part, by the TGF-β1 isoform [134, 138-142]. In fact ANGII stimulates TGF-β secretion in tubular epithelial cells [140], mesangial cells [143], and interstitial fibroblasts [144]. Cells stimulated with ANGII are shown to activate TGF-β1 gene transcription [139] and stimulate the expression of its TGF-βRII receptor [145]. Moreover ANGII increases TGF-β concentration by increasing the availability of its active form, as will be explained later. ANGII may also act directly by favoring the phosphorylation of Smad2 and Smad3 in a TGF-β-independent fashion [146, 147]. While ANGII did not appear to directly increase TGF-β secretion in podocytes, it did induce TGF-βRII expression as well as Smad activation indicating contribution of the TGF-β system in ANGII-induced podocytopathy [148]. On the other hand, the diabetic state is a potent stimulator of intrarenal RAAS, positively affecting several components: the precursor angiotensinogen [149], the enzymatic conversion [149-151], and inhibiting degradation enzymes such as ACE2 [152]. Interestingly, TGF-β itself can induce angiotensinogen gene expression [153], indicating a positive feedback loop that can be highly amplified in the diabetic state.

Oxidative stress is another mainstream pathway in the development of diabetic renal injury. Reactive oxygen species (ROS) are directly increased by hyperglycemia as glucose overdrives the Kreb's cycle and the mitochondrial electron transport system [154]. Concomitantly, they are possibly induced by depletion of endogenous antioxidants, activation of NADPH oxidase, and uncoupling of the Nitric Oxide Synthase eNOS among others [155-157]. When human mesangial cells were incubated with glucose oxidase (GO) - an enzyme that continuously generates hydrogen peroxide from glucose - the promoter activity, mRNA expression, bioactivity and protein production of TGF-β1 were all stimulated [158]. This may be the result of a direct activation of intracellular signaling pathways such as the MAPK and JAK-STAT in the diabetic kidney [157]. However oxidative stress also appears to be the common link leading to the activation of pathogenic mechanisms in diabetes: the polyol pathway, the hexosamine biosynthesis pathway (HBP), the protein kinase C (PKC) system, and advanced glycation endproducts (AGE) [154]. Superoxide can inhibit GAPDH thus leading to the accumulation of upstream metabolites and consequent activation of these pathways of glucose overutilization (see figure 1) [154]. The HBP has been shown to mediate its effects through an upregulation of TGF-β [159-165]. D-glucosamine surpasses the effect of high glucose in increasing fibronectin and proteoglycans synthesis as well as activation of the TGF-β promoter and consequently TGF-β production [163, 165]. By inhibiting glutamine:fructose-6-phosphate aminotransferase (GFAT), the rate limiting enzyme in the HBP, via biochemical and molecular means, researchers have proven that the effect of high glucose on the cytokine is partly mediated by the HBP [160, 163].

Moreover the hexosamines and TGF-β do not have an additive effect on the stimulation of fibronectin and laminin synthesis [159]. To further support this notion the addition of TGF-β antibodies blocks the effect of high glucose and glucosamine on fibronectin expression [159].

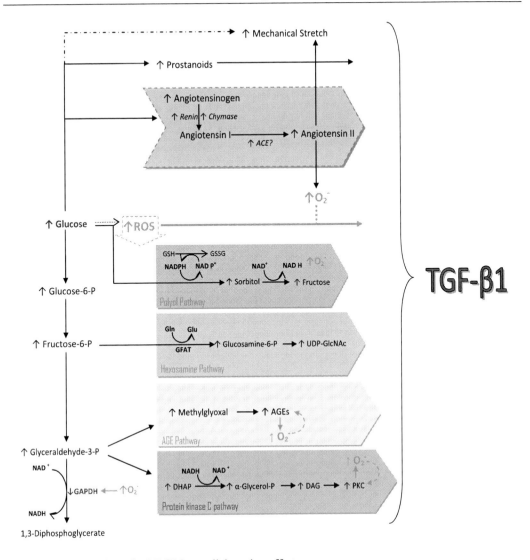

Figure 1. Upregulation of TGF-β1 is a collaborative effort.

Early nonenzymatic modifications of proteins such as amadori-glucose adducts of albumin are capable of increasing TGF-β expression in mesangial cells and glomerular endothelial cells [166, 167]. AGEs have also been shown to contribute to the stimulus for chronic TGF-β upregulation. The increased fibronectin message induced by glycated LDL in cultured mesangial cells is prevented by an anti-TGF-β antibody [168]. Current evidence indicates that signaling cascades activated upon binding of the glycated-ligands to the receptor RAGE are the origin of the growth factor induction. The signal may be directed through the RAAS system since candesartan, an antagonist of the type 1 angiotensin receptor (AT1R), completely inhibited TGF-β overexpression, Smad2 phosphorylation and TGF-β-inducible promoter activity in AGE-exposed mesangial cells [169]. Alternatively, the AGEs could be activating the Smad system via TGF-β dependent and independent pathways [170]. In mesangial cells, tubular epithelial cells, and vascular smooth muscle cells AGEs induce Smad phosphorylation and nuclear translocation in two intervals. First a short one, present in TGF-βRI and TGF-βRII mutant cells, that is mediated by ERK/p38 MAPK signaling. The second occurs after 24 h concurrently with increased TGF-β secretion in the medium that is also inhibited by anti-TGF-β antibody [170].

Finally oxidative stress has also been shown to contribute to the activation of the protein kinase C (PKC) pathway in diabetic nephropathy. PKC signaling contributes to various aspects of the disease process, including upregulation of TGF-β expression [171]. Inhibiting the beta isoform by the PKC inhibitor ruboxistaurin mesylate or KO of the same isoform in rodents is capable of mitigating the upregulation of TGF-β that would have normally been seen in the diabetic kidney [172-174]. In mesangial cells, PKC-β induces TGF-β expression in a p38MAPK/ERK or PI3Kinase/Akt dependent pathways [175-177]. In either case the end-effect is activation of the transcription factor AP1 known to bind to the TGF-β promoter and induce its transcription [175-177]. Thus inhibition of PKC-β appears to be a promising therapy of diabetic kidney disease. In a small clinical study the addition of ruboxistaurin to a standard ACE inhibitor or AT1R antagonist treatment of patients with diabetic nephropathy did not lead to the drop in estimated glomerular filtration rate and increase in urinary TGF-β seen in the control group [178].

It is concluded that the hemodynamic and metabolic processes that activate a myriad of pathogenic mechanisms in the diabetic kidney lead in one way or another to the upregulation of TGF-β expression or signaling.

Molecular Bioactivation of TGF-β in Diabetic Nephropathy

TGF-β is secreted from cells in an inactive latent form. The mature homodimeric TGF-β is non-covalently associated with a dimer of the propetide or latency-associated peptide (LAP) that is encoded by the same gene. Together they form the small latent complex (SLC) a form that is unable to engage the receptors. The SLC can also associate with one of the four latent TGF-β binding proteins (LTBPs) forming the large latent complex (LLC). LTBPs, except for LTBP-2, form covalent bonds with the SLC. They may regulate the deposition of the LLC into the ECM where TGF-β is stored until needed, and appear to have structural and functional similarities with the fibrillins as architectural elements of the ECM [7]. In the kidney, tubular epithelial cells secrete the SLC, while glomerular parenchymal and arteriolar cells secrete the LLC, thus indicating potential differences in the activation and functional regulation of TGF-β between the two renal compartments [25].

Administration of LAP decreases fibronectin expression from mesangial cells cultured in high glucose media [179] indicating that activation of latent TGF-β is essential for it to conduce its pathologic effect. Physiologically, this activation can result from the deglycosylation of the latent complex [180] or from the action of proteases such as plasmin [181]. $\alpha_v\beta_6$ integrins have been suggested to activate the LLC by inducing traction on the complex and activating TGF-β by conformational change [182]. Nonetheless the thrombospondin-induced activation appears to be particularly important in diabetes. Thrombospondin-1 (TSP-1) is a matricellular glycoprotein expressed by a number of cells including platelets, vascular smooth muscle cells and mesangial cells [183, 184]. Although still controversial, it is generally accepted that TSP-1 binds and activates latent TGF-β [184-187]. Two sites in the TSP-1 protein are necessary for this role. The first (GGWSHW—amino acids 418–423, or generically the WXXW motif) binds TGF-β perhaps to orient it appropriately, while the second sequence (KRFK—amino acids 412–415) induces a conformational change of LAP to free an active TGF-β [188-191]. In diabetic glomeruli and tubulointerstitial compartments TSP-1 is found to be expressed in the vicinity of phosphorylated Smads, indicating that it may be activating local TGF-β [192]. Its glomerular expression seems to be concentrated in the mesangial areas [193]. In fact in vitro studies indicate that high glucose induces mRNA and protein expression of TSP-1 in mesangial cells [194, 195]. Interfering with TSP-1-dependent activation of latent TGF-β abrogates glucose-induced accumulation of fibronectin [196]. The mechanisms involved in increasing thrombospondin in mesangial cells are possibly mediated by PKC signaling [197] leading to the nuclear accumulation of Upstream Stimulatory Factor 2 (USF2) [198]. Recent data from microarrays indicate that a similar pattern of upregulation could be present in podocytes treated with high glucose [199]. Furthermore TSP-1 is probably needed for diabetic tubulointerstitial fibrosis. High glucose and AGEs can upregulate TSP-1 in proximal and distal tubular epithelial cells [200, 201]. Blocking the matricellular protein with a specific antibody abrogates high-glucose-induced fibronectin deposition [200]. Daniel and coworkers recently developed a TSP-1-deficient diabetic mouse model, confirming TSP-1's role in vivo, with improved glomerular indices and albuminuria compared to control diabetic mice [202].

Activation of latent TGF-β may be due to direct effect of the oxidative stress that accumulates in diabetic kidney tissues. Evidence clearly indicates that ROS are capable of releasing TGF-β from its latent complex in cell-free models [203]. The cell and tissue-based evidence is less straight-forward and is mostly derived from studies on radiation therapy [204]. Ionizing radiation results in the rapid activation of LTGF-β and is known to lead to the generation of ROS by interacting with water and other oxygen-containing molecules [205, 206]. Interestingly some evidence points that ROS-dependent activation is isoform-specific, as only LTGF-β1 is rendered functional in vitro [207]. The effect may also be cell-specific; cultured mesangial cells, for instance, fail to activate their latent cytokine after exposure to radiation [208]. Certainly the current data on ROS-dependent activation are far from complete, but remain a preliminary indicator of a possible alternative joining forces with other diabetic signals that will culminate in increased levels of the TGF-β1 system: at the ligand expression, activation, and responsiveness in a diseased kidney.

TGF-β is A Pluripotent Growth Factor in the Kidney

TGF-β sustains a multitude of effects in the diabetic kidney that reflect its increased expression in both early and late stages of the disease. In that sense, the cytokine is found to contribute to the deranged vascular autoregulation [209]. It can interfere with IP3/Ca^{++} transients and attenuate cellular contraction [99, 209]. Furthermore, TGF-β1 can upregulate eNOS and enhance arginine resynthesis leading to increased vasodilatory NO [209].

Early on, the focus on TGF-β was led by its activities as a profibrogenic cytokine [22]. The growth factor is capable of replicating, if not in total, the matrix deposition and turnover seen in almost all kidney cells (mesangial cells, podocytes, endothelial cells, vascular smooth muscle cells, interstitial fibroblasts, and tubular epithelial cells) when exposed to high glucose [49, 82, 86, 87, 210]. Whilst many Smad-dependent and independent pathways have been shown to lead to the transcriptional modulation of fibrogenic genes, recent evidence indicates that TGF-β may also mediate its renal effects through mirco RNAs (miRNAs). These small non-coding RNAs function mostly as post-transcriptional repressors of multiple targets at a time [211]. Using cell culture systems, TGF-β has been shown responsible for the upregulation of miRNAs detected in diabetic animal models [211]. miR-192 may thus contribute to the deposition of col1A2 in the mesangial space [212], whilst miR-377 increases fibronectin, p21-activated kinase 1 (PAK1), and superoxide dismutases (SOD1/SOD2) [213]. Other preliminary data suggest that miR-216a may be involved in TGF-β autoregulation controlling its response in disease states [214]. Many other noncoding RNAs are hypothesized to be involved in diabetic nephropathy and will certainly be the focus of future interest [215]. Their versatility and adaptability are certainly fitting with the characteristics of TGF-β signaling in diabetes.

A specific miRNA family, the miR-200s, seems to be of particular importance in MDCK cells that have undergone epithelial-mesenchymal transition (EMT) in response to TGF-β [216]. EMT is in fact a well-established effect of the cytokine in different tissues and cancer types. A number of groups accordingly believe it to be the mechanism for the tubluointersitial fibrosis observed in diabetes [217]. Yet this remains to be a controversial issue. The origin of the myofibroblasts may also be the local fibroblast, or circulating fibrocytes and bone-marrow derived cells recruited into the interstitium [218]. TGF-β is known to activate fibroblasts into their secreting counterparts [218]; however its role in recruiting circulating cells is less straightforward but may be mediated by its capacity to induce the secretion of several chemokines from resident renal cells [219, 220].

In parallel, TGF-β has a growth regulatory effect on kidney cells. Mesangial cells demonstrate increased proliferation for the first 72 h of their culture in high ambient glucose, but this mitogenic activity arrests after the accumulation of glucose-induced TGF-β, manifesting as cellular hypertophy [221]. In fact, diabetes-induced renal expression of TGF-β may be responsible, at least in part, for diabetic renal hypertrophy. The antimitotic and hypertrophic growth effects in the kidney in diabetes are partially mediated by the cell cycle inhibitory $p27^{Kip1}$ [222]. Additionally, in endothelial cells, tubular epithelial cells, and podocytes, TGF-β can induce apoptosis [20, 223, 224], perhaps contributing through this effect to the tubular atrophy and the progressive loss of glomerular and peritubular microvasculature seen in the late stages of diabetic nephropathy. In podocytes the apoptotic effects are thought to be amplified by Smad7 signals leading to $p27^{Kip1}$ and p21 implicated pathways [20, 225]. It should be noted that the growth inhibitory effect in podocytes is dependent on the high concentration of the cytokine to which the cells are exposed, indicating the presence of a threshold above which the apoptosis cascade is initiated [226]. Whether or not the podocytes are ever exposed to that threshold in vivo is difficult to determine. Recent work indicates that the podocytes have alternative responses to TGF-β such as induction of de novo secretion of monocyte chemoattractant protein-1 (MCP-1). The addition of an anti-MCP-1 inhibitory antibody interfered with TGF-β's capacity to rapidly 'heal' a monolayer of podocytes in culture. An active MCP-1/CCR2 signaling has thus been shown to be responsible at least in part for the increased podocyte motility seen with TGF-β [227]. Combined with the apoptosis-independent downregulation of α3β1 integrin [228] these findings provide a good explanation for the decreased adhesion and podocyturia observed in diabetic kidney disease [229].

CCN2: More than Just a Sidekick?

CCN2, formally known as connective tissue growth factor (CTGF), is a member of a family of matricellular proteins that share a motif of four modules including: an insulin-like growth factor-binding protein domain; a von Willebrand factor type-C repeat; a thrombospondin type-1 repeat; and a C-terminal module [230]. This cysteine-rich peptide has been identified as an inducer of kidney fibrosis, and is found to be upregulated in human diabetic kidneys [231]. Similar increases are detected at the mRNA and protein level in animal models, whereby CCN2 seems to accumulate reaching high levels with the progression of diabetic nephropathy [232, 233]. This expression appears to be concentrated in the glomeruli [234], and may involve a cross-talk between podocytes and mesangial cells. Podocyte specific overexpression of CCN2 resulted in worsening of glomerular disease and albuminuria, with noted upregulation of CCN2 in mesangial cells as well [235]. Tubular expression is mostly concentrated in the proximal tubules with a less conspicuous expression in the distal tubules [236]. Inihibition studies confirm the pathogenic role of the growth factor in diabetic nephropathy. Treatment of diabetic mice with anti-sense oligonucleotides directed towards CCN2 ameliorated albuminuria as well as matrix deposition and histological findings [237]. The upregulation of CCN2 in general and in diabetes in particular is traditionally seen as dependent on TGF-β stimuli. The latter can directly induce CCN2 expression by binding to a TGF-β response element present in the promoter region of CCN2 [238]. By that CCN2 can parallel the upregulation of TGF-β seen in response to high glucose. Nonetheless, other TGF-β-independent pathways are also involved. Mesangial cells exposed to cyclical stretch respond by CCN2 upregulation as early as 4 h [234, 239]. Consequently the initial rapid effect is less likely to be induced by TGF-β, as the latter requires 24-48 h to respond to the stretch stimulus [240]. Other cytokines such as TNF-α can also induce CCN2 levels in mesangial cell cultures. The effect occurs without mRNA increase and is most likely the result of upregulation of matrix proteases, releasing bound CCN2 [241]. Furthermore CCN2 is capable of inducing its own expression in mesangial cells [234]. On the other hand, tubular epithelial cells are more likely to express CCN2 upon exposure to growth-factor-enriched glomerular ultrafiltrate rather than a direct effect of hyperglycemia. In this experiment however, proximal tubular cells did not respond to the glycemic stimulus with TGF-β induction [236]. As a downstream growth factor, CCN2 possibly mediates its effects through multiple paths. One such mechanism is the potentiation of TGF-β/Smad signaling. CCN2 may bind TGF-β ligand facilitating its interaction with the TGF-βRII [242]. Moreover, it also binds to BMP-7 leading to inhibition of its signaling ability [243]. BMP7, as will be elaborated on later, is a known inhibitor of TGF-β in the diabetic kidney. The third possible mechanism for facilitating TGF-β signaling involves the Tyrosine receptor kinase A (TrkA) and p75^{NTR} receptor complex. Present in mesangial cells, this receptor induces phosphorylation of a number of downstream targets upon binding to CCN2 [244]. As such CCN2 can induce the expression of TIEG-1 (TGF-β immediate early gene-1) which then represses the transcription of the inhibitory Smad7 [245]. Otherwise, the (TrkA)/p75^{NTR} receptor activation also leads to the secretion of pathogenic cytokines like MCP-1, RANTES, and fracktalkine known to contribute to inflammatory fibrogenic aspects of kidney disease [246]. CCN2's modules allow it to bind and interact with a number of other targets including integrins. In mesangial cells that target is the β3-integrin, and the result is an upregulation of fibronectin [247]. Even so, integrin binding may induce other cellular processes such as activation of the focal adhesion kinases, motility, and adhesion changes. While CCN2 has been found to replicate a number of TGF-β effects such as mesangial matrix expansion, mesangial cell hypertrophy, and tubulointerstial fibrosis [248], the idea that it acts as a pathogenic factor in diabetic nephropathy completely independent of TGF-β is still questionable. Transgenic mice overexpressing CCN2 in the podocytes fail to produce any histological or "clinical" findings, as renal structure and function remained comparable to controls despite significant increase in expression [235]. With that CCN2 appears to require the presence of other diabetic factors to reach its pathogenic potential [248].

Bone Morphogenetic Proteins in Diabetic Nephropathy: "Sibling Rivalry"

The Bone Morphogenetic Proteins (BMPs), mainly BMP-7 and perhaps BMP-2, are the other members of the TGF-β family whose downregulation is implicated in diabetic nephropathy. BMP-7 is of particular importance in kidney embryology. BMP-7 knockout mice die soon after birth as a result of poor renal development [249]. In normal adult kidney BMP-7 is highly expressed in distal convoluted tubules and outer medullary collecting ducts as well as glomerular cells and particularly the podocyte [250, 251]. However BMP-7 receptor distribution in the kidney does not exactly parallel that of the ligand; it is also localized in tubular segments and glomeruli but shows more mesangial than podocytic pattern of distribution [252]. This could implicate the presence of paracrine and autocrine signals in the kidney [253]. Upon engagement of the TypeI/TypeII receptor complex, BMP-7 usually induces phosphorylation of the Smad1, 5, and 8 proteins. Stimulation of mesangial cells and podocytes with BMP-7 favors the activation of Smad5 over Smad1 [254, 255]. Whether or not these data reflect a cell or tissue specific pattern of signaling is still to be clearly proven. In vivo studies are complicated by the fact that Smad activation is not as faithful as originally thought; Smad1 for example may be activated by TGF-β1 as well [253]. The involvement of BMP-7 in the pathophysiology of diabetic kidney disease is supported by the downregulation of this factor in the glomerulus and medulla of rodent diabetic models [256, 257]. In fact, in the STZ-treated rats, tubular BMP-7 was reduced by half after 15–16 weeks from the onset of diabetes, and reached a 90% drop by 30–32 weeks [257]. In addition, diabetes induces further reduction of BMP-7 activity by downregulating its receptors and modulating its antagonists. There is deceased renal expression of BMP Type II receptor and some of the type I receptors in diabetes [257]. As previously noted, CCN2 can interfere with BMP-7 receptor binding. Moreover BMP-7 is further regulated in vivo by noggin, chordin and follistatin, a group of proteins that bind and subsequently inhibit BMP-7 activity [7]. Although all 4 are expressed in the kidney, only follistatin has been shown to increase in diabetes [253, 257]. Noggin expression is however upregulated in podocytes treated with high glucose or TGF-β [253]. In preliminary work, Inhibin, a member of the TGF-β family and an inhibitor of the BMP receptor, is also upregulated in the diabetic kidney [253]. Bringing further evidence to the role of BMP-7 in diabetic nephropathy are the systemic replacement and transgenic overexpression studies conducted in rodent models of the disease. In their BMP-7 transgenic mice, Wang et al. show that this growth factor is capable of preventing progression of diabetic nephropathy [258]. The maintenance of its expression reduced albuminuria, glomerular sclerosis, and podocyte loss [258]. BMP-7 has also been shown to have a therapeutic potential partially reverting kidney hypertrophy and improving histology, albuminuria and glomerular filtration rate towards normal [256]. These results were further supported in the STZ-treated CD1-mice, a model of severe type 1 diabetic nephropathy, where BMP-7 administration was particularly helpful in improving the tubulointerstitial fibrosis prominent in these animals [259]. On the cellular level, BMP-7 has been shown to prevent TGF-β-induced mesangial ECM accumulation and tubular cell EMT [255, 260]. The mechanisms of this BMP-7/TGF-β rivalry involve interference with TGF-β signaling. In mesangial cells, BMP-7 induction of Smad5 results in the upregulation of the inhibitory Smad6 [255]. The latter prevents Smad3, the main fibrogenic signal in diabetic nephropathy, from translocating into the nucleus [255]. In addition Smad5 signaling appears to mediate the anti-apoptotic effects that BMP-7 has on podocytes. It reverts Caspase-3 activity induced by TGF-β or high ambient glucose [251, 254]. BMP-7 may also sustain TGF-β-independent actions, as it suppresses TNF-α-induced expression of interleukins (IL)-6 and -8, and MCP-1 in proximal tubular epithelial cells [261].

Other bone morphogenetic proteins, such as BMP-2 and BMP-4, may be linked to fibrotic nephropathies as well. In a unilateral ureteral obstruction model, BMP-2 was found to improve renal interstitial fibrosis. The authors propose that BMP-2 activates Smad7, which then results in TGF-βRI degradation [262]. BMP-4, on the other hand, has been postulated to contribute to the ameliorating renal damage due to mesangial proliferation caused by aldosterone [263]. Both BMP-2 and BMP-4 are known to be the favored targets for binding and inhibition by Gremlin [264]. Accordingly, it can be postulated that when upregulated in the diabetic kidney [265, 266], Gremlin abrogates the protective effect of these BMPs, resulting in a stronger TGF-β signal, and further fibrosis and disease.

Vascular Endothelial Growth Factor-VEGF

Vascular endothelial growth factor A (VEGF-A) or VEGF, is another growth factor that has accumulated increasing interest over the last few years, catapulted by its original characterization as a "Vascular Permeability Factor". The foremost theory was that if VEGF is upregulated in the diabetic glomeruli, its induction of vascular permeability would explain the observed albuminuria [267]. This homodimeric glycoprotein belongs to a mammalian gene family, also including VEGF-B, -C, -D, -E, and placenta growth factor (PlGF) [268]. Alternative splicing of the eight exons of the VEGF-A gene results in the generation of 12 different isoforms that have been divided into two families (Figure 2). Proximal splice-site selection (PSS) in exon 8 results in a pro-angiogenic set of isoforms $VEGF_{xxx}$ (xxx is the number of amino acids), whilst distal splice-site selection (DSS) results in the anti-angiogenic $VEGF_{xxx}b$ isoforms [269].

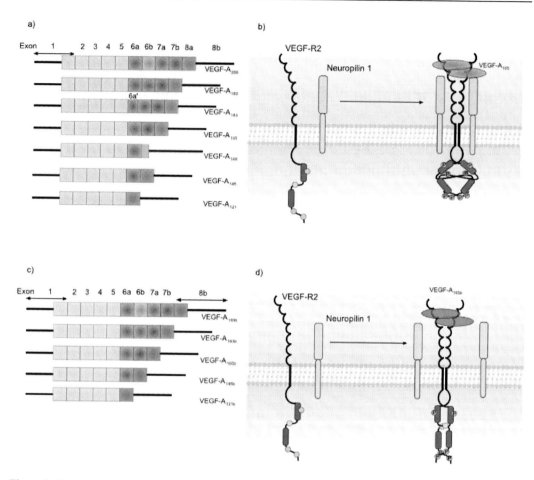

Figure 2. The angiogenic and antiangiogenic VEGF splice variants.

a) Splicing of exons 6 and 7 in congruence with proximal splice-site selection of exon 8 of the VEGF-A gene results in the generation of 7 different angiogenic isoforms. b) VEGF-A$_{165}$ engages VEGF-R2 resulting in receptor dimerization, and phosphorylation of Tyrosine residues. A conformational change in the intracellular portion of the receptor exposes the kinase domain for downstream signaling. c) Distal splice-site selection of exon 8 results in the VEGF-A$_{xxx}$b set of growth factors. d) These ligands can bind to VEGF-R2 with the same affinity, but cannot bind the co-receptor neuropilin 1. VEGF-A$_{165}$b results in weak and incomplete phosphorylation of the Tyrosines, moreover it doesn't expose the kinase domain completely resulting in inefficient transient activity. Whilst the first set results in endothelial proliferation, migration, vasodilatation and capillary permeability, the b variants do not. Both however seem protective to the podocyte

Further variation occurs within each of the two sets secondary to the splicing at exons 6 and 7. This in turn defines the binding of the cytokine to heparin and heparan-sulfate proteoglycans and accordingly whether it is secreted freely or remains bound to the cell surface or ECM [269]. The VEGF signal is transduced upon binding to 2 main receptors, VEGF-R1 or fms-like tyrosine kinase (Flt-1), VEGF-R2 or fetal liver kinase 1 (Flk-1/KDR). These tyrosine kinase receptors will accordingly dimerize, get phosphorylated, and initiate further downstream signaling [268]. In addition a soluble form of VEGF-R1 has been dubbed as regulator of VEGF availability. Originally believed to result from alternative splicing of the VEGF-R1 gene, recent evidence indicates that it may also be produced via ectodomain shedding upon binding of VEGF-A or PlGF to the membrane bound receptor [270]. Neuropilin-1 and -2, receptors for the collapsin/semaphorin family, contribute to the VEGF signaling by acting as isoform-specific co-receptors [268]. Going back to the PSS vs. DSS variation, VEGF$_{165}$b has been shown to inhibit VEGF$_{165}$-induced endothelial proliferation, migration and vasodilatation [269]. It appears to do so by competing with the angiogenic isoform for receptor binding, only to induce an inefficient VEGF-R autophosphorylation. This leads to a poorly activated kinase. Moreover VEGF$_{165}$b cannot bind to neuropilin 1 which could add further variation in the resulting downstream signal [269]. Since the ability to and the interest in differentiating between the PSS and DSS isoforms is only recent, most of the studies we will be reviewing, unless specified, assess for a role of the pro-angiogenic isoforms or detect both.

VEGF in Experimental Diabetic Nephropathy

VEGF is Upregulated in the Diabetic Rodent Kidney

Experimental evidence from rodent diabetic models indicates an association between VEGF and the disease pathology. In the rodent STZ model of type 1 diabetes, VEGF was found to be upregulated at 2-3 weeks and up to 32 weeks of diabetes [56, 271-277]. However, a shorter 1 week timeframe resulted in downregulation of the cytokine [278]. Whilst this paradoxical effect may suggest a physiological response dependent on the stage of diabetes, technical differences related to experimental design cannot be ruled out. This particular study used the rat as model of disease. Nonetheless the positive correlation with diabetes is supported by a concomitant upregulation of VEGF-R2 and VEGF-R1 [271-274, 277] and increased signaling as evidenced by increased phosphorylation of VEGF-R2 [56, 277]. Upregulation of VEGF was confirmed in the Wistar rat model of spontaneous type 1 diabetes [279].

Similarly, VEGF is generally upregulated in the kidneys of type 2 diabetic animals. The *db/db* mice show increased VEGF expression and activity irrespective of the background of the mouse, C57BLKS strain or FVB [280, 281]. In the Zucker diabetic fatty rat, VEGF mRNA increased progressively up to 7 months of disease and was coupled with an upregulation of VEGF-R2 and VEGF-R1 expression [273, 282]. These findings were reversed upon correction of hyperglycemia with insulin therapy [273]. On the other hand, in the Otsuka Long-Evans Tokushima fatty rat VEGF increased early on in the disease, and remained elevated, although lower in the later period [283, 284].

Evidence from Overexpression and Inhibition Studies

The ability of a certain growth factor to reproduce features of the disease puts a high mark in its involvement in the pathophysiology of the disease. In VEGF's case, only a few preliminary studies are currently available for review. Nonetheless, they stand to suggest the involvement of VEGF in diabetic nephropathy. One of the earlier attempts to put VEGF to the test involved infusing VEGF into the isolated perfused rat kidney [285]. The result was a vasodilation mediated by nitric oxide. But there was no apparent increase in protein excretion rate, possibly because the perfused kidney already has increased protein excretion and is not amenable to pharmacologic manipulation. Sison et al. utilized a podocyte-specific conditional overexpression mouse [286]; VEGF$_{164}$ (corresponding to VEGF$_{165}$ in humans) the most abundant and active of the angiogenic VEGF isoforms, was accordingly overexpressed only in adult mice and upon treatment with doxycycline. The investigators noted a marked nephrotic range proteinuria within one day of induction, without changes in the glomeruli examined by electron microscopy. Yet, following 4 weeks of continuous VEGF overexpression, glomeruli showed evidence of foot process effacement, GBM thickening, and nodular sclerosis [286]. All are reminiscent of diabetic changes. Recently Veron et al. continued the work studying the added effect of VEGF-A overexpression on STZ-diabetes [287]. The diabetic transgenic mice had increased proteinuria, GBM thickening, as well as podocyte effacement and fusion when compared to the diabetic controls. Moreover, the authors reported similar mesangial expansion between both groups, but 50% increase in glomerular volume in the transgenics. Surprisingly, however, conditional podocyte-specific-silencing of all VEGF-A isoforms did not reverse glomerular pathology. Knockdown-diabetic mice showed severe mesangial sclerosis, thickening of the GBM, and effacement of the foot processes. They also presented with decreased glomerular volume, increased proteinuria and a higher mortality rate when compared to their diabetic controls. In their abstract the authors do not specify the level of knockdown obtained in their model [287]. Complete knockout of the VEGF gene in adult mice has been described to result in proteinuria and other glomerular and systemic changes suggestive of renal thrombotic microangiopathy [288].

These results are even more unexpected in that they come to contradict the findings of the antagonism of the VEGF protein. In fact a number of studies have been able to demonstrate that the inhibition of VEGF activity can prevent albuminuria without altering the metabolic derangements of diabetes. In the STZ-treated rat, neutralizing VEGF with an anti-VEGF antibody has been shown to decrease albuminuria by as much as 50% after 6 weeks of follow up [289]. No analogous findings were detected with the administration of an isotype-matched irrelevant antibody, and hyperglycemia was not affected [289]. Flyvbjerg et al. used the same antibody to inhibit VEGF activity in the *db/db* mouse model of type 2 diabetes [290]. After 2 months of treatment, albuminuria was reduced by two thirds compared to the respective controls. Moreover, there was significant improvement in thickening of the glomerular basement membrane and prevention of glomerular hyperfiltration [291]. Recently Gnudi's group developed a transgenic mouse model to overexpress sFlt-1 (a natural inhibitor of VEGF) specifically at the podocyte level with an inducible expression system [277]. This provided a localized specific inhibition of VEGF, independent of antibody pharmacodynamics and localization. Albuminuria was found to be decreased by more than 50% after 10 weeks of sustained s-Flt1 overexpression. This effect occurred despite no significant difference in VEGF-A and VEGF-R2 expression with VEGF inhibition. Moreover, the decrease in VEGF-R2 activation noted in the transgenic diabetic mice was not statistically significant [277]. This raises the possibility of the involvement of other VEGF receptors in the induction of diabetic nephropathy.

Indeed, our experiments with the VEGF receptor kinase inhibitor SU5416 suggest that the decrease of VEGF signaling is essential for the reversal of diabetic renal pathology [280]. SU5416 is a nonpeptide inhibitor that targets the phosphorylation of all three VEGF receptors. Diabetic *db/db* mice treated with this small molecule inhibitor for 8 weeks after the onset of hyperglycemia showed significant improvement in some features of the kidney disease. In fact, albumin excretion rate was brought down to the nondiabetic control levels. Moreover by assaying for VEGF-R1 activation, we showed a decrease in receptor phosphorylation in SU5416 treated diabetic kidneys. This not only confirms the stringency of the design, but also indicates a possible role of VEGF-R1 in diabetic kidney disease, and possibly even podocyte pathology, where the receptor seems to be localized in vivo [280].

VEGF in Human Diabetic Kidney Disease

Making a case for the role of VEGF in human diabetic nephropathy has been less straightforward than expected. Publications on the subject have brought a mix of negative and positive results. We have selected to review these findings in that order (negative then positive) focusing on intrarenal VEGF, circulating and urinary VEGF, and genetics of VEGF.

Intrarenal VEGF

In one of the earliest studies assaying VEGF protein and mRNA expression in human renal biopsies, Shulman et al. concluded a downregulation of VEGF expression in diabetic kidneys [292]. The conclusion may have been influenced by a selection bias towards patients with advanced renal disease. Three out of the five biopsies had notable mesangial matrix nodules [292]. Likewise a later study reviewing archival renal biopsies noted a 40% drop in glomerular VEGF expression when comparing a cohort of diabetics with proteinuria to their matched controls [293]. Contrary to original suspicions, VEGF was having an inverse relationship with proteinuria. This finding was replicated in a study that focused on the glomeruli [294]. In the microdissected samples collected from 17 type 2 diabetic patients, the authors also found an inverse relationship between VEGF expression and the magnitude of mesangial matrix expansion. Specifically, the decrease in $VEGF_{165}$ and not the $VEGF_{121}$ isoform, correlated with the glomerular histology [294].

Most of the biopsies examined above were collected from patients with relatively advanced diabetic nephropathy. It is well established that progression of glomerular disease is associated with a dwindling of podocyte numbers. Since podocytes are a strong source of VEGF, the decrease in expression may be the result of loss of growth factor secreting cells with disease advancement. Indeed, in an attempt to explain their microarray findings [295] Baelde and coworkers found that VEGF levels correlated with the decreased expression of podocyte-specific genes (nephrin, podocin, and WT1) as well as podocyte numbers [296]. This may also explain why Shulman et al. originally noted that VEGF mRNA and protein expression levels were stronger in the glomeruli with preserved architecture compared to the sclerotic ones [292]. Nonetheless, the validity of such a hypothesis has been challenged by a recent study that examined biopsies at both early and late stages of diabetic nephropathy. While the authors do not correlate their findings with podocyte numbers, they do note a decrease in VEGF expression even before the development of renal failure [297].

In contrast, some human studies have detected increased intrarenal VEGF expression and activity. In situ hybridization performed on renal specimens from 18 type 2 diabetic nephropathy patients showed increase in VEGF mRNA expression. These findings were concomitant with glomerular neovascularization and a higher mesangial matrix index [298]. Not only VEGF expression, but also VEGF receptor activity was found to be elevated in glomeruli from 52 archival biopsies of type 2 diabetic patients [299]. Whilst the VEGF increase was sustained across different stages of diabetes in this study, VEGF receptor activity decreased with progression. Receptor-bound VEGF and Akt phosphorylation were lower in glomeruli with severe disease characterized by glomerular capillary rarefaction [299]. It is possible that VEGF plays a dual role, whereby its original increase contributes to glomerular pathology in an autocrine manner but as disease progresses the dissociation between its levels and the paracrine bioactivity at the target endothelial cells impairs endothelial healing, and thus leads to the accumulation of capillary injury.

Circulating and Urinary VEGF

To study the effect of VEGF in diabetic nephropathy a number of researchers have attempted to link its serum levels with the development of albuminuria. Nonetheless this method is hurdled by a few limitations. Circulating VEGF levels likely originate from a number of different organs, and may be contributed to by other diseases usually associated with diabetes, such as atherosclerosis for example [300]. VEGF-C has been reported to be elevated in individuals with hypertension [301]. Moreover VEGF is more of a paracrine-acting cytokine than a systemic hormone, limiting its effects to the local microcirculation. In a case report, elevated serum VEGF level secondary to POEMS syndrome (polyneuropathy, organomegaly, endocrinopathy, monoclonal gammopathy, and skin changes) was not associated with signs of diabetic nephropathy [302]. Accordingly, plasma VEGF levels did not correlate with the urinary albumin-to-creatinine ratio or the serum creatinine in Japanese elderly patients with type 2 diabetes [303]. Similarly no correlation was found with microvascular disease in normoalbuminuric non-hypertensive type 1 diabetic patients from the EUCLID placebo-controlled clinical trial of the ACE inhibitor lisinopril [304].

Even so, VEGF levels were elevated in a cohort of type 1 diabetic patients with nephropathy from the Steno Diabetes Center (Denmark) [305]. The results were attributed to the higher levels in nephropathic men, as women with or without albuminuria did not have increased levels of the cytokine. While the authors do not give details on the lipid status of their patients, atherosclerosis, more common in men, may have been a factor to consider. Age is another confounder that can influence the VEGF findings. Circulating VEGF concentrations increased in patients with type 1 diabetes with the onset of disease in childhood, but were particularly evident in the pubertal children and young adults compared to the pre-pubertal patients [306]. In this study, serum VEGF was independently associated with albumin excretion rate after multivariate analysis [306]. Circulating VEGF has also been suggested as a predictor of microalbuminuria and incipient diabetic nephropathy in adolescents and young adults [307]. Normoalbuminuric diabetic children and adolescents were followed for 8 years, and the odds ratio for the development of microalbuminuria after adjustment for confounding variables was 4.1 [307].

Urinary VEGF (uVEGF) levels may be the more meaningful measurement to study in a renal disease process. It is noteworthy, however, that the cellular source of VEGF in the urine is yet to be precisely identified, as it can be filtered from the plasma or secreted by the kidney.

All in all, the data associating urinary VEGF with diabetic nephropathy remain more or less incongruous. One of the earlier studies did not detect a statistical difference between diabetic patients with proteinuria and the disease-free controls. Nonetheless, uVEGF levels tended to be higher with diabetes [308]. While larger or more recent studies were able to show a significant increase in cytokine levels with type 2 diabetes, results with insulin-dependent diabetes remain negative [309, 310].

In a study of 154 subjects divided into 4 well represented groups: non-diabetic healthy controls, a normoalbuminuric diabetic group, a microalbuminuric diabetic group and an overt proteinuric diabetic group, urinary VEGF concentration was higher in all diabetic subjects compared with controls [311]. Moreover, uVEGF increased with the severity of diabetic nephropathy and correlated positively with albumin-to-creatinine ratio [311]. The same investigators were able to replicate their findings in a separate cohort, adding that sFLT-1 was also associated with albuminuria [312]. However it was found to lag behind the rise in albuminuria, leaving a period of relatively unopposed VEGF action [312]. In a recent longitudinal study, uVEGF was significantly correlated with the change in albumin excretion rate induced by treatment with an AT1R blocker [313]. Urinary levels decreased significantly with the treatment only in the patients who had a 50% reduction in albumin excretion rate [313].

VEGF Genetics

Moving from bench to bedside, Ray et al. attempted to study the role of two VEGF-A polymorphisms that had been proven to substantially increase the gene's promoter activity [314]. While one of the polymorphisms was found predictive of retinopathy, neither correlated with renal disease [314]. Likewise, a survey of type 2 diabetes for insertion/deletion polymorphism at position −2549 in the promoter region of the VEGF gene [315], and a single nucleotide polymorphisms (SNPs) study in type 1 diabetes from the Diabetes Control and Complications Trial (DCCT)/Epidemiology of Diabetes Interventions and Complications (EDIC) failed to show a connection with albuminuria, while assoctiations with retinopathy were put forward [316]. On the contrary, the same deletion at position −2549 in the promoter region in type 1 diabetic patients was associated with susceptibility to diabetic nephropathy and not retinopathy [317]. In another SNPs study of patients with type 1 diabetes in Ireland, alteration of cytosine to thymine at position 1499 in the VEGF gene was associated with a twofold excess risk of developing diabetic nephropathy [318]. However, all of these studies except for the DCCT/EDIC trial used a case-control design and were limited at least by a small sample number. Variations in the ethnic background as well as the type of diabetes are also factors that may have resulted in such contradictory results.

VEGF in the Cellular Pathogenesis of Diabetic Kidney Disease

Despite the controversy surrounding VEGF's role in human diabetic nephropathy, in vitro studies paint a decent picture of the pathophysiology centered around the podocyte. The podocyte is a rich source of renal VEGF, and the levels are even higher when the cells are exposed to high glucose [87, 199, 319], TGF-β [87], angiotensin II [148, 275], or are stimulated by Hypoxia-Inducible Factor (HIF) [320]. For glomerular proteinuria to occur, blood proteins have to traverse three main layers: the endothelium, the glomerular basement membrane (GBM), and the podocyte slit-diaphragm. Podocyte-derived VEGF, may potentially dysregulate the barrier properties of each of these layers.

The Endothelium

The role of the glomerular endothelium in the maintenance of physiologic normoalbuminuria is still a matter of debate. Proponents of the endothelial barrier suggest that a number of proteinuric diseases including diabetes are associated with a certain level of endothelial dysfunction. While the endothelial cell relatively large fenestrae certainly do not constitute much of a barrier to albumin, the glycocalyx gel covering the cells and extending into their fenestrae may hinder albumin traversal [321]. Irrespective of the extent of its contribution to albuminuria, the glomerular endothelium is evidently affected by VEGF in diabetes. With the podocyte as the main source of the growth factor, the cross-talk between the two cells is vulnerable to the pathological setting of disease [322]. VEGF upregulation leads to glomerular endothelial permeability. A plausible mechanism involves signaling through VEGF-R2 leading to activation of RhoA GTPase. Upon phosphorylation of the myosin light chain kinase, actin cytoskeletal rearrangement is induced resulting in an increase in the paracellular gap between endothelial cells [323]. Moreover, in the setting of diabetes VEGF deviates from its protective role, oscillating between the two extremes of endothelial proliferation and apoptosis. VEGF normally induces the release of NO that relaxes the vascular tone, decreases glomerular pressure, and maintains vascular integrity. In diabetes, NO production is impaired resulting in an "uncoupling of VEGF from NO" and the resultant endothelial cell proliferation, that may explain the neovascularization in the kidney [324]. On the other hand, in the presence of TGF-β, VEGF's signaling is converted into apoptosis [325] possibly causing the glomerular vascular atrophy seen in the later stages of the disease.

The GBM

The GBM is a specialized basal lamina composed of many matrix proteins, and predominantly type IV collagen. In a healthy adult kidney the GBM collagen includes the restricted α3, α4, and α5 collagen IV chains rather than the ubiquitous α1 and α2 chains. The thicker GBM in both type 1 and type 2 diabetes is actually leakier to albumin, reflecting an altered composition and architecture of the GBM in the diabetic state. In fact, the correlation between GBM thickening and proteinuria results more from the composition of the matrix rather than its volume. The podocyte, a primary source of the restricted collagen chains, responds to VEGF signaling in tissue culture by preferentially depositing α3 collagen IV and not α5 [326]. This effect was suppressed by SU5416, an inhibitor of VEGF receptors. In diabetes this effect will probably be amplified due to the presence of a VEGF autocrine loop that is apparently activated by TGF-β [326]. The role of VEGF in GBM thickening and dysfunction has been corroborated in vivo, when the treatment of diabetic mice with SU5416 largely prevented the histological findings in the GBM as well as prevented the albuminuria [280]. It remains to be seen if in mice the increase in endogenous podocyte-derived VEGF also regulates the composition of the GBM.

The Podocyte

The podocyte and its slit diaphragm are the last elements of the glomerular filtration barrier and are also affected in diabetes. Decreased podocyte number due to detachment and/or apoptosis, effacement of the foot processes, and decreased slit pore density along the GBM have all been reported to occur. A large element of the podocytopathy encountered in diabetic kidney disease could be mediated by high levels of podocyte-derived VEGF. In our study with SU5416, VEGF inhibition partially restored slit pore density in diabetic mice [280]. Similarly nephrin expression, when assayed by immunofluorescence, was decreased in diabetes via VEGF dependent mechanisms. Improvement of these findings with SU5416 was paralleled with a decrease in albuminuria [280]. While not specific VEGF inhibitors, tumstatin, endostatin and NM-3 (all antiangiogenic agents) prevented VEGF upregulation in the diabetic kidney [272, 274, 327]. Concomitantly, all three studies noted restoration of nephrin expression with treatment. Thus, VEGF may mediate its effects of the podocyte via downregulation of nephrin, and accordingly deregulation of the slit diaphragm structure.

Nonetheless, exogenous VEGF is yet to replicate all the features of diabetic podocytopathy in vitro. On the contrary, in both mouse and human immortalized podocyte cultures, VEGF has been shown to act as a survival factor possibly through nephrin phosphorylation [328, 329]. These findings do not necessarily discredit the animal studies. The effect of the cytokine on podocytes may be dependent on the milieu it is signaling in. Other growth factors and mediators could contribute to modifying the presentation and the downstream signals of VEGF. Moreover, VEGF upregulation in diabetic rodent kidneys may be a survival response to promote cell healing in the face of increased stresses in diabetes. Exaggeration of this defense reaction in disease may be "too much of a good thing", leading to the pathogenic effects of VEGF in the kidney. Cell culture studies designed to replicate the VEGF concentration and milieu may be essential for further elucidation of its role.

A Possible Role for Antiangiogenic Isforms?

Denys-Drash syndrome (DDS) is a rare disorder resulting from mutations in the Wilms' tumor-1 (*WT1*) gene. From a nephrological stand-point the disease is characterized by a typical nodular, "cannon ball" mesangial sclerosis. It also shows evidence of swollen, non-fenestrated endothelial cells, thickened GBM, and effacement of the foot processes [330]. Schumacher et al. showed that DDS podocytes are characterized by high levels of the proangiogenic isoform $VEGF_{165}$, but completely lack the inhibitory isoform $VEGF_{165}b$ [330]. While it is evident that a balance in the two isoforms is necessary for proper renal development [331, 332], little has been done to study their role in disease and particularly diabetic nephropathy. The antiangiogenic isoform appears to be the higher isoform in renal development and adulthood [332]. Unlike its counterpart, $VEGF_{165}b$ does not increase endothelial permeability. Surprisingly, however, both are protective to the podocyte and maintain its survival [332]. Moreover, different growth factors may differentially upregulate a splice variant in the human immortalized podocyte. Insulin-like growth factor 1 (IGF1) induces the proangiogenic isoform, while TGF-β favors splicing of VEGF$_{165}$b [333]. These findings certainly add a layer of complexity to our understanding of the role of VEGF in the kidney, and may turn out to be a reason for the inconsistencies faced in researching the role of VEGF in diabetic nephropathy. In so far as diabetic retinopathy has been linked with a differential splicing that increases the angiogenic isoforms [334], it would be interesting to check whether the balance between the two variants is also swayed in nephropathy.

Conclusions on Therapeutic Targets

As we uncover more and more the complexities surrounding the role of growth factors in diabetic nephropathy, numerous molecular targets for intervention will definitely unfold -- whether at the expression level, local availability, receptor binding, or downstream signaling. Many therapeutic agents can be envisioned with respect to the TGF-β system. One could antagonize the cytokine with soluble receptors or antibodies; inhibit TGF-β type-I receptor from signaling; or utilize BMP-7's inherent antagonism. CCN2 is seen as a suitable target, since it appears to be the fibrogenic arm of TGF-β in diabetic nephropathy. Inhibiting the fibrotic effects of CCN2 would avoid interference with TGF-β's other essential effects.

With the discrepancy between animal and human studies on the role of VEGF, interfering with its signaling in patients comes with a cautionary note. Low VEGF itself has been associated with renal disease such as with anti-VEGF therapy in certain human cancers. Inhibition of VEGF activity or signaling in human diabetes seems to require a delicate balancing act that may shift in the other, unfavorable direction. Clarifying the VEGF mechanisms further in diabetic nephropathy is necessary. In diabetes, higher than normal podocyte-derived VEGF levels may cause albuminuria and the aim of therapy should be to lower the elevated VEGF level down to the normal range but not to below normal. In turn, antiangiogenic VEGF isoforms may find their place in the treatment of diabetic nephropathy. Because of their endogenous nature and the lack of side effects they may outweigh other chemical therapies [269].

But with these growth factors widely distributed in organs and tissues, with their involvement in essential metabolic processes, and the fine balance in their regulation, systemic therapies may be associated with unexpected side effects. We may have to consider a more pinpoint approach limited to the kidney in diabetes. The miRNAs hold an important potential as therapeutic targets. Packaged in liposomes, viral vectors, and nanoparticles they can potentially be delivered locally in the renal arteries [335]. Otherwise they can also be conjugated to aptamers, lipids, peptides, proteins, or polymers that home into the kidney [336]. Identifying their roles in diabetes may uncover a number of targets downstream from the cytokines.

References

[1] Rossing, P., *Diabetic nephropathy: worldwide epidemic and effects of current treatment on natural history.* Curr Diab Rep, 2006. 6(6): p. 479-83.

[2] Mathiesen, E.R., et al., *Randomised controlled trial of long term efficacy of captopril on preservation of kidney function in normotensive patients with insulin dependent diabetes and microalbuminuria.* BMJ, 1999. 319(7201): p. 24-25.

[3] Lewis, E.J., et al., *The effect of angiotensin-converting-enzyme inhibition on diabetic nephropathy. The collaborative study group.* N Engl J Med, 1993. 329(20): p. 1456-1462.

[4] Ficociello, L.H., et al., *Determinants of progression from microalbuminuria to proteinuria in patients who have type 1 diabetes and are treated with angiotensin-converting enzyme inhibitors.* Clin J Am Soc Nephrol, 2007. 2(3): p. 461-9.

[5] Mathiesen, E.R., et al., *Randomised controlled trial of long term efficacy of captopril on preservation of kidney function in normotensive patients with insulin dependent diabetes and microalbuminuria.* BMJ, 1999. 319(7201): p. 24-5.

[6] Burney, B.O., R.G. Kalaitzidis, and G.L. Bakris, *Novel therapies of diabetic nephropathy.* Curr Opin Nephrol Hypertens, 2009. 18(2): p. 107-11.

[7] Derynck, R. and K.o. Miyazono, *The TGF-[beta] family.* Cold Spring Harbor monograph series. 2008, Cold Spring Harbor, N.Y.: Cold Spring Harbor Laboratory Press.

[8] Sun, P.D. and D.R. Davies, *The cysteine-knot growth-factor superfamily.* Annu Rev Biophys Biomol Struct, 1995. 24: p. 269-91.

[9] Schmierer, B. and C.S. Hill, *TGF[beta]-SMAD signal transduction: molecular specificity and functional flexibility.* Nat Rev Mol Cell Biol, 2007. 8(12): p. 970-982.

[10] Mogensen, C.E., *The kidney and hypertension in diabetes mellitus.* 6th ed. 2004, Boston: Kluwer Academic Publishers. p.

[11] Massague, J., L. Attisano, and J.L. Wrana, *The TGF-beta family and its composite receptors.* Trends Cell Biol, 1994. 4: p. 172-178.

[12] Wieser, R., et al., *Signaling activity of transforming growth factor-beta type II receptors lacking specific domains in the cytoplasmic region.* Mol Cell Biol, 1993. 13: p. 7239-7247.

[13] Wrighton, K.H., X. Lin, and X.-H. Feng, *Phospho-control of TGF-[beta] superfamily signaling.* Cell Res. 19(1): p. 8-20.

[14] Lee, M.K., et al., *TGF-beta activates Erk MAP kinase signaling through direct phosphorylation of ShcA.* EMBO J, 2007. 26(17): p. 3957-67.

[15] Lawler, S., et al., *The type II transforming growth factor-beta receptor autophosphorylates not only on serine and threonine but also on tyrosine residues.* J Biol Chem, 1997. 272(23): p. 14850-9.

[16] Sekelsky, J.J., et al., *Genetic characterization and cloning of mothers against dpp, a gene required for decapentaplegic function in Drosophila melanogaster.* Genetics, 1995. 139: p. 1347-1358.

[17] Liu, F., et al., *A human Mad protein acting as a BMP-regulated transcriptional activator.* Nature, 1996. 381: p. 620-623.

[18] Derynck, R., et al., *Nomenclature: Vertebrate Mediators of TGF[beta] Family Signals.* Cell, 1996. 87(2): p. 173-173.

[19] Shi, Y. and J. Massagué, *Mechanisms of TGF-[beta] Signaling from Cell Membrane to the Nucleus.* Cell, 2003. 113(6): p. 685-700.

[20] Schiffer, M., et al., *Apoptosis in podocytes induced by TGF-beta and Smad7.* J Clin Invest, 2001. 108(6): p. 807-16.

[21] Zhang, Y.E., *Non-Smad pathways in TGF-beta signaling.* Cell Res, 2009. 19(1): p. 128-39.

[22] Sharma, K. and F.N. Ziyadeh, *Hyperglycemia and diabetic kidney disease: the case for transforming growth factor-beta as a key mediator.* Diabetes, 1995. 44(10): p. p1139-46.

[23] Thompson, N.L., et al., *Expression of transforming growth factor-beta1 in specific cells and tissues of adult and neonatal mice.* J Cell Biol, 1989. 108: p. 661-669.

[24] Ando, T., et al., *Localization of TGF-beta and its receptors in the kidney.* Miner Electrolyte Metab, 1998. 24(2-3): p. 149-53.

[25] Ando, T., et al., *Localization of transforming growth factor-beta and latent transforming growth factor-beta binding protein in rat kidney.* Kidney Int, 1995. 47(3): p. 733-739.

[26] MacKay, K., et al., *Expression of transforming growth factor-beta1 and beta2 in rat glomeruli.* Kidney Int, 1990. 38: p. 1095-1100.

[27] Wilson, H.M., et al., *Transforming growth factor-beta isoforms and glomerular injury in nephrotoxic nephritis.* Kidney Int, 2000. 57(6): p. 2434-44.

[28] Horikoshi, S., et al., *Water deprivation stimulates transforming growth factor-beta 2 accumulation in the juxtaglomerular apparatus of mouse kidney.* J Clin Invest, 1991. 88(6): p. 2117-2122.

[29] MacKay, K., et al., *Transforming growth factor-beta: Murine glomerular receptors and responses of isolated glomerular cells.* J Clin Invest, 1989. 83: p. 160-167.

[30] Uchida, K., et al., *Localization of Smad6 and Smad7 in the rat kidney and their regulated expression in the anti-Thy-1 nephritis.* Mol Cell Biol Res Commun, 2000. 4(2): p. 98-9105.

[31] Furuse, Y., et al., *Activation of the Smad pathway in glomeruli from a spontaneously diabetic rat model, OLETF rats.* Nephron Exp Nephrol, 2004. 98(3): p. e100-8.

[32] Schiffer, M., et al., *Inhibitory Smads and TGF-{beta} Signaling in Glomerular Cells.* J Am Soc Nephrol, 2002. 13(11): p. 2657-2666.

[33] Banas, M.C., et al., *Localization of TGF-beta signaling intermediates Smad2, 3, 4, and 7 in developing and mature human and mouse kidney.* J Histochem Cytochem, 2007. 55(3): p. 275-85.

[34] Ostendorf, T., et al., *The Effects of Platelet-Derived Growth Factor Antagonism in Experimental Glomerulonephritis Are Independent of the Transforming Growth Factor-{beta} System.* J Am Soc Nephrol, 2002. 13(3): p. 658-667.

[35] Isono, M., et al., *Smad pathway is activated in the diabetic mouse kidney and Smad3 mediates TGF-beta-induced fibronectin in mesangial cells.* Biochem Biophys Res Commun, 2002. 296(5): p. 1356-65.

[36] Erman, A., et al., *Renin-angiotensin system blockade prevents the increase in plasma transforming growth factor beta 1, and reduces proteinuria and kidney hypertrophy in*

the streptozotocin-diabetic rat. J Renin Angiotensin Aldosterone Syst, 2004. 5(3): p. 146-51.

[37] Sharma, K., et al., *Neutralization of TGF-beta by anti-TGF-beta antibody attenuates kidney hypertrophy and the enhanced extracellular matrix gene expression in STZ-induced diabetic mice.* Diabetes, 1996. 45(4): p. 522-30.

[38] Bollineni, J.S. and A.S. Reddi, *Transforming growth factor-beta1 enhances glomerular collagen synthesis in diabetic rats.* Diabetes, 1993. 42(11): p. 1673-1677.

[39] Sharma, K. and F.N. Ziyadeh, *Renal hypertrophy is associated with upregulation of TGF-beta 1 gene expression in diabetic BB rat and NOD mouse.* Am J Physiol, 1994. 267(6 Pt 2): p. F1094-01.

[40] Shankland, S.J., et al., *Expression of transforming growth factor-beta 1 during diabetic renal hypertrophy.* Kidney Int, 1994. 46(2): p. 430-42.

[41] Nakamura, T., et al., *mRNA expression of growth factors in glomeruli from diabetic rats.* Diabetes, 1993. 42: p. 450-456.

[42] Yang, C.-W., et al., *Overexpression of transforming growth factor-beta1 mRNA is associated with up-regulation of glomerular tenascin and laminin gene expression in nonobese diabetic mice.* J Am Soc Nephrol, 1995. 5: p. 1610-1617.

[43] Yamamoto, T., et al., *Expression of transforming growth factor beta is elevated in human and experimental diabetic nephropathy.* Proc Natl Acad Sci USA, 1993. 90: p. 1814-1818.

[44] Park, I.S., et al., *Expression of transforming growth factor-beta and type IV collagen in early streptozotocin-induced diabetes.* Diabetes, 1997. 46(3): p. 473-80.

[45] Gilbert, R.E., et al., *Expression of transforming growth factor-beta1 and type IV collagen in the renal tubulointerstitium in experimental diabetes: effects of ACE inhibition.* Diabetes, 1998. 47(3): p. 414-422.

[46] Pankewycz, O.G., et al., *Renal TGF-beta regulation in spontaneously diabetic NOD mice with correlations in mesangial cells.* Kidney Int, 1994. 46(3): p. 748-758.

[47] Hill, C., et al., *The renal expression of transforming growth factor-beta isoforms and their receptors in acute and chronic experimental diabetes in rats.* Endocrinology, 2000. 141(3): p. 1196-1208.

[48] Powell, D.W., et al., *Renal tubulointerstitial fibrosis in OVE26 type 1 diabetic mice.* Nephron Exp Nephrol, 2009. 111(1): p. e11-9.

[49] Isono, M., et al., *Stimulation of TGF-beta type II receptor by high glucose in mouse mesangial cells and in diabetic kidney.* Am J Physiol Renal Physiol, 2000. 278(5): p. F830-F838.

[50] Zheng, S., et al., *Development of late-stage diabetic nephropathy in OVE26 diabetic mice.* Diabetes, 2004. 53(12): p. 3248-57.

[51] Hong, S.W., et al., *Increased glomerular and tubular expression of transforming growth factor-beta1, its type II receptor, and activation of the Smad signaling pathway in the db/db mouse.* Am J Pathol, 2001. 158(5): p. 1653-1663.

[52] Gonzalez-Albarran, O., et al., *Role of systolic blood pressure on the progression of kidney damage in an experimental model of type 2 diabetes mellitus, obesity, and hypertension (Zucker rats).* Am J Hypertens, 2003. 16(11 Pt 1): p. 979-985.

[53] Shinomiya, K., et al., *A role of oxidative stress-generated eicosanoid in the progression of arteriosclerosis in type 2 diabetes mellitus model rats.* Hypertens Res, 2002. 25(1): p. 91-98.

[54] Ziyadeh, F.N., et al., *Long-term prevention of renal insufficiency, excess matrix gene expression, and glomerular mesangial matrix expansion by treatment with monoclonal antitransforming growth factor-beta antibody in db/db diabetic mice.* Proc Natl Acad Sci U S A, 2000. 97(14): p. 8015-8020.

[55] Chen, S., et al., *Reversibility of established diabetic glomerulopathy by anti-TGF-beta antibodies in db/db mice.* Biochem Biophys Res Commun, 2003. 300(1): p. 16-22.

[56] Wang, A., et al., *Interference with TGF-beta signaling by Smad3-knockout in mice limits diabetic glomerulosclerosis without affecting albuminuria.* Am J Physiol Renal Physiol, 2007. 293(5): p. F1657-65.

[57] Reeves, W.B. and T.E. Andreoli, *Transforming growth factor beta contributes to progressive diabetic nephropathy.* Proc Natl Acad Sci U S A, 2000. 97(14): p. 7667-7669.

[58] Ziyadeh, F.N., *Different roles for TGF-beta and VEGF in the pathogenesis of the cardinal features of diabetic nephropathy.* Diabetes Res Clin Pract, 2008. 82 Suppl 1: p. S38-41.

[59] Benigni, A., et al., *Add-on anti-TGF-beta antibody to ACE inhibitor arrests progressive diabetic nephropathy in the rat.* J Am Soc Nephrol, 2003. 14(7): p. 1816-24.

[60] Benigni, A., et al., *Beneficial effect of TGFbeta antagonism in treating diabetic nephropathy depends on when treatment is started.* Nephron Exp Nephrol, 2006. 104(4): p. e158-68.

[61] Kim, H.W., et al., *Heterozygous mice for TGF-betaIIR gene are resistant to the progression of streptozotocin-induced diabetic nephropathy.* Kidney Int, 2004. 66(5): p. 1859-65.

[62] Sugaru, E., et al., *SMP-534 ameliorates progression of glomerular fibrosis and urinary albumin in diabetic db/db mice.* Am J Physiol Renal Physiol, 2006. 290(4): p. F813-20.

[63] Petersen, M., et al., *Oral administration of GW788388, an inhibitor of TGF-beta type I and II receptor kinases, decreases renal fibrosis.* Kidney Int, 2008. 73(6): p. 705-15.

[64] Juarez, P., et al., *Soluble betaglycan reduces renal damage progression in db/db mice.* Am J Physiol Renal Physiol, 2007. 292(1): p. F321-9.

[65] Russo, L.M., et al., *Evidence for a role of transforming growth factor (TGF)-beta1 in the induction of postglomerular albuminuria in diabetic nephropathy: amelioration by soluble TGF-beta type II receptor.* Diabetes, 2007. 56(2): p. 380-8.

[66] Fujimoto, M., et al., *Mice lacking Smad3 are protected against streptozotocin-induced diabetic glomerulopathy.* Biochem Biophys Res Commun, 2003. 305(4): p. 1002-7.

[67] Yoshioka, K., et al., *Transforming growth factor-beta protein and mRNA in glomeruli in normal and diseased human kidneys.* Lab Invest, 1993. 68(2): p. 154-163.

[68] Yamamoto, T., et al., *Expression of transforming growth factor-beta isoforms in human glomerular diseases.* Kidney Int, 1996. 49: p. 461-469.

[69] Iwano, M., et al., *Quantification of glomerular TGFbeta1 mRNA in patients with diabetes mellitus.* Kidney Int, 1996. 49: p. 1120-1126.

[70] Sharma, K., et al., *Increased renal production of transforming growth factor-beta1 in patients with type II diabetes.* Diabetes, 1997. 46(5): p. 854-9.

[71] McGowan, T.A., et al., *Stimulation of urinary TGF-beta and isoprostanes in response to hyperglycemia in humans.* Clin J Am Soc Nephrol, 2006. 1(2): p. 263-8.

[72] Sato, H., et al., *Increased excretion of urinary transforming growth factor beta 1 in patients with diabetic nephropathy.* Am J Nephrol, 1998. 18(6): p. 490-4.

[73] Chaturvedi, N., et al., *Circulating and urinary transforming growth factor beta1, Amadori albumin, and complications of type 1 diabetes: the EURODIAB prospective complications study.* Diabetes Care, 2002. 25(12): p. 2320-7.

[74] Ewens, K.G., et al., *Assessment of 115 candidate genes for diabetic nephropathy by transmission/disequilibrium test.* Diabetes, 2005. 54(11): p. 3305-18.

[75] Granier, C., et al., *Gene and protein markers of diabetic nephropathy.* Nephrol Dial Transplant, 2008. 23(3): p. 792-9.

[76] Ng, D.P., J.H. Warram, and A.S. Krolewski, *TGF-beta 1 as a genetic susceptibility locus for advanced diabetic nephropathy in type 1 diabetes mellitus: an investigation of multiple known DNA sequence variants.* Am J Kidney Dis, 2003. 41(1): p. 22-8.

[77] Wong, T.Y., et al., *Association of transforming growth factor-beta (TGF-beta) T869C (Leu 10Pro) gene polymorphisms with type 2 diabetic nephropathy in Chinese.* Kidney Int, 2003. 63(5): p. 1831-5.

[78] Patel, A., et al., *The TGF-beta 1 gene codon 10 polymorphism contributes to the genetic predisposition to nephropathy in Type 1 diabetes.* Diabet Med, 2005. 22(1): p. 69-73.

[79] Buraczynska, M., et al., *TGF-beta1 and TSC-22 gene polymorphisms and susceptibility to microvascular complications in type 2 diabetes.* Nephron Physiol, 2007. 106(4): p. p69-75.

[80] McKnight, A.J., et al., *Resequencing of genes for transforming growth factor beta1 (TGFB1) type 1 and 2 receptors (TGFBR1, TGFBR2), and association analysis of variants with diabetic nephropathy.* BMC Med Genet, 2007. 8: p. 5.

[81] Prasad, P., et al., *Association of TGFbeta1, TNFalpha, CCR2 and CCR5 gene polymorphisms in type-2 diabetes and renal insufficiency among Asian Indians.* BMC Med Genet, 2007. 8: p. 20.

[82] Ziyadeh, F.N., et al., *Stimulation of collagen gene expression and protein synthesis in murine mesangial cells by high glucose is mediated by autocrine activation of transforming growth factor- beta.* J Clin Invest, 1994. 93: p. 536-542.

[83] Hoffman, B., et al., *Transcriptional activation of TGF-b1 by high glucose.* J. Am. Soc. Nephrol, 1995. 6: p. 1041 (abstract).

[84] Montero, A., et al., *F(2)-isoprostanes mediate high glucose-induced TGF-beta synthesis and glomerular proteinuria in experimental type I diabetes.* Kidney Int, 2000. 58(5): p. 1963-72.

[85] Rocco, M.V., et al., *Elevated glucose stimulates TGF- beta gene expression and bioactivity in proximal tubule.* Kidney Int, 1992. 41: p. 107-114.

[86] Han, D.C., et al., *High glucose stimulates proliferation and collagen type I synthesis in renal cortical fibroblasts: mediation by autocrine activation of TGF-beta.* J Am Soc Nephrol, 1999. 10(9): p. 1891-1899.

[87] Iglesias-de la Cruz, M.C., et al., *Effects of high glucose and TGF-beta1 on the expression of collagen IV and vascular endothelial growth factor in mouse podocytes.* Kidney Int, 2002. 62(3): p. 901-13.

[88] Hostetter, T.H., *Hyperfiltration and glomerulosclerosis.* Semin Nephrol, 2003. 23(2): p. 194-199.

[89] Levine, D.Z., et al., *Modulation of single-nephron GFR in the db/db mouse model of type 2 diabetes mellitus.* Am J Physiol Regul Integr Comp Physiol, 2006. 290(4): p. 975-981.

[90] Hayashi, K., et al., *Impaired myogenic responsiveness of the afferent arteriole in streptozotocin-induced diabetic rats: role of eicosanoid derangements.* J Am Soc Nephrol, 1992. 2(11): p. 1578-1586.

[91] Anderson, S., H.G. Rennke, and B.M. Brenner, *Therapeutic advantage of converting enzyme inhibitors in arresting progressive renal disease associated with systemic hypertension in the rat.* J Clin Invest, 1986. 77(6): p. 1993-2000.

[92] Riser, B.L., et al., *Mesangial cell stretch stimulates the formation of transforming growth factor- beta and extracellular matrix synthesis.* J Am Soc Nephrol, 1992. 3: p. 642 (abstract).

[93] Riser, B.L., et al., *Cyclic stretching force selectively up-regulates transforming growth factor-beta isoforms in cultured rat mesangial cells.* Am J Pathol, 1996. 148: p. 1915-1923.

[94] Yasuda, T., et al., *Regulation of extracellular matrix by mechanical stress in rat glomerular mesangial cells.* J Clin Invest, 1996. 98: p. 1991-2000.

[95] Durvasula, R.V., et al., *Activation of a local tissue angiotensin system in podocytes by mechanical strain.* Kidney Int, 2004. 65(1): p. 30-9.

[96] Ohno, M., et al., *Fluid shear stress induces endothelial transforming growth factor beta-1 transcription and production. Modulation by potassium channel blockade.* J Clin Invest, 1995. 95: p. 1363-1369.

[97] Gruden, G., et al., *Mechanical stretch-induced fibronectin and transforming growth factor-beta1 production in human mesangial cells is p38 mitogen-activated protein kinase-dependent.* Diabetes, 2000. 49(4): p. 655-61.

[98] Forbes, J.M., K. Fukami, and M.E. Cooper, *Diabetic nephropathy: where hemodynamics meets metabolism.* Exp Clin Endocrinol Diabetes, 2007. 115(2): p. 69-84.

[99] Chen, S., G. Wolf, and F.N. Ziyadeh, *The renin-angiotensin system in diabetic nephropathy.* Contrib Nephrol, 2001(135): p. 212-21.

[100] Scharschmidt, L.A., E. Lianos, and M.J. Dunn, *Arachidonate metabolites and the control of glomerular function.* Fed Proc, 1983. 42(14): p. 3058-3063.

[101] Baylis, C., *Effects of administered thromboxanes on the intact, normal rat kidney.* Ren Physiol, 1987. 10(2): p. 110-121.

[102] Ledbetter, S., et al., *Altered steady-state mRNA levels of basement membrane proteins in diabetic mouse kidneys and thromboxane synthase inhibition.* Diabetes, 1990. 39: p. 196-203.

[103] Gambardella, S., et al., *Renal hemodynamics and urinary excretion of 6-keto-prostaglandin F1 alpha and thromboxane B2 in newly diagnosed type I diabetic patients.* Diabetes, 1988. 37: p. 1044-1048.

[104] Craven, P.A. and F.R. DeRubertis, *Protein kinase C is activated in glomeruli from streptozotocin diabetic rats.* J Clin Invest, 1989. 83: p. 1667-1675.

[105] Craven, P.A., M.A. Caines, and F.R. DeRubertis, *Sequential alterations in glomerular prostaglandin and thromboxane synthesis in diabetic rats: Relationship to the hyperfiltration of early diabetes.* Metabolism, 1987. 36: p. 95-103.

[106] Sebekova, K., et al., *Renal effects of S18886 (Terutroban), a TP receptor antagonist, in an experimental model of type 2 diabetes.* Diabetes, 2007. 56(4): p. 968-74.

[107] Awad, A.S., et al., *Increased renal production of angiotensin II and thromboxane B2 in conscious diabetic rats.* Am J Hypertens, 2005. 18(4 Pt 1): p. 544-8.

[108] Dai, F., et al., *Diabetes-induced endothelial dysfunction in streptozotocin-treated rats: role of prostaglandin endoperoxides and free radicals.* J Am Soc Nephrol, 1993. 4(6): p. 1327-1336.

[109] Uriu, K., et al., *Acute and chronic effects of thromboxane A2 inhibition on the renal hemodynamics in streptozotocin-induced diabetic rats.* Kidney Int, 1994. 45(3): p. 794-802.

[110] Uriu, K., et al., *Effect of Acute Thromboxane A2 Inhibition on the Renal Hemodynamics in a Spontaneously Non-Insulin-Dependent Diabetic Rat, Otsuka Long-Evans Tokushima Fatty Rat.* Journal of Diabetes and its Complications, 1999. 13(4): p. 182-186.

[111] Wilkes, B.M., et al., *Reduced glomerular thromboxane receptor sites and vasoconstrictor responses in diabetic rats.* Kidney Int, 1992. 41(4): p. 992-9.

[112] Morinelli, T.A., et al., *Thromboxane A2/prostaglandin H2 receptors in streptozotocin-induced diabetes: effects of insulin therapy in the rat.* Prostaglandins, 1993. 45(5): p. 427-38.

[113] Cediel, E., et al., *Role of endothelin-1 and thromboxane A2 in renal vasoconstriction induced by angiotensin II in diabetes and hypertension.* Kidney Int Suppl, 2002(82): p. 2-7.

[114] Ajayi, A.A., et al., *Alteration in endothelin receptor sub-type responsiveness and in the endothelin-TXA2 mimetic U46619 interaction, in type-2 hypertensive diabetic Zucker rats.* Diabetes Research and Clinical Practice, 2004. 63(3): p. 155-169.

[115] Studer, R.K., F.R. DeRubertis, and P.A. Craven, *Nitric oxide suppresses increases in mesangial cell protein kinase C, transforming growth factor beta, and fibronectin synthesis induced by thromboxane.* J Am Soc Nephrol, 1996. 7(7): p. 999-1005.

[116] Studer, R.K., P.A. Craven, and F.R. DeRubertis, *Thromboxane stimulation of mesangial cell fibronectin synthesis is signalled by protein kinase C and modulated by cGMP.* Kidney Int, 1994. 46(4): p. 1074-82.

[117] Negrete, H., et al., *Role for transforming growth factor beta in thromboxane-induced increases in mesangial cell fibronectin synthesis.* Diabetes, 1995. 44(3): p. 335-9.

[118] Studer, R.K., et al., *Protein kinase C signals thromboxane induced increases in fibronectin synthesis and TGF-beta bioactivity in mesangial cells.* Kidney Int, 1995. 48: p. 422-430.

[119] Patel, A., et al., *Effects of a fixed combination of perindopril and indapamide on macrovascular and microvascular outcomes in patients with type 2 diabetes mellitus (the ADVANCE trial): a randomised controlled trial.* Lancet, 2007. 370(9590): p. 829-40.

[120] Patel, A., et al., *Intensive blood glucose control and vascular outcomes in patients with type 2 diabetes.* N Engl J Med, 2008. 358(24): p. 2560-72.

[121] Navar, L.G. and L. Rosivall, *Contribution of the renin-angiotensin system to the control of intrarenal hemodynamics.* Kidney Int, 1984. 25(6): p. 857-868.

[122] Epstein, M. and J.R. Sowers, *Diabetes mellitus and hypertension.* Hypertension, 1992. 19(5): p. 403-418.

[123] Zatz, R., et al., *Prevention of diabetic glomerulopathy by pharmacological amelioration of glomerular capillary hypertension.* J Clin Invest, 1986. 77: p. 1925-1930.

[124] Mitchell, K.D. and L.G. Navar, *Interactive effects of angiotensin II on renal hemodynamics and tubular reabsorptive function.* Kidney Int Suppl, 1990. 30: p. S69-73.

[125] Blantz, R.C. and F.B. Gabbai, *Effect of angiotensin II on glomerular hemodynamics and ultrafiltration coefficient.* Kidney Int Suppl, 1987. 20: p. S108-11.

[126] Bjorck, S. and M. Aurell, *Diabetes mellitus, the renin-angiotensin system, and angiotensin-converting enzyme inhibition.* Nephron, 1990. 55 Suppl 1: p. 10-20.

[127] Wolf, G. and E. Neilson, *Angiotensin II as a renal growth factor.* J Am Soc Nephrol, 1993. 3(9): p. 1531-1540.

[128] Ravid, M., et al., *Long-term stabilizing effect of angiotensin-converting enzyme inhibition on plasma creatinine and on proteinuria in normotensive type II diabetic patients.* Ann Intern Med, 1993. 118(8): p. 577-581.

[129] Remuzzi, A., et al., *Prevention of renal injury in diabetic MWF rats by angiotensin II antagonism.* Exp Nephrol, 1998. 6(1): p. 28-38.

[130] Wolf, G., U. Haberstroh, and E.G. Neilson, *Angiotensin II stimulates the proliferation and biosynthesis of type I collagen in cultured murine mesangial cells.* Am J Pathol, 1992. 140: p. 95-107.

[131] Wolf, G., et al., *Angiotensin II stimulates cellular hypertrophy of LLC-PK1 cells through the AT1 receptor.* Nephrol Dial Transplant, 1993. 8(2): p. 128-33.

[132] Wolf, G. and E.G. Neilson, *Angiotensin II induces cellular hypertrophy in cultured murine proximal tubular cells.* Am J Physiol, 1990. 259(5 Pt 2): p. F768-77.

[133] Anderson, P.W., Y.S. Do, and W.A. Hsueh, *Angiotensin II causes mesangial cell hypertrophy.* Hypertension, 1993. 21(1): p. 29-35.

[134] Wolf, G., et al., *Angiotensin II induces alpha3(IV) collagen expression in cultured murine proximal tubular cells.* Proc Assoc Am Physicians, 1999. 111(4): p. 357-64.

[135] Singh, R., et al., *Role of angiotensin II in glucose-induced inhibition of mesangial matrix degradation.* Diabetes, 1999. 48(10): p. 2066-73.

[136] Wolf, G., *Growth factors and the development of diabetic nephropathy.* Curr Diab Rep, 2003. 3(6): p. 485-90.

[137] Wolf, G., P.D. Killen, and E.G. Neilson, *Intracellular signaling of transcription and secretion of type IV collagen after angiotensin II-induced cellular hypertrophy in cultured proximal tubular cells.* Cell Reg, 1991. 2: p. 219-227.

[138] Wolf, G. and F.N. Ziyadeh, *Renal tubular hypertrophy induced by angiotensin II.* Semin Nephrol, 1997. 17(5): p. 448-54.

[139] Wolf, G., et al., *Angiotensin II-stimulated expression of transforming growth factor beta in renal proximal tubular cells: attenuation after stable transfection with the c-mas oncogene.* Kidney Int, 1995. 48(6): p. 1818-27.

[140] Wolf, G., et al., *Angiotensin II-induced hypertrophy of cultured murine proximal tubular cells is mediated by endogenous transforming growth factor-beta.* J Clin Invest, 1993. 92(3): p. 1366-72.

[141] Fakhouri, F., et al., *Angiotensin II activates collagen type I gene in the renal cortex and aorta of transgenic mice through interaction with endothelin and TGF-beta.* J Am Soc Nephrol, 2001. 12(12): p. 2701-10.

[142] Tharaux, P.L., et al., *Angiotensin II activates collagen I gene through a mechanism involving the MAP/ER kinase pathway.* Hypertension, 2000. 36(3): p. 330-6.

[143] Kagami, S., et al., *Angiotensin II stimulates extracellular matrix protein synthesis through induction of transforming growth factor-beta expression in rat glomerular mesangial cells.* J Clin Invest, 1994. 93(6): p. 2431-7.

[144] Ruiz-Ortega, M. and J. Egido, *Angiotensin II modulates cell growth-related events and synthesis of matrix proteins in renal interstitial fibroblasts.* Kidney Int, 1997. 52(6): p. 1497-510.

[145] Wolf, G., F.N. Ziyadeh, and R.A. Stahl, *Angiotensin II stimulates expression of transforming growth factor beta receptor type II in cultured mouse proximal tubular cells.* J Mol Med, 1999. 77(7): p. 556-64.

[146] Wang, W., et al., *Essential role of Smad3 in angiotensin II-induced vascular fibrosis.* Circ Res, 2006. 98(8): p. 1032-1039.

[147] Rodriguez-Vita, J., et al., *Angiotensin II activates the Smad pathway in vascular smooth muscle cells by a transforming growth factor-beta-independent mechanism.* Circulation, 2005. 111(19): p. 2509-2517.

[148] Chen, S., et al., *Angiotensin II stimulates {alpha}3(IV) collagen production in mouse podocytes via TGF-{beta} and VEGF signalling: implications for diabetic glomerulopathy.* Nephrol. Dial. Transplant., 2005. 20(7): p. 1320-1328.

[149] Singh, R., et al., *Mechanism of increased angiotensin II levels in glomerular mesangial cells cultured in high glucose.* J Am Soc Nephrol, 2003. 14(4): p. 873-880.

[150] Huang, X.R., et al., *Chymase is upregulated in diabetic nephropathy: implications for an alternative pathway of angiotensin II-mediated diabetic renal and vascular disease.* J Am Soc Nephrol, 2003. 14(7): p. 1738-1747.

[151] Vidotti, D.B., et al., *High glucose concentration stimulates intracellular renin activity and angiotensin II generation in rat mesangial cells.* Am J Physiol Renal Physiol, 2004. 286(6): p. F1039-45.

[152] Tikellis, C., et al., *Characterization of renal angiotensin-converting enzyme 2 in diabetic nephropathy.* Hypertension, 2003. 41(3): p. 392-7.

[153] Brezniceanu, M.L., et al., *Transforming growth factor-beta 1 stimulates angiotensinogen gene expression in kidney proximal tubular cells.* Kidney Int, 2006. 69(11): p. 1977-85.

[154] Brownlee, M., *Biochemistry and molecular cell biology of diabetic complications.* Nature, 2001. 414(6865): p. 813-20.

[155] DeRubertis, F.R., et al., *Attenuation of renal injury in db/db mice overexpressing superoxide dismutase: evidence for reduced superoxide-nitric oxide interaction.* Diabetes, 2004. 53(3): p. 762-8.

[156] Kakkar, R., et al., *Antioxidant defense system in diabetic kidney: a time course study.* Life Sci, 1997. 60(9): p. 667-79.

[157] Lee, H.B., et al., *Reactive Oxygen Species-Regulated Signaling Pathways in Diabetic Nephropathy.* J Am Soc Nephrol, 2003. 14(90003): p. S241-245.

[158] Iglesias-de la Cruz, M.C., et al., *Hydrogen peroxide increases extracellular matrix mRNA through TGF-beta in human mesangial cells.* Kidney Int, 2001. 59(1): p. 87-95.

[159] Singh, L.P., et al., *Hexosamines and TGF-beta1 use similar signaling pathways to mediate matrix protein synthesis in mesangial cells.* Am J Physiol Renal Physiol, 2004. 286(2): p. F409-16.

[160] Weigert, C., et al., *Glutamine:fructose-6-phosphate aminotransferase enzyme activity is necessary for the induction of TGF-beta1 and fibronectin expression in mesangial cells.* Diabetologia, 2003. 46(6): p. 852-5.

[161] James, L.R., et al., *Overexpression of GFAT activates PAI-1 promoter in mesangial cells.* Am J Physiol Renal Physiol, 2000. 279(4): p. F718-27.

[162] Weigert, C., et al., *Overexpression of glutamine:fructose-6-phosphate-amidotransferase induces transforming growth factor-beta1 synthesis in NIH-3T3 fibroblasts.* FEBS Lett, 2001. 488(1-2): p. 95-9.

[163] Kolm-Litty, V., et al., *High glucose-induced transforming growth factor beta1 production is mediated by the hexosamine pathway in porcine glomerular mesangial cells.* J Clin Invest, 1998. 101(1): p. 160-169.

[164] Burt, D.J., et al., *P38 mitogen-activated protein kinase mediates hexosamine-induced TGFbeta1 mRNA expression in human mesangial cells.* Diabetologia, 2003. 46(4): p. 531-537.

[165] Daniels, M.C., D.A. McClain, and E.D. Crook, *Transcriptional regulation of transforming growth factor beta1 by glucose: investigation into the role of the hexosamine biosynthesis pathway.* Am J Med Sci, 2000. 319(3): p. 138-42.

[166] Chen, S., et al., *Glycated albumin stimulates TGF-beta 1 production and protein kinase C activity in glomerular endothelial cells.* Kidney Int, 2001. 59(2): p. 673-681.

[167] Ziyadeh, F.N., et al., *Glycated albumin stimulates fibronectin gene expression in glomerular mesangial cells: involvement of the transforming growth factor-beta system.* Kidney Int, 1998. 53: p. 631-638.

[168] Ha, H., et al., *Role of glycated low density lipoprotein in mesangial extracellular matrix synthesis.* Kidney Int Suppl, 1997. 60: p. S54-S59.

[169] Fukami, K., et al., *AGEs activate mesangial TGF-beta-Smad signaling via an angiotensin II type I receptor interaction.* Kidney Int, 2004. 66(6): p. 2137-47.

[170] Li, J.H., et al., *Advanced glycation end products activate Smad signaling via TGF-beta-dependent and independent mechanisms: implications for diabetic renal and vascular disease.* FASEB J, 2004. 18(1): p. 176-8.

[171] Noh, H. and G.L. King, *The role of protein kinase C activation in diabetic nephropathy.* Kidney Int Suppl, 2007(106): p. S49-53.

[172] Koya, D., et al., *Characterization of protein kinase C beta isoform activation on the gene expression of transforming growth factor-beta, extracellular matrix components, and prostanoids in the glomeruli of diabetic rats.* J Clin Invest, 1997. 100: p. 115-126.

[173] Ohshiro, Y., et al., *Reduction of diabetes-induced oxidative stress, fibrotic cytokine expression, and renal dysfunction in protein kinase Cbeta-null mice.* Diabetes, 2006. 55(11): p. 3112-20.

[174] Koya, D., et al., *Amelioration of accelerated diabetic mesangial expansion by treatment with a PKC beta inhibitor in diabetic db/db mice, a rodent model for type 2 diabetes.* FASEB J, 2000. 14(3): p. 439-47.

[175] Wu, D., et al., *PKC-beta1 mediates glucose-induced Akt activation and TGF-beta1 upregulation in mesangial cells.* J Am Soc Nephrol, 2009. 20(3): p. 554-66.

[176] Weigert, C., et al., *AP-1 proteins mediate hyperglycemia-induced activation of the human TGF-beta1 promoter in mesangial cells.* J Am Soc Nephrol, 2000. 11(11): p. 2007-16.

[177] Isono, M., et al., *Extracellular signal-regulated kinase mediates stimulation of TGF-beta1 and matrix by high glucose in mesangial cells.* J Am Soc Nephrol, 2000. 11(12): p. 2222-30.

[178] Gilbert, R.E., et al., *Effect of ruboxistaurin on urinary transforming growth factor-beta in patients with diabetic nephropathy and type 2 diabetes.* Diabetes Care, 2007. 30(4): p. 995-6.

[179] Nomura, K., et al., *Transforming growth factor-beta-1 latency-associated peptide and soluble betaglycan prevent a glucose-induced increase in fibronectin production in cultured human mesangial cells.* Nephron, 2002. 91(4): p. 606-11.

[180] Miyazono, K. and C.H. Heldin, *Role for carbohydrate structures in TGF-beta 1 latency.* Nature, 1989. 338(6211): p. 158-60.

[181] Flaumenhaft, R., et al., *Basic fibroblast growth factor-induced activation of latent transforming growth factor beta in endothelial cells: Regulation of plasminogen activator activity.* J Cell Biol, 1992. 118: p. 901-909.

[182] Munger, J.S., et al., *The integrin alpha v beta 6 binds and activates latent TGF beta 1: a mechanism for regulating pulmonary inflammation and fibrosis.* Cell, 1999. 96(3): p. 319-28.

[183] Zhu, Y., H.K. Usui, and K. Sharma, *Regulation of transforming growth factor beta in diabetic nephropathy: implications for treatment.* Semin Nephrol, 2007. 27(2): p. 153-60.

[184] Bornstein, P., *Thrombospondins as matricellular modulators of cell function.* J Clin Invest, 2001. 107(8): p. 929-934.

[185] Abdelouahed, M., et al., *Activation of platelet-transforming growth factor beta-1 in the absence of thrombospondin-1.* J Biol Chem, 2000. 275(24): p. 17933-17936.

[186] Bailly, S., et al., *Analysis of small latent transforming growth factor-beta complex formation and dissociation by surface plasmon resonance. Absence of direct interaction with thrombospondins.* J Biol Chem, 1997. 272(26): p. 16329-16334.

[187] Grainger, D.J. and E.K. Frow, *Thrombospondin 1 does not activate transforming growth factor beta1 in a chemically defined system or in smooth-muscle-cell cultures.* Biochem J, 2000. 350 Pt 1: p. 291-8.

[188] Murphy-Ullrich, J.E. and M. Poczatek, *Activation of latent TGF-beta by thrombospondin-1: mechanisms and physiology.* Cytokine Growth Factor Rev, 2000. 11(1-2): p. 59-69.

[189] Ribeiro, S.M., et al., *The activation sequence of thrombospondin-1 interacts with the latency-associated peptide to regulate activation of latent transforming growth factor-beta.* J Biol Chem, 1999. 274(19): p. 13586-13593.

[190] Schultz-Cherry, S., et al., *Regulation of transforming growth factor-beta activation by discrete sequences of thrombospondin 1.* J Biol Chem, 1995. 270(13): p. 7304-7310.

[191] Yevdokimova, N., N.A. Wahab, and R.M. Mason, *Thrombospondin-1 is the key activator of TGF-beta1 in human mesangial cells exposed to high glucose.* J Am Soc Nephrol, 2001. 12(4): p. 703-712.

[192] Hohenstein, B., et al., *Correlation of enhanced thrombospondin-1 expression, TGF-beta signalling and proteinuria in human type-2 diabetic nephropathy.* Nephrol Dial Transplant, 2008. 23(12): p. 3880-7.

[193] Wahab, N.A., et al., *Glomerular expression of thrombospondin-1, transforming growth factor beta and connective tissue growth factor at different stages of diabetic*

nephropathy and their interdependent roles in mesangial response to diabetic stimuli. Diabetologia, 2005. 48(12): p. 2650-60.

[194] Murphy, M., et al., *Suppression subtractive hybridization identifies high glucose levels as a stimulus for expression of connective tissue growth factor and other genes in human mesangial cells.* J Biol Chem, 1999. 274(9): p. 5830-5834.

[195] Tada, H. and S. Isogai, *The fibronectin production is increased by thrombospondin via activation of TGF-beta in cultured human mesangial cells.* Nephron, 1998. 79(1): p. 38-43.

[196] Poczatek, M.H., et al., *Glucose stimulation of transforming growth factor-beta bioactivity in mesangial cells is mediated by thrombospondin-1.* Am J Pathol, 2000. 157(4): p. 1353-63.

[197] Tada, H., et al., *High glucose levels enhance TGF-beta1-thrombospondin-1 pathway in cultured human mesangial cells via mechanisms dependent on glucose-induced PKC activation.* J Diabetes Complications, 2001. 15(4): p. 193-7.

[198] Wang, S., et al., *Glucose Up-regulates Thrombospondin 1 Gene Transcription and Transforming Growth Factor-{beta} Activity through Antagonism of cGMP-dependent Protein Kinase Repression via Upstream Stimulatory Factor 2.* J. Biol. Chem., 2004. 279(33): p. 34311-34322.

[199] Han, S.H., et al., *Gene expression patterns in glucose-stimulated podocytes.* Biochem Biophys Res Commun, 2008. 370(3): p. 514-8.

[200] Yung, S., et al., *Elevated glucose induction of thrombospondin-1 up-regulates fibronectin synthesis in proximal renal tubular epithelial cells through TGF-beta1 dependent and TGF-beta1 independent pathways.* Nephrol Dial Transplant, 2006. 21(6): p. 1504-13.

[201] Yang, Y.L., et al., *Thrombospondin-1 mediates distal tubule hypertrophy induced by glycated albumin.* Biochem J, 2004. 379(Pt 1): p. 89-97.

[202] Daniel, C., et al., *Thrombospondin-1 is an endogenous activator of TGF-beta in experimental diabetic nephropathy in vivo.* Diabetes, 2007. 56(12): p. 2982-9.

[203] Barcellos-Hoff, M.H. and T.A. Dix, *Redox-mediated activation of latent transforming growth factor-beta 1.* Mol Endocrinol, 1996. 10(9): p. 1077-83.

[204] Lawrence, D.A., *Latent-TGF-β: An overview.* Molecular and Cellular Biochemistry, 2001. 219(1): p. 163-170.

[205] Ehrhart, E.J., et al., *Latent transforming growth factor beta1 activation in situ: quantitative and functional evidence after low-dose gamma-irradiation.* FASEB J, 1997. 11(12): p. 991-1002.

[206] Riley, P.A., *Free radicals in biology: oxidative stress and the effects of ionizing radiation.* Int J Radiat Biol, 1994. 65(1): p. 27-33.

[207] Jobling, M.F., et al., *Isoform-specific activation of latent transforming growth factor beta (LTGF-beta) by reactive oxygen species.* Radiat Res, 2006. 166(6): p. 839-48.

[208] O'Malley, Y., et al., *Radiation-induced alterations in rat mesangial cell Tgfb1 and Tgfb3 gene expression are not associated with altered secretion of active Tgfb isoforms.* Radiat Res, 1999. 152(6): p. 622-8.

[209] Tsuchida, K., B. Cronin, and K. Sharma, *Novel aspects of transforming growth factor-Beta in diabetic kidney disease.* Nephron, 2002. 92(1): p. 7-21.

[210] Li, J.H., et al., *Role of TGF-beta signaling in extracellular matrix production under high glucose conditions.* Kidney Int, 2003. 63(6): p. 2010-9.

[211] Saal, S. and S.J. Harvey, *MicroRNAs and the kidney: coming of age.* Curr Opin Nephrol Hypertens, 2009.

[212] Kato, M., et al., *MicroRNA-192 in diabetic kidney glomeruli and its function in TGF-beta-induced collagen expression via inhibition of E-box repressors.* Proc Natl Acad Sci U S A, 2007. 104(9): p. 3432-7.

[213] Wang, Q., et al., *MicroRNA-377 is up-regulated and can lead to increased fibronectin production in diabetic nephropathy.* FASEB J, 2008. 22(12): p. 4126-35.

[214] Kato, M., et al., *Roles of renal microRNA-216a (miR-216a) in TGF-beta signaling and diabetic nephropathy.* FASEB J., 2008. 22(1_MeetingAbstracts): p. 603.4-.

[215] Muhonen, P. and H. Holthofer, *Epigenetic and microRNA-mediated regulation in diabetes.* Nephrol. Dial. Transplant., 2009. 24(4): p. 1088-1096.

[216] Gregory, P.A., et al., *The miR-200 family and miR-205 regulate epithelial to mesenchymal transition by targeting ZEB1 and SIP1.* Nat Cell Biol, 2008. 10(5): p. 593-601.

[217] Simonson, M.S., *Phenotypic transitions and fibrosis in diabetic nephropathy.* Kidney Int, 2007. 71(9): p. 846-54.

[218] Qi, W., et al., *The renal cortical fibroblast in renal tubulointerstitial fibrosis.* Int J Biochem Cell Biol, 2006. 38(1): p. 1-5.

[219] Wada, T., et al., *Fibrocytes: a new insight into kidney fibrosis.* Kidney Int, 2007. 72(3): p. 269-73.

[220] Wang, W.-m., et al., *PPAR-[gamma] agonists inhibit TGF-[beta]1-induced chemokine expression in human tubular epithelial cells.* Acta Pharmacol Sin, 2008. 30(1): p. 107-112.

[221] Wolf, G., et al., *High glucose-induced proliferation in mesangial cells is reversed by autocrine TGF-beta.* Kidney Int, 1992. 42: p. 647-656.

[222] Wolf, G., et al., *High glucose stimulates expression of p27Kip1 in cultured mouse mesangial cells: relationship to hypertrophy.* Am J Physiol, 1997. 273(3 Pt 2): p. F348-F356.

[223] Miyajima, A., et al., *Antibody to transforming growth factor-beta ameliorates tubular apoptosis in unilateral ureteral obstruction.* Kidney Int, 2000. 58(6): p. 2301-13.

[224] Choi, M.E. and B.J. Ballermann, *Inhibition of capillary morphogenesis and associated apoptosis by dominant negative mutant transforming growth factor-beta receptors.* J Biol Chem, 1995. 270(36): p. 21144-50.

[225] Wada, T., et al., *The cyclin-dependent kinase inhibitor p21 is required for TGF-[beta]1-induced podocyte apoptosis.* Kidney Int, 2005. 68(4): p. 1618-1629.

[226] Wu, D.T., et al., *TGF-{beta} Concentration Specifies Differential Signaling Profiles of Growth Arrest/Differentiation and Apoptosis in Podocytes.* J Am Soc Nephrol, 2005. 16(11): p. 3211-3221.

[227] Lee, E.Y., et al., *Monocyte chemoattractant protein-1/CCR2 loop, inducible by TGF-{beta}, increases podocyte motility and albumin permeability.* Am J Physiol Renal Physiol, 2009.

[228] Dessapt, C., et al., *Mechanical forces and TGF{beta}1 reduce podocyte adhesion through {alpha}3{beta}1 integrin downregulation.* Nephrol. Dial. Transplant., 2009: p. gfp204.

[229] Toyoda, M., et al., *Podocyte Detachment and Reduced Glomerular Capillary Endothelial Fenestration in Human Type 1 Diabetic Nephropathy.* Diabetes, 2007. 56(8): p. 2155-2160.

[230] Cortes, P. and C.E. Mogensen, *The diabetic kidney.* 2006, Totowa, N.J.: Humana Press. xviii, 564 p.

[231] Ito, Y., et al., *Expression of connective tissue growth factor in human renal fibrosis.* Kidney Int, 1998. 53(4): p. 853-61.

[232] Wahab, N.A., et al., *Role of connective tissue growth factor in the pathogenesis of diabetic nephropathy.* Biochem J, 2001. 359(Pt 1): p. 77-87.

[233] Roestenberg, P., et al., *Temporal expression profile and distribution pattern indicate a role of connective tissue growth factor (CTGF/CCN-2) in diabetic nephropathy in mice.* Am J Physiol Renal Physiol, 2006. 290(6): p. F1344-54.

[234] Riser, B.L., et al., *Regulation of connective tissue growth factor activity in cultured rat mesangial cells and its expression in experimental diabetic glomerulosclerosis.* J Am Soc Nephrol, 2000. 11(1): p. 25-38.

[235] Yokoi, H., et al., *Overexpression of connective tissue growth factor in podocytes worsens diabetic nephropathy in mice.* Kidney Int, 2008. 73(4): p. 446-55.

[236] Wang, S., et al., *Connective tissue growth factor in tubulointerstitial injury of diabetic nephropathy.* Kidney Int, 2001. 60(1): p. 96-105.

[237] Guha, M., et al., *Specific down-regulation of connective tissue growth factor attenuates progression of nephropathy in mouse models of type 1 and type 2 diabetes.* FASEB J, 2007. 21(12): p. 3355-68.

[238] Grotendorst, G.R., H. Okochi, and N. Hayashi, *A novel transforming growth factor beta response element controls the expression of the connective tissue growth factor gene.* Cell Growth Differ, 1996. 7(4): p. 469-80.

[239] Hishikawa, K., B.S. Oemar, and T. Nakaki, *Static pressure regulates connective tissue growth factor expression in human mesangial cells.* J Biol Chem, 2001. 276(20): p. 16797-803.

[240] Riser, B.L., et al., *Cyclic stretching force selectively up-regulates transforming growth factor-beta isoforms in cultured rat mesangial cells.* Am J Pathol, 1996. 148(6): p. 1915-23.

[241] Cooker, L.A., et al., *TNF-alpha, but not IFN-gamma, regulates CCN2 (CTGF), collagen type I, and proliferation in mesangial cells: possible roles in the progression of renal fibrosis.* Am J Physiol Renal Physiol, 2007. 293(1): p. F157-65.

[242] Abreu, J.G., et al., *Connective-tissue growth factor (CTGF) modulates cell signalling by BMP and TGF-beta.* Nat Cell Biol, 2002. 4(8): p. 599-604.

[243] Nguyen, T.Q., et al., *CTGF inhibits BMP-7 signaling in diabetic nephropathy.* J Am Soc Nephrol, 2008. 19(11): p. 2098-107.

[244] Wahab, N.A., B.S. Weston, and R.M. Mason, *Connective tissue growth factor CCN2 interacts with and activates the tyrosine kinase receptor TrkA.* J Am Soc Nephrol, 2005. 16(2): p. 340-51.

[245] Abdel Wahab, N., B.S. Weston, and R.M. Mason, *Modulation of the TGF[beta]/Smad signaling pathway in mesangial cells by CTGF/CCN2.* Experimental Cell Research, 2005. 307(2): p. 305-314.

[246] Wu, S.H., et al., *Signal transduction involved in CTGF-induced production of chemokines in mesangial cells.* Growth factors, 2008. 26(4): p. 192-200.

[247] Crean, J.K., et al., *The role of p42/44 MAPK and protein kinase B in connective tissue growth factor induced extracellular matrix protein production, cell migration, and actin cytoskeletal rearrangement in human mesangial cells.* J Biol Chem, 2002. 277(46): p. 44187-94.

[248] Mason, R.M., *Connective tissue growth factor(CCN2), a pathogenic factor in diabetic nephropathy. What does it do? How does it do it?* J Cell Commun Signal, 2009.

[249] Dudley, A.T., K.M. Lyons, and E.J. Robertson, *A requirement for bone morphogenetic protein-7 during development of the mammalian kidney and eye.* Genes Dev, 1995. 9(22): p. 2795-807.

[250] Simon, M., et al., *Expression of bone morphogenetic protein-7 mRNA in normal and ischemic adult rat kidney.* AM J Physiol, 1999. 276(3 Pt 2): p. 382-389.

[251] De Petris, L., et al., *Bone morphogenetic protein-7 delays podocyte injury due to high glucose.* Nephrol Dial Transplant, 2007. 22(12): p. 3442-50.

[252] Bosukonda, D., et al., *Characterization of receptors for osteogenic protein-1/bone morphogenetic protein-7 (OP-1/BMP-7) in rat kidneys.* Kidney Int, 2000. 58(5): p. 1902-11.

[253] Mitu, G. and R. Hirschberg, *Bone morphogenetic protein-7 (BMP7) in chronic kidney disease.* Front Biosci, 2008. 13: p. 4726-39.

[254] Mitu, G.M., S. Wang, and R. Hirschberg, *BMP7 is a podocyte survival factor and rescues podocytes from diabetic injury.* Am J Physiol Renal Physiol, 2007. 293(5): p. F1641-8.

[255] Wang, S. and R. Hirschberg, *BMP7 antagonizes TGF-beta -dependent fibrogenesis in mesangial cells.* Am J Physiol Renal Physiol, 2003. 284(5): p. 1006-1013.

[256] Wang, S., et al., *Bone morphogenic protein-7 (BMP-7), a novel therapy for diabetic nephropathy.* Kidney Int, 2003. 63(6): p. 2037-49.

[257] Wang, S.N., J. Lapage, and R. Hirschberg, *Loss of tubular bone morphogenetic protein-7 in diabetic nephropathy.* J Am Soc Nephrol, 2001. 12(11): p. 2392-9.

[258] Wang, S., et al., *Renal bone morphogenetic protein-7 protects against diabetic nephropathy.* J Am Soc Nephrol, 2006. 17(9): p. 2504-12.

[259] Sugimoto, H., et al., *Renal fibrosis and glomerulosclerosis in a new mouse model of diabetic nephropathy and its regression by bone morphogenic protein-7 and advanced glycation end product inhibitors.* Diabetes, 2007. 56(7): p. 1825-33.

[260] Zeisberg, M., et al., *BMP-7 counteracts TGF-[beta]1-induced epithelial-to-mesenchymal transition and reverses chronic renal injury.* Nat Med, 2003. 9(7): p. 964-968.

[261] Gould, S.E., et al., *BMP-7 regulates chemokine, cytokine, and hemodynamic gene expression in proximal tubule cells.* Kidney Int, 2002. 61(1): p. 51-60.

[262] Yang, Y.L., et al., *Bone morphogenetic protein-2 antagonizes renal interstitial fibrosis by promoting catabolism of type I transforming growth factor-beta receptors.* Endocrinology, 2009. 150(2): p. 727-40.

[263] Otani, H., et al., *Antagonistic effects of bone morphogenetic protein-4 and -7 on renal mesangial cell proliferation induced by aldosterone through MAPK activation.* Am J Physiol Renal Physiol, 2007. 292(5): p. F1513-1525.

[264] Michos, O., et al., *Gremlin-mediated BMP antagonism induces the epithelial-mesenchymal feedback signaling controlling metanephric kidney and limb organogenesis.* Development, 2004. 131(14): p. 3401-10.

[265] Roxburgh, S.A., et al., *Allelic depletion of grem1 attenuates diabetic kidney disease.* Diabetes, 2009.

[266] Dolan, V., et al., *Expression of gremlin, a bone morphogenetic protein antagonist, in human diabetic nephropathy.* Am J Kidney Dis, 2005. 45(6): p. 1034-9.

[267] Chen, S. and F.N. Ziyadeh, *Vascular endothelial growth factor and diabetic nephropathy.* Curr Diab Rep, 2008. 8(6): p. 470-6.

[268] Ferrara, N., *Role of vascular endothelial growth factor in regulation of physiological angiogenesis.* Am J Physiol Cell Physiol, 2001. 280(6): p. C1358-66.

[269] Harper, S.J. and D.O. Bates, *VEGF-A splicing: the key to anti-angiogenic therapeutics?* Nat Rev Cancer, 2008. 8(11): p. 880-7.

[270] Rahimi, N., T.E. Golde, and R.D. Meyer, *Identification of ligand-induced proteolytic cleavage and ectodomain shedding of VEGFR-1/FLT1 in leukemic cancer cells.* Cancer Res, 2009. 69(6): p. 2607-14.

[271] Cooper, M.E., et al., *Increased renal expression of vascular endothelial growth factor (VEGF) and its receptor VEGFR-2 in experimental diabetes.* Diabetes, 1999. 48(11): p. 2229-39.

[272] Ichinose, K., et al., *Antiangiogenic endostatin peptide ameliorates renal alterations in the early stage of a type 1 diabetic nephropathy model.* Diabetes, 2005. 54(10): p. 2891-2903.

[273] Chou, E., et al., *Decreased cardiac expression of vascular endothelial growth factor and its receptors in insulin-resistant and diabetic States: a possible explanation for impaired collateral formation in cardiac tissue.* Circulation, 2002. 105(3): p. 373-9.

[274] Yamamoto, Y., et al., *Tumstatin peptide, an inhibitor of angiogenesis, prevents glomerular hypertrophy in the early stage of diabetic nephropathy.* Diabetes, 2004. 53(7): p. 1831-1840.

[275] Lee, E.-Y., et al., *Angiotensin II receptor blocker attenuates overexpression of vascular endothelial growth factor in diabetic podocytes.* Exp Mol Med, 2004. 36(1): p. 65-70.

[276] Ho, C., et al., *Simvastatin alleviates diabetes-induced VEGF-mediated nephropathy via the modulation of Ras signaling pathway.* Ren Fail, 2008. 30(5): p. 557-65.

[277] Ku, C.H., et al., *Inducible overexpression of sFlt-1 in podocytes ameliorates glomerulopathy in diabetic mice.* Diabetes, 2008. 57(10): p. 2824-33.

[278] Singh, A.K., et al., *Vascular factors altered in glucose-treated mesangial cells and diabetic glomeruli. Changes in vascular factors impair endothelial cell growth and matrix.* Lab Invest, 2004. 84(5): p. 597-606.

[279] Braun, L., et al., *The regulation of the induction of vascular endothelial growth factor at the onset of diabetes in spontaneously diabetic rats.* Life Sci, 2001. 69(21): p. 2533-2542.

[280] Sung, S.H., et al., *Blockade of vascular endothelial growth factor signaling ameliorates diabetic albuminuria in mice.* J Am Soc Nephrol, 2006. 17(11): p. 3093-104.

[281] Wang, Z., et al., *Regulation of renal lipid metabolism, lipid accumulation, and glomerulosclerosis in FVBdb/db mice with type 2 diabetes.* Diabetes, 2005. 54(8): p. 2328-35.

[282] Hoshi, S., et al., *Podocyte injury promotes progressive nephropathy in zucker diabetic fatty rats.* Lab Invest, 2002. 82(1): p. 25-35.

[283] Tsuchida, K., et al., *Suppression of transforming growth factor beta and vascular endothelial growth factor in diabetic nephropathy in rats by a novel advanced glycation end product inhibitor, OPB-9195.* Diabetologia, 1999. 42(5): p. 579-88.

[284] Cha, D.R., et al., *Vascular endothelial growth factor is increased during early stage of diabetic nephropathy in type II diabetic rats.* J Endocrinol, 2004. 183(1): p. 183-94.

[285] Klanke, B., et al., *Effects of vascular endothelial growth factor (VEGF)/vascular permeability factor (VPF) on haemodynamics and permselectivity of the isolated perfused rat kidney.* Nephrol Dial Transplant, 1998. 13(4): p. 875-885.

[286] Sison K, F.I., Quaggin SE, *Podocyte-specific increase in VEGF-A production leads to rapid alterations in glomerular permeability and features of diabetic nephropathy* Presented at the 38th Annual American Society of Nephrology Meeting. Philadelphia; November 10-13, 2005. [abstract F-FC193].

[287] Veron, D., et al., *VEGF-A Dysregulation Alters the Glomerular Phenotype of Streptozotocin Diabetic Mice.* Presented at the 38th Annual American Society of Nephrology Meeting. Philadelphia; November 4-9, 2008.

[288] Eremina, V., et al., *VEGF inhibition and renal thrombotic microangiopathy.* N Engl J Med, 2008. 358(11): p. 1129-36.

[289] de Vriese, A.S., et al., *Antibodies against vascular endothelial growth factor improve early renal dysfunction in experimental diabetes.* J Am Soc Nephrol, 2001. 12(5): p. 993-1000.

[290] Flyvbjerg, A., et al., *Amelioration of long-term renal changes in obese type 2 diabetic mice by a neutralizing vascular endothelial growth factor antibody.* Diabetes, 2002. 51(10): p. 3090-4.

[291] Schrijvers, B.F., et al., *A neutralizing VEGF antibody prevents glomerular hypertrophy in a model of obese type 2 diabetes, the Zucker diabetic fatty rat.* Nephrol Dial Transplant, 2006. 21(2): p. 324-9.

[292] Shulman, K., et al., *Expression of vascular permeability factor (VPF/VEGF) is altered in many glomerular diseases.* J Am Soc Nephrol, 1996. 7(5): p. 661-666.

[293] Bailey, E., et al., *Vascular endothelial growth factor mRNA expression in minimal change, membranous, and diabetic nephropathy demonstrated by non-isotopic in situ hybridisation.* J Clin Pathol, 1999. 52(10): p. 735-738.

[294] Bortoloso, E., et al., *Quantitave and qualitative changes in vascular endothelial growth factor gene expression in glomeruli of patients with type 2 diabetes.* Eur J Endocrinol, 2004. 150(6): p. 799-807.

[295] Baelde, H.J., et al., *Gene expression profiling in glomeruli from human kidneys with diabetic nephropathy.* Am J Kidney Dis, 2004. 43(4): p. 636-50.

[296] Baelde, H.J., et al., *Reduction of VEGF-A and CTGF expression in diabetic nephropathy is associated with podocyte loss.* Kidney Int, 2007. 71(7): p. 637-45.

[297] Lindenmeyer, M.T., et al., *Interstitial vascular rarefaction and reduced VEGF-A expression in human diabetic nephropathy.* J Am Soc Nephrol, 2007. 18(6): p. 1765-76.

[298] Kanesaki, Y., et al., *Vascular endothelial growth factor gene expression is correlated with glomerular neovascularization in human diabetic nephropathy.* Am J Kidney Dis, 2005. 45(2): p. 288-294.

[299] Hohenstein, B., et al., *Local VEGF activity but not VEGF expression is tightly regulated during diabetic nephropathy in man.* Kidney Int, 2006. 69(9): p. 1654-61.

[300] Kimura, K., et al., *Serum VEGF--as a prognostic factor of atherosclerosis.* Atherosclerosis, 2007. 194(1): p. 182-8.

[301] Machnik, A., et al., *Macrophages regulate salt-dependent volume and blood pressure by a vascular endothelial growth factor-C-dependent buffering mechanism.* Nat Med, 2009. 15(5): p. 545-52.

[302] Baba, T., et al., *No nephropathy in Type 2 diabetic patient with POEMS syndrome with an elevated plasma VEGF.* Diabet Med, 2004. 21(3): p. 292-294.

[303] Shimada, K., et al., *Plasma vascular endothelial growth factor in Japanese Type 2 diabetic patients with and without nephropathy.* J Diabetes Complications, 2002. 16(6): p. 386-90.

[304] Chaturvedi, N., et al., *Circulating plasma vascular endothelial growth factor and microvascular complications of type 1 diabetes mellitus: the influence of ACE inhibition.* Diabet Med, 2001. 18(4): p. 288-94.

[305] Hovind, P., et al., *Elevated vascular endothelial growth factor in type 1 diabetic patients with diabetic nephropathy.* Kidney Int Suppl, 2000. 75: p. S56-61.

[306] Chiarelli, F., et al., *Vascular endothelial growth factor (VEGF) in children, adolescents and young adults with Type 1 diabetes mellitus: relation to glycaemic control and microvascular complications.* Diabet Med, 2000. 17(9): p. 650-656.

[307] Santilli, F., et al., *Increased vascular endothelial growth factor serum concentrations may help to identify patients with onset of type 1 diabetes during childhood at risk for developing persistent microalbuminuria.* J Clin Endocrinol Metab, 2001. 86(8): p. 3871-3876.

[308] Honkanen, E.O., A.M. Teppo, and C. Gronhagen-Riska, *Decreased urinary excretion of vascular endothelial growth factor in idiopathic membranous glomerulonephritis.* Kidney Int, 2000. 57(6): p. 2343-9.

[309] Lenz, T., et al., *Vascular endothelial growth factor in diabetic nephropathy.* Kidney Blood Press Res, 2003. 26(5-6): p. 338-343.

[310] De Mattia, G., et al., *Endothelial dysfunction and oxidative stress in type 1 and type 2 diabetic patients without clinical macrovascular complications.* Diabetes Res Clin Pract, 2008. 79(2): p. 337-42.

[311] Kim, N.H., et al., *Plasma and urinary vascular endothelial growth factor and diabetic nephropathy in Type 2 diabetes mellitus.* Diabet Med, 2004. 21(6): p. 545-551.

[312] Kim, N.H., et al., *Vascular endothelial growth factor (VEGF) and soluble VEGF receptor FLT-1 in diabetic nephropathy.* Kidney Int, 2005. 67(1): p. 167-77.

[313] Chen, H.B., et al., *The protective effect of the RAS inhibitor on diabetic patients with nephropathy in the context of VEGF suppression.* Acta Pharmacol Sin, 2009. 30(2): p. 242-50.

[314] Ray, D., et al., *Association of the VEGF gene with proliferative diabetic retinopathy but not proteinuria in diabetes.* Diabetes, 2004. 53(3): p. 861-864.

[315] Buraczynska, M., et al., *Association of the VEGF gene polymorphism with diabetic retinopathy in type 2 diabetes patients.* Nephrol Dial Transplant, 2007. 22(3): p. 827-32.

[316] Al-Kateb, H., et al., *Multiple variants in vascular endothelial growth factor (VEGFA) are risk factors for time to severe retinopathy in type 1 diabetes: the DCCT/EDIC genetics study.* Diabetes, 2007. 56(8): p. 2161-2168.

[317] Yang, B., et al., *Polymorphisms of the vascular endothelial growth factor and susceptibility to diabetic microvascular complications in patients with type 1 diabetes mellitus.* J Diabetes Complications, 2003. 17(1): p. 1-6.

[318] McKnight, A.J., et al., *Association of VEGF-1499C-->T polymorphism with diabetic nephropathy in type 1 diabetes mellitus.* J Diabetes Complications, 2007. 21(4): p. 242-5.

[319] Hoshi, S., et al., *High glucose induced VEGF expression via PKC and ERK in glomerular podocytes.* Biochem Biophys Res Commun, 2002. 290(1): p. 177-84.

[320] Chuang, P.Y. and J.C. He, *Signaling in regulation of podocyte phenotypes.* Nephron Physiol, 2009. 111(2): p. p9-15.

[321] Jeansson, M. and B. Haraldsson, *Morphological and functional evidence for an important role of the endothelial cell glycocalyx in the glomerular barrier.* Am J Physiol Renal Physiol, 2006. 290(1): p. F111-6.

[322] Eremina, V., H.J. Baelde, and S.E. Quaggin, *Role of the VEGF--a signaling pathway in the glomerulus: evidence for crosstalk between components of the glomerular filtration barrier.* Nephron Physiol, 2007. 106(2): p. p32-7.

[323] Zeng, L., et al., *HMG CoA reductase inhibition modulates VEGF-induced endothelial cell hyperpermeability by preventing RhoA activation and myosin regulatory light chain phosphorylation.* FASEB J, 2005. 19(13): p. 1845-7.

[324] Nakagawa, T., *Uncoupling of the VEGF-endothelial nitric oxide axis in diabetic nephropathy: an explanation for the paradoxical effects of VEGF in renal disease.* Am J Physiol Renal Physiol, 2007. 292(6): p. F1665-72.

[325] Ferrari, G., et al., *VEGF, a prosurvival factor, acts in concert with TGF-beta1 to induce endothelial cell apoptosis.* Proc Natl Acad Sci U S A, 2006. 103(46): p. 17260-5.

[326] Chen, S., et al., *Podocyte-derived vascular endothelial growth factor mediates the stimulation of alpha3(IV) collagen production by transforming growth factor-beta1 in mouse podocytes.* Diabetes, 2004. 53(11): p. 2939-49.

[327] Ichinose, K., et al., *2-(8-hydroxy-6-methoxy-1-oxo-1h-2-benzopyran-3-yl) propionic acid, an inhibitor of angiogenesis, ameliorates renal alterations in obese type 2 diabetic mice.* Diabetes, 2006. 55(5): p. 1232-42.

[328] Foster, R.R., et al., *Vascular endothelial growth factor and nephrin interact and reduce apoptosis in human podocytes.* Am J Physiol Renal Physiol, 2005. 288(1): p. F48-57.

[329] Guan, F., et al., *Autocrine VEGF-A system in podocytes regulates podocin and its interaction with CD2AP.* Am J Physiol Renal Physiol, 2006. 291(2): p. F422-8.

[330] Schumacher, V.A., et al., *Impaired glomerular maturation and lack of VEGF165b in Denys-Drash syndrome.* J Am Soc Nephrol, 2007. 18(3): p. 719-29.

[331] Ferguson, J.K., et al., *Podocyte specific over-expression of VEGF-A165b, unlike VEGF-A165, does not cause collapsing glomerulopathy.* FASEB J., 2008. 22(1_MeetingAbstracts): p. 926.16-.

[332] Bevan, H.S., et al., *The alternatively spliced anti-angiogenic family of VEGF isoforms VEGFxxxb in human kidney development.* Nephron Physiol, 2008. 110(4): p. p57-67.

[333] Nowak, D.G., et al., *Expression of pro- and anti-angiogenic isoforms of VEGF is differentially regulated by splicing and growth factors.* J Cell Sci, 2008. 121(Pt 20): p. 3487-95.

[334] Perrin, R.M., et al., *Diabetic retinopathy is associated with a switch in splicing from anti- to pro-angiogenic isoforms of vascular endothelial growth factor.* Diabetologia, 2005. 48(11): p. 2422-7.
[335] Jeong, J.H., et al., *siRNA conjugate delivery systems.* Bioconjug Chem, 2009. 20(1): p. 5-14.
[336] Nishina, K., et al., *Efficient in vivo delivery of siRNA to the liver by conjugation of alpha-tocopherol.* Mol Ther, 2008. 16(4): p. 734-40.
[337] Landau, D., et al., *A novel somatostatin analogue prevents early renal complications in the nonobese diabetic mouse.* Kidney Int, 2001. 60(2): p. 505-512.
[338] Gronbaek, H., et al., *Inhibitory effects of octreotide on renal and glomerular growth in early experimental diabetes in mice.* J Endocrinol, 2002. 172(3): p. 637-643.
[339] Gronbaek, H., et al., *Effect of octreotide on experimental diabetic renal and glomerular growth: importance of early intervention.* J Endocrinol, 1995. 147(1): p. 95-9102.
[340] Flyvbjerg, A., et al., *Octreotide administration in diabetic rats: Effects on renal hypertrophy and urinary albumin excretion.* Kidney Int, 1992. 41: p. 805-812.
[341] Flyvbjerg, A., et al., *Somatostatin analogue administration prevents increase in kidney somatomedin C and initial renal growth in diabetic and uninephrectomized rats.* Diabetologia, 1989. 32: p. 261-265.
[342] Segev, Y., et al., *Growth hormone receptor antagonism prevents early renal changes in nonobese diabetic mice.* J Am Soc Nephrol, 1999. 10(11): p. 2374-2381.
[343] Chen, N.Y., W.Y. Chen, and J.J. Kopchick, *A growth hormone antagonist protects mice against streptozotocin induced glomerulosclerosis even in the presence of elevated levels of glucose and glycated hemoglobin.* Endocrinology, 1996. 137(11): p. 5163-5165.
[344] Chen, N.Y., et al., *Effects of streptozotocin treatment in growth hormone (GH) and GH antagonist transgenic mice.* Endocrinology, 1995. 136(2): p. 660-667.
[345] Bellush, L.L., et al., *Protection against diabetes-induced nephropathy in growth hormone receptor/binding protein gene-disrupted mice.* Endocrinology, 2000. 141(1): p. 163-8.
[346] Segev, Y., et al., *Systemic and renal growth hormone-IGF1 axis involvement in a mouse model of type 2 diabetes.* Diabetologia, 2007. 50(6): p. 1327-34.
[347] Bacci, S., et al., *Role of insulin-like growth factor (IGF)-1 in the modulation of renal haemodynamics in Type I diabetic patients.* Diabetologia, 2000. 43(7): p. 922-926.
[348] Verrotti, A., et al., *Growth hormone and IGF-I in diabetic children with and without microalbuminuria.* Diabetes Nutr Metab, 1999. 12(4): p. 271-276.
[349] Cummings, E.A., et al., *Contribution of growth hormone and IGF-I to early diabetic nephropathy in type 1 diabetes.* Diabetes, 1998. 47(8): p. 1341-1346.
[350] Sen, A. and A. Buyukgebiz, *Albumin excretion rate, serum insulin-like growth factor-I and glomerular filtration rate in type I diabetes mellitus at puberty.* J Pediatr Endocrinol Metab, 1997. 10(2): p. 209-15.
[351] Hoogenberg, K., et al., *Insulin-like growth factor I and altered renal hemodynamics in growth hormone deficiency, acromegaly, and type I diabetes mellitus.* Transplant Proc, 1994. 26(2): p. 505-507.
[352] Spagnoli, A., et al., *Evaluation of the components of insulin-like growth factor (IGF)-IGF binding protein (IGFBP) system in adolescents with type 1 diabetes and persistent*

microalbuminuria: relationship with increased urinary excretion of IGFBP-3 18 kD N-terminal fragment. Clin Endocrinol (Oxf), 1999. 51(5): p. 587-96.
[353] Serri, O., et al., *Somatostatin analogue, octreotide, reduces increased glomerular filtration rate and kidney size in insulin-dependent diabetes.* JAMA, 1991. 265: p. 888-892.
[354] Tack, I., et al., *Autocrine activation of the IGF-I signaling pathway in mesangial cells isolated from diabetic NOD mice.* Diabetes, 2002. 51(1): p. 182-8.
[355] Schreiber, B.D., M.L. Hughes, and G.C. Groggel, *Insulin-like growth factor-1 stimulates production of mesangial cell matrix components.* Clin Nephrol, 1995. 43(6): p. 368-74.
[356] Oemar, B.S., et al., *Regulation of insulin-like growth factor I receptors in diabetic mesangial cells.* J Biol Chem, 1991. 266(4): p. 2369-73.
[357] Moran, A., et al., *Effects of IGF-I and glucose on protein and proteoglycan synthesis by human fetal mesangial cells in culture.* Diabetes, 1991. 40(10): p. 1346-54.
[358] Horney, M.J., et al., *Elevated glucose increases mesangial cell sensitivity to insulin-like growth factor I.* AM J Physiol, 1998. 274(6 Pt 2): p. F1045-53.
[359] Doi, T., et al., *Insulinlike growth factor-1 is a progression factor for human mesangial cells.* Am J Pathol, 1989. 134(2): p. 395-404.
[360] Conti, F.G., et al., *Studies on binding and mitogenic effect of insulin and insulin-like growth factor I in glomerular mesangial cells.* Endocrinology, 1988. 122(6): p. 2788-95.
[361] Abrass, C.K., et al., *Insulin and insulin-like growth factor I binding to cultured rat glomerular mesangial cells.* Endocrinology, 1988. 123(5): p. 2432-9.
[362] Reddy, G.R., et al., *Identification of the glomerular podocyte as a target for growth hormone action.* Endocrinology, 2007. 148(5): p. 2045-55.
[363] Bridgewater, D.J., et al., *Insulin-like growth factors inhibit podocyte apoptosis through the PI3 kinase pathway.* Kidney Int, 2005. 67(4): p. 1308-14.
[364] Senthil, D., et al., *Regulation of protein synthesis by IGF-I in proximal tubular epithelial cells.* Am J Physiol Renal Physiol, 2002. 283(6): p. F1226-36.
[365] Hirschberg, R., *Bioactivity of glomerular ultrafiltrate during heavy proteinuria may contribute to renal tubulo-interstitial lesions: evidence for a role for insulin-like growth factor I.* J Clin Invest, 1996. 98(1): p. 116-24.
[366] Schrijvers, B.F., A.S. De Vriese, and A. Flyvbjerg, *From hyperglycemia to diabetic kidney disease: the role of metabolic, hemodynamic, intracellular factors and growth factors/cytokines.* Endocr Rev, 2004. 25(6): p. 971-1010.
[367] Kelly, D.J., et al., *Aminoguanidine ameliorates overexpression of prosclerotic growth factors and collagen deposition in experimental diabetic nephropathy.* J Am Soc Nephrol, 2001. 12(10): p. 2098-107.
[368] Nakagawa, H., et al., *Immunohistochemical characterization of glomerular PDGF B-chain and PDGF beta-receptor expression in diabetic rats.* Diabetes Res Clin Pract, 2000. 48(2): p. 87-98.
[369] Nakamura, T., et al., *mRNA expression of growth factors in glomeruli from diabetic rats.* Diabetes, 1993. 42(3): p. 450-6.
[370] Young, B.A., et al., *Cellular events in the evolution of experimental diabetic nephropathy.* Kidney Int, 1995. 47(3): p. 935-944.

[371] Riley, S.G., et al., *Augmentation of kidney injury by basic fibroblast growth factor or platelet-derived growth factor does not induce progressive diabetic nephropathy in the Goto Kakizaki model of non-insulin-dependent diabetes.* J Lab Clin Med, 1999. 134(3): p. 304-12.

[372] Lassila, M., et al., *Imatinib attenuates diabetic nephropathy in apolipoprotein E-knockout mice.* J Am Soc Nephrol, 2005. 16(2): p. 363-73.

[373] Uehara, G., et al., *Glomerular expression of platelet-derived growth factor (PDGF)-A, -B chain and PDGF receptor-alpha, -beta in human diabetic nephropathy.* Clinical and Experimental Nephrology, 2004. 8(1): p. 36-42.

[374] Langham, R.G., et al., *Over-expression of platelet-derived growth factor in human diabetic nephropathy.* Nephrology Dialysis Transplantation, 2003. 18(7): p. 1392-6.

[375] Fagerudd, J.A., et al., *Urinary excretion of TGF-beta1, PDGF-BB and fibronectin in insulin-dependent diabetes mellitus patients.* Kidney Int Suppl, 1997. 63: p. S195-S197.

[376] Choudhury, G.G., et al., *PI-3-kinase and MAPK regulate mesangial cell proliferation and migration in response to PDGF.* AM J Physiol, 1997. 273(6 Pt 2): p. 931-938.

[377] Throckmorton, D.C., et al., *PDGF and TGF-beta mediate collagen production by mesangial cells exposed to advanced glycosylation end products.* Kidney Int, 1995. 48(1): p. 111-117.

[378] Mizuno, S. and T. Nakamura, *Suppressions of chronic glomerular injuries and TGF-beta 1 production by HGF in attenuation of murine diabetic nephropathy.* Am J Physiol Renal Physiol, 2004. 286(1): p. F134-43.

[379] Kagawa, T., et al., *Hepatocyte growth factor gene therapy slows down the progression of diabetic nephropathy in db/db mice.* Nephron Physiol, 2006. 102(3-4): p. p92-102.

[380] Cruzado, J.M., et al., *Regression of advanced diabetic nephropathy by hepatocyte growth factor gene therapy in rats.* Diabetes, 2004. 53(4): p. 1119-27.

[381] Dai, C., et al., *Intravenous administration of hepatocyte growth factor gene ameliorates diabetic nephropathy in mice.* J Am Soc Nephrol, 2004. 15(10): p. 2637-47.

[382] Kulseng, B., et al., *Elevated hepatocyte growth factor in sera from patients with insulin-dependent diabetes mellitus.* Acta Diabetol, 1998. 35(2): p. 77-80.

[383] Nakamura, S., et al., *Hepatocyte growth factor as a potential index of complication in diabetes mellitus.* J Hypertens, 1998. 16(12 Pt 2): p. 2019-2026.

[384] Randers, E., et al., *Serum hepatocyte growth factor levels in patients with chronic renal disease--effect of GFR and pathogenesis.* Scand J Clin Lab Invest, 2001. 61(8): p. 615-9.

[385] Dai, C. and Y. Liu, *Hepatocyte growth factor antagonizes the profibrotic action of TGF-beta1 in mesangial cells by stabilizing Smad transcriptional corepressor TGIF.* J Am Soc Nephrol, 2004. 15(6): p. 1402-12.

[386] Li, Y., et al., *hepatocyte growth factor is a downstream effector that mediates the antifibrotic action of peroxisome proliferator-activated receptor-gamma agonists.* J Am Soc Nephrol, 2006. 17(1): p. 54-65.

[387] Esposito, C., et al., *Hepatocyte growth factor (HGF) modulates matrix turnover in human glomeruli.* Kidney Int, 2005. 67(6): p. 2143-50.

[388] Fornoni, A., et al., *Hepatocyte growth factor, but not insulin-like growth factor I, protects podocytes against cyclosporin A-induced apoptosis.* Am J Pathol, 2001. 158(1): p. 275-80.

[389] Toba, H., et al., *Chronic treatment with recombinant human erythropoietin exerts renoprotective effects beyond hematopoiesis in streptozotocin-induced diabetic rat.* Eur J Pharmacol, 2009. 612(1-3): p. 106-14.

[390] Tong, Z., et al., *Promoter polymorphism of the erythropoietin gene in severe diabetic eye and kidney complications.* Proc Natl Acad Sci U S A, 2008. 105(19): p. 6998-7003.

[391] Singh, D.K., P. Winocour, and K. Farrington, *Mechanisms of disease: the hypoxic tubular hypothesis of diabetic nephropathy.* Nat Clin Pract Nephrol, 2008. 4(4): p. 216-26.

[392] Wolf, G., et al., Leptin stimulates proliferation and TGF-beta expression in renal glomerular endothelial cells: potential role in glomerulosclerosis. Kidney Int, 1999. 56(3): p. 860-72.

[393] Han, D.C., et al., Leptin stimulates type I collagen production in db/db mesangial cells: *glucose uptake and TGF-beta type II receptor expression. Kidney Int, 2001. 59(4): p. 1315-23.*

In: Advances in Pathogenesis of Diabetic Nephropathy
Editor: Sharma S. Prabhakar

ISBN: 978-1-61122-134-3
© 2012 Nova Science Publishers, Inc.

ChapterVIII

Role of Activated Renin-Angiotensin System in the Pathogenesis of Diabetic Nephropathy

Hiroyuki Kobori[1,], Lisa M. Harrison-Bernard[2] and L. Gabriel Navar[1]*

[1]Department of Physiology, and Hypertension and Renal Center of Excellence, Tulane University School of Medicine, New Orleans, LA, US
[2]Department of Physiology, Louisiana State University Health Sciences Center, New Orleans, LA, US

Abstract

Diabetes mellitus is one of the most prevalent diseases and is associated with increased incidence of structural and functional derangements in the kidneys, eventually leading to end-stage renal disease in a significant fraction of afflicted individuals. The renoprotective effects of RAS blockade have been established; however, the mechanistic pathways have not been fully elucidated. In this chapter, the role of an activated RAS in the pathogenesis of diabetic nephropathy is discussed with a focus on 8 themes: 1) Renal functional changes in diabetes, 2) Systemic and intrarenal RAS, 3) ACE and ACE2 in diabetes, 4) ACE-independent mechanisms of angiotensin II formation, 5) Mediators responsible for intrarenal RAS activation in diabetic kidneys, 6) RAS polymorphisms and susceptibility to diabetic nephropathy, 7) Clinical outcomes of RAS blockade in diabetic nephropathy, and 8) Potential of urinary AGT as an early biomarker of intrarenal RAS status in diabetic nephropathy. This analysis provides mechanistic explanations in support of the hypothesis that an activated intrarenal RAS contributes to the pathogenesis

---

[*] Correspondence to:Hiroyuki Kobori, MD, PhD, FJSIM, FAHA, FASN, FJSH, Associate Professor of Departments of Medicine and Physiology, Director of the Molecular Core in Hypertension and Renal Center of Excellence, Tulane University Health Sciences Center, 1430 Tulane Avenue, #SL39/M720, New Orleans, LA 70112-2699, USA Tel: +1-504-988-2591,Fax: +1-504-988-0911, E-mail: hkobori@tulane.edu.

of diabetic nephropathy, and that urinary AGT levels provide an index of intrarenal RAS activity.

Abbreviations

ACE:	angiotensin converting enzyme
AGT:	angiotensinogen
ARB:	angiotensin II type 1 receptor blocker
AT1:	angiotensin II type 1
AT2:	angiotensin II type 2
BMK:	big MAP kinase
ERK:	extracellular signal-regulated kinase
GFR:	glomerular filtration rate
I/D:	insertion/deletion
JNK:	c-Jun N-terminal kinase
MAP:	mitogen-activated protein
NFkB:	nuclear factor kappa beta
NOS:	nitric oxide synthase
RAS:	renin-angiotensin system
ROS:	reactive oxygen species
TGF:	transforming growth factor

Introduction

Diabetes affects 29 million Americans, 230 million people worldwide, is the 6th leading cause of death in the US, and is associated with increased incidence of functional and structural alterations in the kidneys eventually leading to end-stage renal failure. Diabetic nephropathy is the most common cause of end-stage renal failure in the US, accounting for 45% of patients starting dialysis [1,2]. Type 2 diabetes mellitus is the most common endocrine disease accounting for 90-95% of all diagnosed cases of diabetes and affecting 8% of the US population [3,4]. Obesity has been identified as the principal risk factor associated with the rising prevalence of type 2 diabetes [5] The incidence of obesity and diabetes has reached epidemic proportions, justifying the enormous effort to identify novel pathways and molecules involved in prevention and treatment. This chronic and debilitating disease is characterized by progressive albuminuria, declining GFR, renal functional and structural deterioration and increased risk for cardiovascular disease.

Glomerular histology reveals thickening of the glomerular basement membrane and mesangial cell expansion. At the latter stages of the disease, glomerulosclerosis, arteriolar hyalinosis, and tubulointerstitial fibrosis develop [6]. About 20-40% of patients with diabetes develop microalbuminuria, and a significant portion of those go on to develop overt diabetic nephropathy. The prevalence of diabetes in the United States of America is predicted to reach 9% of the population by 2025 [7].

Elevated plasma glucose concentration is the principal factor associated with renal damage in both type 1 [8] and type 2 [9] diabetes. Although the underlying genetic predisposition to this microvascular complication remains elusive, many studies have shown that various renal cell types cultured in high glucose medium or stimulated by high glucose exhibit increased oxidative stress and the typical features of cellular hypertrophy, cell proliferation, and excessive production of extracellular matrix that are characteristic of diabetic nephropathy [10,11]. Altered glomerular mesangial cell function in high glucose exposure plays a central role in the pathogenesis of progressive diabetic glomerulopathy.

The detailed mechanisms responsible for the development and progression of diabetic nephropathy have yet to be fully elucidated. However, the renoprotective effect of drugs that block or interfere with the RAS indicate that inappropriate activation of RAS contributes to diabetic nephropathy [12,13]. ACE inhibitors reduce proteinuria in patients with diabetes [12]. In a large-scale clinical study, captopril, an ACE inhibitor, provided protection against deterioration in renal function in diabetic nephropathy patients with type 1 diabetes [13]. Similarly, losartan, an ARB, conferred significant renal benefits in diabetic nephropathy patients with type 2 diabetes [14]. Thus, the renoprotective effects of ACE inhibitors and ARBs have been established in various studies. Combination therapy with ACE inhibitors and ARBs provides greater renoprotection than with ACE inhibitors alone in diabetic renal disease [15,16] suggesting that ACE-independent pathways for angiotensin II formation may be of significance. Figure 1 depicts the various pathways for angiotensin II formation. Upregulation of chymase-dependent angiotensin II generation in diabetes has been reported in mesangial and vascular smooth muscle cells of humans with diabetic nephropathy [17]. Although these studies suggest that angiotensin II-dependent mechanisms contribute to the development of diabetic nephropathy, the precise derangements in angiotensin II regulation of renal function in diabetes mellitus remain poorly defined. Studies attempting to characterize the contribution of the RAS in diabetes mellitus have yielded conflicting data, in part because the intrarenal RAS and the systemic RAS can be differentially regulated [18]. In contrast to the encouraging results from studies in type 2 diabetes, recent clinical trials in type 1 diabetes indicate that treatment with ACE inhibitors or ARBs did not slow the progression of nephropathy [19]. However, exclusion of patients with elevated blood pressure may have led to selection of patients less prone to progression of renal disease [20] and a lower risk for developing large increases in albuminuria or reductions in GFR.

1) Renal Functional Changes in Diabetes

The pathophysiology of diabetic nephropathy is complex [6], but the basic mechanisms that eventually lead to nephropathy are thought to be similar in types 1 and 2 diabetes although type 2 is often presented in a complex setting of the metabolic syndrome [21]. Early stages of type 1 and type 2 diabetes mellitus are characterized by glomerular hyperfiltration [6,22,23].

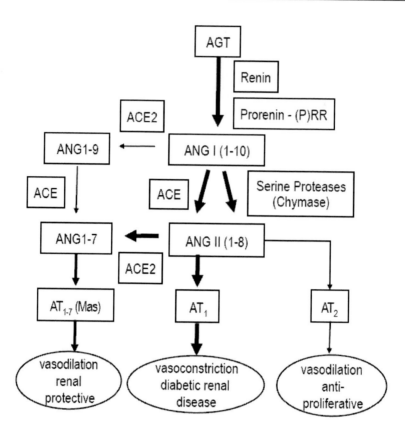

Figure 1. Enzymes in the RAS cascade.

The initiation and progression of diabetic nephropathy has been shown to be initially associated with increases in glomerular capillary pressure and flow. Increases in glomerular transcapillary hydraulic pressure lead to progressive albuminuria in diabetic rats [24]. In addition to these hemodynamic alterations, genetic susceptibility is also crucial for the development of diabetic nephropathy [25]. The earliest renal manifestations in diabetes are nephromegaly and glomerular hypertrophy, which are associated with afferent arteriolar vasodilation, renal hyperperfusion, and glomerular hyperfiltration [26,27]. GFR is increased by 20-40% above normal values.

Renal afferent arteriolar dilation is the major vascular alteration leading to diabetic hyperfiltration [28]; however, the mechanisms mediating the reduced preglomerular vascular tone have not been fully resolved. Several studies indicate a direct impairment of the renal vasculature related to increased activity of potassium channels [26,29]. Increased nitric oxide activity has also been suggested as partially responsible for the reduced renal vascular tone [26,30,31]. The demonstration that there is increased endothelial NOS expression associated with greater diameters in afferent arterioles of diabetic models prompted consideration of the role of nitric oxide in mediating the hyperfiltration phase [32,33]. Functional studies showed increased urinary excretion of nitric oxide metabolites in diabetic rats compared to control rats and that the hyperfiltration was prevented by treating with NOS inhibitors [34]. Increased tubular fluid nitric oxide activity has also been reported [35]. In studies where renal blood flow was measured continuously in diabetic rats, the onset of diabetes induced with streptozotocin was associated with increased renal blood flow and impaired autoregulation by 14-day after induction. These changes were prevented in rats where NOS was blocked with L-nitro-arginine methyl ester supporting a role for nitric oxide in mediating the early renal vasodilation in diabetes [36]. Likewise, the increases in GFR observed after induction of diabetes were prevented by L-nitro-arginine methyl ester treatment [33,37]. The increased nitric oxide activity is due predominantly to augmented endothelial NOS and not inducible NOS [33]. The hyperfiltration response was restored by treatment with the superoxide dismutase mimetic, tempol, suggesting an enhanced role for increased superoxide under conditions of NOS blockade [37]. These results are supported by studies showing that renal cortical superoxide production increased in diabetic rats which may offset the increased nitric oxide production [38]. Some of the increased nitric oxide production may be due to increased activity of neuronal NOS because diabetic rats are more sensitive than control rats to selective inhibition of neuronal NOS, and neuronal NOS inhibition reduces GFR in db/db mice [35,3,9]. These and other studies suggest that during the early phases of diabetes, there is increased intrarenal nitric oxide production mediated by increased endothelial NOS and neuronal NOS thus shifting the balance toward an augmented nitric oxide influence which contributes to the renal vasodilation and hyperfiltration [40]. As the duration of the diabetes increases, other factors including augmented superoxide levels and increased RAS activity suppress nitric oxide bioavailability leading to progressive nitric oxide deficiency caused by endothelial dysfunction thus reducing renal function back to and below normal levels. With further progression, there is accumulation of TGF beta and other cytokines along with advanced glycation products thus leading to deterioration of renal function and the development of diabetic nephropathy [10,31,40].

Nevertheless, there is still some uncertainty on the overall role of augmented nitric oxide activity in the early phase of diabetic because microcirculation studies have failed to demonstrate that there is a greater nitric oxide-mediated influence in normal afferent arterioles of diabetic rats as reflected by their responses to NOS inhibition [41]. Blocking superoxide activity resulted in restoration of the responses to NOS inhibition. Similarly, cortical and medullary blood flow were reduced to a lesser extent by NOS inhibition in diabetic rats than in control rats suggesting that there is a reduced rather than augmented nitric oxide-dependent influence in early experimental diabetes [42]. Furthermore, some reports indicate that renal production of nitric oxide is reduced in early diabetes [43]. Thus, there are conflicting data on the role of nitric oxide in mediating the early hyperfiltration phase, but the bulk of the evidence suggests that it contributes, at least in part, to the early vasodilatory phase. However, the counterbalancing influences of angiotensin II and nitric oxide on the renal microvasculature exert differential influences on afferent and efferent arterioles [44]. Once ROS are activated, they may in turn suppress the modulatory influence of nitric oxide on angiotensin II-induced afferent arteriolar constriction [44]. In the absence of endothelial NOS, the db/db diabetic mouse has an accelerated nephropathy [45].

The possible contribution of tubular glomerular feedback mechanisms in mediating hyperfiltration by alterations in proximal tubular reabsorption or increases in tubular nitric oxide levels has also been suggested [23,27,35]. Various other possible mediators including kinins, atrial natriuretic peptides, autonomic nervous system, and prostaglandins have been suggested [11]. The possible role of RAS activation has also been suggested [46]. However, it is not clear how increased intrarenal RAS activation could lead to a condition of afferent arteriolar vasodilation. Indeed, it appears that low angiotensin II levels may be contributing to the hyperfiltration state because angiotensin II infusion decreased GFR in hyperfiltering patients [46]. Nevertheless, there are complex contributions of the RAS that contribute to the altered renal hemodynamics in the various stages of diabetes [6,47-49]. In the next stage, GFR may remain elevated or may decrease to within the normal range [6,24]. The progressive expansion of the glomerular mesangium causes a reduction in the glomerular filtering surface area. In addition, GFR falls as a result of nephron loss due to tubulointerstitial fibrosis. As the disease progresses, GFR continues to decline due to worsening hypertension and a complex contributions of various cytokines and growth factors [10]. In the final stages of diabetic nephropathy, progressive renal failure leads to end-stage renal disease with GFR declining to 15 ml/min or lower. The average time for progression to ESRD is about 20 to 25 years [6,50].

2) Systemic and Intrarenal RAS

The role of the RAS on BP regulation and sodium and fluid homeostasis is well recognized [51,52]. Figure 1 demonstrates the cascade of events and enzymes responsible for the formation, degradation, and action of angiotensin peptides. The biologically active peptides that are formed from AGT include angiotensin II and angiotensin 1-7. The balance between the vasoconstrictor actions of angiotensin II mediated by the AT1 receptor are countered by the vasodilator actions of angiotensin II mediated by the AT2 receptor [53] and angiotensin 1-7 acting on G protein-coupled receptor, Mas [54]. Formation of angiotensin II is dependent upon the substrate availability of AGT and angiotensin I and the activities of renin, ACE, ACE2, and ACE-independent enzymatic pathways including serine proteases, chymase, tonin, cathepsin G, trypsin, and kallikrein. The actions of angiotensin II are determined by the signaling via AT1 and AT2 receptors and the putative angiotensin 1-7 receptor, Mas [55].

In recent years, the focus of interest on the RAS has shifted to a main emphasis on the role of the local/tissue RAS in specific tissues [56]. Emerging evidence has demonstrated the importance of the tissue RAS in the brain [57], heart [58], adrenal glands [59], vasculature [60,61] as well as the kidneys [18]. In particular, renal RAS is unique because all of the components necessary to generate intrarenal angiotensin II are present along the nephron in both interstitial and intratubular compartments (Figure 2) [52,55]. The presence of the AGT gene in the proximal tubules has been shown using in situ hybridization [62]. AGT mRNA is expressed primarily in the proximal convoluted tubules and proximal straight tubules with small amounts in glomeruli and vasa recta and the renal vasculature [63]. As shown by immunohistochemistry, renal AGT protein is abundant in the proximal convoluted tubules [64-66]. There is strong positive immunostaining for AGT protein in proximal convoluted tubules and proximal straight tubules (Figure 3), and weak positive staining in glomeruli and vasa recta; however, distal tubules and collecting ducts are negative [67]. The synthesized AGT in the kidney is secreted into the lumen leading to angiotensin I generation. Low but measurable renin concentrations have been detected in proximal tubule fluid in rats [68]. Renin mRNA and renin-like activity have been demonstrated in cultured proximal tubular cells [69-71]. There is abundant expression of ACE mRNA [72] and protein [73,74] on brush border membranes of proximal tubules of human kidney. ACE has also been measured in proximal and distal tubular fluid but is greater in proximal tubule fluid [75]. Therefore, all of major components to generate angiotensin II are expressed within the kidneys [18,52]..

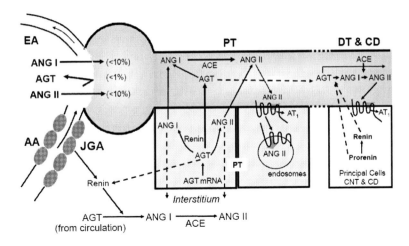

Intratubular/Interstitial RAS

Figure 2. Intrarenal RAS components and urinary angiotensinogen as a potential biomarker for intrarenal RAS status. PT: proximal tubules, DT: distal tubules, CD: collecting ducts.

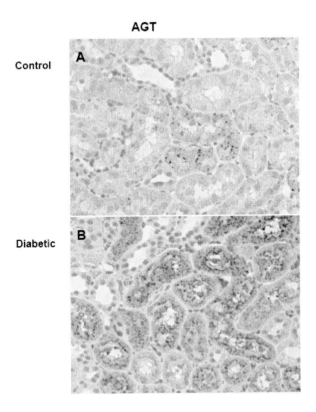

Figure 3. Immunohistochemical distribution of AGT in the rat renal cortex illustrating prominent proximal tubular localization. Distal tubules exhibited negative staining. Representative light photomicrographs illustrating the immunohistochemical distribution of AGT in kidneys from control (A) and type 2 diabetic rats (B). AGT immunoreactivity was more intense in kidneys from diabetic rats (B) compared with control rats (A).

In addition to renin in the granules of juxtaglomerular apparatus of the afferent arterioles, renin is also present in the principal cells of connecting tubules and collecting ducts [76-79]. Thus, AGT secreted from the proximal tubule cells into the tubular fluid may spill over into distal nephron segments where it can be acted on by renin to form angiotensin I, and then converted to angiotensin II by ACE present in the lumen of collecting ducts.

The recently discovered (pro)renin receptor is also abundantly expressed in the kidney vasculature and tubules [80,81]. The (pro)renin receptor binds prorenin with higher affinity than renin and markedly increases the catalytic efficiency of angiotensin I formation from AGT. In addition, activation of the (pro)renin receptor stimulates intracellular signaling with activation of ERK [80]. The mesangial localization of (pro)renin receptor has given rise to suggestions that it may contribute to angiotensin I generation and possible renal injury to the glomerulus. The presence of the (pro)renin receptor on the luminal side of distal nephron and collecting duct segments provides a possible role for the (pro)renin receptor to serve as an anchor for prorenin secreted by the principal cells thus increasing the efficacy of formation of angiotensin I from proximally delivered AGT [81].

There are two major types of angiotensin II receptors, AT1 receptors and AT2 receptors, but there is much less AT2 receptor expression in adult kidneys [82,83]. AT1 receptor mRNA has been localized to proximal convoluted and straight tubules, thick ascending limb of the loop of Henle, cortical and medullary collecting duct cells, glomeruli, arterial vasculature, vasa recta, and juxtaglomerular cells [63]. In rodents, both subtypes of AT1a receptor and AT1b receptor mRNAs have been demonstrated in the vasculature and glomerulus and in all nephron segments [83]. The AT1a receptor mRNA is the predominant subtype in nephron segments, whereas the AT1b receptor is more abundant than AT1a receptor in the glomerulus [84]. Studies using polyclonal and monoclonal antibodies to the AT1 receptor demonstrate that AT1 receptor protein has been localized on vascular smooth muscle cells throughout the vasculature, including the afferent and efferent arterioles and glomerular mesangial cells [85]. AT1 receptors are also present on proximal tubule brush border and basolateral membranes, thick ascending limb epithelia, distal tubules, collecting ducts, glomerular podocytes, and macula densa cells [82,83,85].

The status of the intrarenal RAS in diabetes has remained somewhat of an enigma [86-88]. It is often stated that the intrarenal RAS is activated in diabetes and that augmented intrarenal angiotensin II is responsible for many or most of the renal functional derangements that occur during the development and progression of diabetes. Furthermore, there are many studies demonstrating the beneficial effects of treating diabetic subjects with ACE inhibitors or ARBs and, in particular, their ability to slow down or arrest the renal injury and the progression toward diabetic nephropathy. Ironically, however, obtaining direct evidence confirming the augmented intrarenal activity of RAS activity and demonstrating its role in mediating diabetes related renal injury has remained elusive. Experimental data related to the RAS status in experimental diabetic models have yielded highly variable results. Thus, although various studies support an association between RAS and diabetic nephropathy, direct measurements have failed to establish that intrarenal angiotensin II is consistently elevated in diabetes [88]. Kidney angiotensinogen levels have been reported to be unchanged or decreased; renin content has been variable and ACE expression has been shown to be increased or unchanged in glomeruli and vessels [87,89]. Zimplemann, et al. [88] demonstrated that renin and ACE mRNA levels were increased in streptozotocin-induced diabetic rats and these increases were prevented by insulin treatment [88]. However, AT1 receptor protein levels were significantly elevated cortex from streptozotocin-induced diabetic rats compared with control rats associated with downregulation of AT2 receptors [87,89]. Cortical collecting ducts of streptozotocin-induced diabetic kidneys displayed a striking increase in AT1 receptor immunostaining intensity relative to control kidneys (Figure 4) [87]. Of interest, it was recently shown that prorenin expression is elevated in the cortical collecting ducts of type 1 diabetic rats [76]. Thus, although the data are somewhat variable, emerging studies suggest that the intrarenal RAS, and in particular, the distal nephron RAS, is upregulated in diabetes. Furthermore, studies in models of type 2 diabetes do show increased intrarenal angiotensin II levels and AGT mRNA which are prevented by treatment with an ARB [90,91]. Zucker diabetic fatty obese rats were shown to have increases in renal cortical AGT (Figure 3) and angiotensin II levels associated with increased oxidative stress and renal injury compared to control lean rats [92,93].

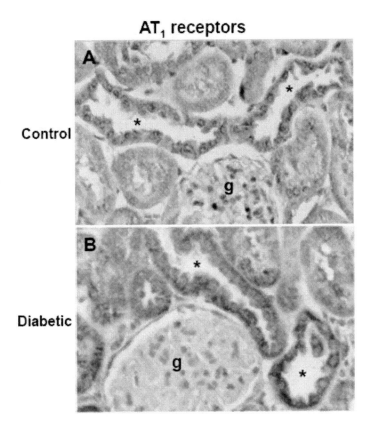

Figure 4. Representative light photomicrographs illustrating the immunohistochemical distribution of AT1 receptors in kidneys from control (A) and type 1 diabetic rats (B) utilizing a monoclonal antibody. In the cortex, immunostaining for AT1 receptor protein was evident in proximal tubules and cortical collecting ducts (asterisks), with fainter staining of glomeruli (g). AT1 receptor immunoreactivity was more intense in cortical collecting ducts in kidneys from diabetic rats (B) compared with control rats (A).

The involvement of (pro)renin receptor in diabetic nephropathy has been suggested by several studies [94,95]. In db/db mice, glomerulosclerosis was reduced by administration of a decoy peptide that inhibits prorenin binding to the (pro)renin receptor [96]. There were also associated decreases in intrarenal angiotensin I and angiotensin II levels [97]. However, an angiotensin-independent direct role of (pro)renin receptor activation was suggested by studies in diabetic AT1a receptor deficient mice. In these mice, (pro)renin receptor blockade but not ACE inhibition reduced the MAP kinase activation and nephropathy [98]. Because prorenin levels are increased in subjects with diabetes [99] and animal models of diabetes [76], the possible role of activated (pro)renin receptor in mediating diabetic nephropathy is of substantial potential importance.

There are many deleterious effects of the activated RAS contributing to the pathophysiology of diabetic nephropathy. Increased intrarenal angiotensin II may contribute to systemic and glomerular hypertension, glomerular and tubulointerstitial fibrosis, and inflammatory processes. Angiotensin II contributes to podocyte foot process broadening, which is followed by foot process effacement and local detachments. These changes subsequently progress to focal segmental glomerulosclerosis and ultrafiltration of proteins. Activation of the RAS may play an important role in macrophage recruitment, and cytokine activation which may contribute to glomerular and tubular inflammation associated with proteinuria [6,92,100,101]. In diabetic rats with hyperglycemia for up to 10 months, the increases in glomerular fractional mesangial area, 15 glomerulosclerosis index and macrophage infiltration were partially reversed by treatment with losartan indicating that regression of well-established structural derangements is possible [102].

3) ACE and ACE2 in Diabetes

Pharmacologic drugs that inhibit the actions of ACE and the AT1 receptor delay the onset and slow the progression of diabetic nephropathy in humans, indicating the importance of the RAS in diabetic renal disease. However, ACE inhibitors and AT1 receptor blockers do not arrest disease progression to end-stage renal failure. Additionally, the demonstration that combined ACE inhibitor plus AT1 receptor blocker lowers BP [103,104] and provides greater renal protection [15,16] than ACE inhibitor alone suggests that ACE inhibitor-dependent suppression of the RAS is incomplete. It has been suggested that dual blockade of RAS with inhibition of ACE and AT1 receptor blockade results in additional reduction in proteinuria in patients with chronic kidney disease [105]. This may be due to the activation of non-ACE dependent pathways of angiotensin II formation and degradation in diabetes.

ACE is a zinc metalloprotease that catalyzes cleavage of the C-terminal dipeptide from angiotensin I to produce the potent vasopressor octapeptide angiotensin II [106]. A new component of the RAS, ACE2, was discovered in 2000 [107,108]. ACE2 is located on the X chromosome and shares 42% homology to ACE. ACE2 enzyme contains 1 catalytic site and is insensitive to ACE inhibitors. ACE2 converts angiotensin I to angiotensin 1-9 and angiotensin II to angiotensin 1-7. Angiotensin 1-7 is a peptide with vasodilator and anti-proliferative properties [109]. ACE2 catalytic efficiency is 400X higher for angiotensin II as a substrate than for angiotensin I [110]. ACE protein is found predominantly in the endothelium of coronary and intrarenal vessels and renal proximal tubule cells. The organ- and cell-specific expression of ACE2 suggests an essential role in the regulation of RAS in the heart and kidney [108]. ACE2 mutant mice develop glomerulosclerosis by 12 months of age [111]; furthermore, deletion of the ACE2 gene accelerates diabetic kidney injury in the Akita mouse [112] suggesting that ACE2 plays a protective role in the diabetic kidney.

Wysocki et al. [113] demonstrated that renal cortical ACE protein expression is reduced, while ACE2 protein expression is elevated in streptozotocin-induced diabetic mice compared to control mice. Additionally, proximal tubule expression of ACE is reduced and ACE2 elevated in streptozotocin-induced type 1 diabetic compared to control mice [114]. Renal cortical ACE protein expression is reduced, while ACE2 protein expression is elevated in young female diabetic db/db compared to control db/m mice [115]. Furthermore, renal cortical ACE activity is significantly decreased while ACE2 activity is significantly increased in adult male type 2 diabetic compared to control mice [116]. ACE/ACE2 ratio in kidney is significantly lower in diabetic compared to control mice [116]. As shown in Figure 5, ACE protein immunohistochemical localization is decreased in the diabetic compared to control kidneys, while ACE2 protein is increased [116]. Elevated ACE2 protein expression is thought to provide a renoprotective effect on diabetic renal injury due to the ability of ACE2 to degrade angiotensin II and generate angiotensin 1-7. Angiotensin 1-7 is a peptide with vasodilator and anti-proliferative properties [109,117]. Therefore, an attenuation of ACE-dependent angiotensin II formation and increased conversion of angiotensin II to angiotensin 1-7 by ACE2 may be part of a renal protective response against the development of diabetic nephropathy at the early stages of diabetes. The pattern of change of intrarenal ACE and ACE2 is similar in mouse models of type I and II diabetes and suggests that hyperglycemia may be the common regulator [115,117].

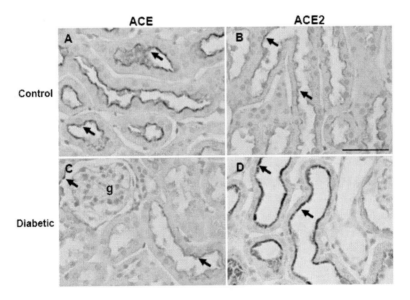

Figure 5. ACE (A, C) and ACE2 (B, D) immunohistochemical localization of renal cortex of control (A-B) and type 2 diabetic (C-D) mice. ACE and ACE2 proteins are localized to the proximal tubule brush border of control and diabetic kidneys. ACE is also expressed in endothelial cells of the renal vasculature and glomerular capillaries. The density of renal cortical ACE protein immunostaining is significantly reduced in diabetic compared to control kidneys. However, ACE2 immunostaining density is significantly greater in diabetic compared to control kidneys. Antibody dilutions for ACE and ACE2 antibodies were 1:1,000 and 1:10,000, respectively. Images were obtained from the mid-cortical region of the kidney using an X100 oil immersion lens. g - glomerulus, arrow – proximal tubule brush border, Bar = 50 microns.

As described earlier, ACE processes the decapeptide angiotensin I to the octapeptide angiotensin II [118-120]. While the carboxypeptidase, ACE2, cleaves only a single amino acid from the C terminals of angiotensin I to form the nonapeptide angiotensin 1-9, ACE2 does not convert angiotensin 1-9 to angiotensin II [107,121-124]. Therefore, it is possible that ACE2 regulates ACE-dependent angiotensin II formation by stimulating an alternative pathway for angiotensin I degradation. ACE2 also directly converts angiotensin II to angiotensin 1-7 [121-124] which has been shown to activate the orphan heterotrimeric G protein-coupled receptor, Mas receptor [54]. Genetic deletion of the G protein-coupled receptor encoded by the Mas protooncogene abolished the binding of angiotensin 1-7 to mouse renal cells [54]. Angiotensin 1-7 is thought to serve as an endogenous antagonist of the angiotensin II induced actions mediated via angiotensin receptors [109,121-125]. Thus, actions of ACE2 could have substantial impact on the balance of angiotensin peptides found in the kidney by diverting the RAS cascade from angiotensin II to angiotensin 1-7. This helps explain the elevated angiotensin II levels in the ACE2 knockout mice [126]. ACE2 is abundantly expressed in renal epithelial cells including proximal tubular cells [107,122,124]. Kidney ACE2 expression is significantly decreased in hypertensive [127] and diabetic rats [128]. Although the pathophysiological significance of ACE2 in renal injury remains to be established, emerging evidence suggests that ACE2 deficiency supports increased intrarenal angiotensin II levels [100].

4) ACE-Independent Mechanisms of Angiotensin II Formation

Tonin, cathepsins and kallikreins are capable of acting on AGT to form angiotensin I or angiotensin II directly (Figure 1) [129]. A growing body of evidence indicates that chymase-dependent pathways play a critical role in forming angiotensin II from angiotensin I in cardiovascular tissues [130-132]. Chymase, a chymotrypsin-like serine protease, is present predominantly in the secretory granules of mast cells [130,131]. Mast cell-derived chymase can convert angiotensin I to angiotensin II in dogs, monkeys, hamsters and humans, but not in rats and mice [130,131]. Chymase has no enzymatic activity in granules, because the optimal pH of chymase is between 7 and 9 whereas the pH in the granule is approximately 5.5 [133]. However, once the mast cells are activated in injured or inflammatory tissues, chymase is released into the extracellular matrix (pH 7.4) and immediately activated [134,135]. Of note, strong chymase inhibitors, such as serine protease inhibitors, are mostly contained in the blood [130-132]. Thus, the chymase activity is inactivated in blood immediately after being released, indicating that chymase has enzymatic activity only in local tissues. In addition to mast cell-derived chymase, a novel rat vascular chymase is constitutively expressed in vascular smooth muscle cells and converts angiotensin I to angiotensin II [136]. Rat vascular chymase expression is increased in vascular smooth muscle cells of spontaneously hypertensive rats [136]. Furthermore, the conditional and targeted overexpression of rat vascular chymase in vascular smooth muscle cells induces hypertension in mice [137]. Chymase-dependent angiotensin II formation was more dominant than ACE-dependent angiotensin II formation in aorta extracts of normotensive rats [138]. There is also angiotensin II-forming chymase in the pulmonary arteries of monocrotaline-induced pulmonary hypertensive rats [139]. These data suggest that vascular chymase plays an important role in vascular angiotensin II formation. In the human heart, chymase is synthesized and stored in endothelial cells and mesenchymal cells and is secreted directly into the interstitium, contributing up to 80% of angiotensin II [140].

ACE-knockout mice have unchanged kidney angiotensin II contents but 14-fold increases in chymase activity, suggesting the possible involvement of chymase and residual ACE activity in angiotensin II generation in the kidney [141]. Intraarterial infusion of [Pro^{11}, D-Ala^{12}]-angiotensin I, which is inactive but yields angiotensin II on digestion by chymase, but not by ACE, induces renal vasoconstriction in dogs [142]. This study also revealed that the angiotensin II-forming activity in dog renal cortex is 20% chymase-dependent in vitro [142]. Further studies showed that intraarterial infusion of a non-specific chymase inhibitor, chemostatin, significantly decreased intrarenal angiotensin II contents in the ischemic kidney [143]. In the ischemic kidneys of two-kidney-one-clip rats and in kidneys of subtotal nephrectomized rats, increases in chymase activity and expression are also observed [144]. Increased chymase expression has been found in rejected kidneys [145] and kidneys of patients with renovascular hypertension [146] and diabetes [17,147]. Collectively, these data support the potential contribution of chymase-dependent intrarenal angiotensin II formation to the progression of renal injury [148].

5) Mediators Responsible for Intrarenal RAS Activation in Diabetic Kidneys

As summarized in Figure 6, high glucose induces de novo synthesis of diacylglycerol in vivo and in vitro [149]. Diacylglycerol activates the protein kinase C pathway [150]. Activation of protein kinase C is one of the major mechanisms involved in high glucose-induced glomerular injury [151] and produces oxidative stress with increased ROS leading to subsequent lipid peroxidation [152-155]. High glucose generates ROS as a result of glucose auto-oxidation, metabolism, and formation of advanced glycation end products [155,156]. All these signaling molecules are involved in MAP kinase signaling pathways in glomerular cells [157]. High glucose-induced diabetic complications have been implicated, in part, to the activation of MAP kinases [157].

Four subfamilies of MAP kinases that are activated by high glucose have been identified as follows: ERK1/2, JNK, p38 kinase, and BMK1 [158]. Each subfamily may be regulated via different signal transduction pathways and modulate specific cell functions [159]. The activated ROS pathways and MAP kinase pathways together stimulate cytokines/chemokines and growth factors, thus inducing macrophage infiltration, inflammation, extracellular matrix expansion which eventually leads to the development and progression on diabetic nephropathy [160-169].

As summarized in Figure 6, angiotensin II stimulates extracellular matrix protein synthesis through induction of TGF beta 1 expression in rat glomerular cells and this induction is via an AT1 receptor-dependent mechanism [170]. Furthermore, TGF beta 1 is known to be an important mediator of hypertrophy and fibrosis in kidney diseases via multiple pathways including G1 phase arrest, cell size enlargement, protein synthesis induction, inhibition of proteinase activity, and extracellular matrix enhancement [101,171].

High glucose-induced ROS/MAP kinase pathways and the intrarenal RAS-dependent TGF beta 1 pathway play key roles in diabetic nephropathy. Previous studies also imply an augmentation of AGT expression by ROS via several pathways (Figure 6).

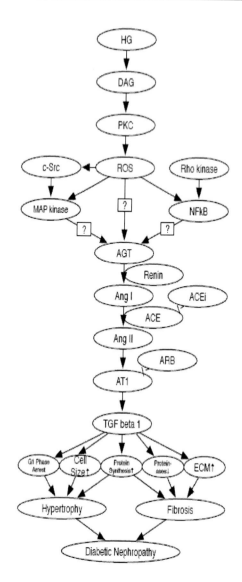

Figure 6. Mediators in the RAS activation in diabetic kidney. HG: high glucose, DAG: diacylglycerol, PKC: protein kinase C, c-Src: a non-receptor tyrosine kinase, ROS: reactive oxygen species, Rho: a small GTPase, MAP: mitogen-activated protein, NFkB: nuclear factor kappa beta, AGT: angiotensinogen, Ang: angiotensin, AT1: Ang II type 1 receptor, TGF: transforming growth factor, ECM: extracellular matrix, ACE: Ang converting enzyme, ACEi: ACE inhibitor, ARB: AT1 receptor blocker.

Hydrogen peroxide induces ERK1/2 and activates JNK via c-Src-dependent mechanisms in vascular smooth muscle cells [172,173]. Hydrogen peroxide also activates c-Src-mediated BMK1 in PC12 cells [174], in glomeruli of diabetic rats and in glomerular mesangial cells under high glucose conditions [175]. In addition, hydrogen peroxide and oxygen radicals activate NFkB in a human T cell line [176] and Rho activates NFkB in 3T3 cells [177]. Interestingly, all of these 3 mediators (MAP kinase, ROS, and NFkB) can activate AGT expression. AGT gene expression is stimulated via p38 kinase pathway in immortalized proximal tubular cells of rat kidney [178], and AGT gene expression is activated via ROS in a proximal tubular cell line [156]. AGT gene expression is activated by NFkB p65 transcription factor in hepatocytes [179]. Moreover, recent findings suggest a possible linkage between MAP kinase activation and NFkB pathways [180,181] thus indicating that the augmentation of AGT expression by ROS may involve several pathways. The demonstration that high glucose augments AGT gene expression in a cell line of rat immortalized renal proximal tubular cells provide s a critical link between diabetes and AGT synthesis [156,178,182-186]. Rat AGT gene has a putative insulin-responsive element in its promoter region [187,188] suggesting that glucose regulates AGT gene expression. However, in vivo evidence demonstrating the linkage between ROS and AGT in the kidneys of type 2 diabetic rats is not yet available although ROS-dependent activation of intrarenal AGT plays an important role in hypertensive rats [189,190]. Blockade of the RAS in prediabetic rats attenuates the development of renal injury in type 2 diabetic rats later in life [90]. Thus, the elevated ROS may synergize with the augmentation of intrarenal AGT and initiate the development of diabetic nephropathy in type 2 diabetic rats [92,93] supporting a critical linkage between ROS/MAP kinase pathways and RAS/TGF beta 1 pathways.

6) RAS Polymorphisms and Susceptibility to Diabetic Nephropathy

A linkage between an I/D polymorphism on the 16th intron of ACE gene and serum ACE activity [191] as well as renal ACE gene expression has been suggested [192]. Healthy subjects with D-allele show higher serum ACE activity and renal ACE gene expression. In patients with diabetic nephropathy, there was an association with D-allele in type 1 diabetes [193,194] and type 2 diabetes [195]. A comprehensive meta-analysis including a total of 14,727 subjects from 47 studies was conducted [196] with 8,663 cases having type 1 or 2 diabetic subjects with incipient (microalbuminuria) or advanced diabetic nephropathy (proteinuria, chronic renal failure, end-stage renal disease). Control subjects (6,064) were predominantly normoalbuminuric. Using a minimal-case definition based on incipient diabetic nephropathy, subjects with the II genotype had a 22% lower risk of diabetic nephropathy than carriers of the D-allele (pooled odds ratio = 0.78, 95% confidence interval = 0.69 - 0.88). While there was a reduced risk of diabetic nephropathy associated with the II genotype among Caucasians with either type 1 or type 2 diabetes, the association was most marked among type 2 diabetic Asians (Chinese, Japanese, Koreans) (odds ratio = 0.65, 95% confidence interval = 0. 51 - 0.83). This odds ratio is significantly different from the odds ratio of 0.90 (95% confidence interval = 0.78 - 1.04) that was obtained for type 2 diabetic Caucasians (P = 0.019). Using a stricter case definition based on advanced diabetic nephropathy, a comparable risk reduction of 24 - 32% was observed among the three subgroups, although statistical significance was reached only among Asians. The results of this meta-analysis support a genetic association of the I/D polymorphism of ACE gene with diabetic nephropathy [196]. Based on these data, the association between diabetic nephropathy and polymorphisms within the ACE gene was examined in a large cohort of Japanese type 2 diabetic patients [197]. Single nucleotide polymorphisms within the ACE gene were genotyped using invader assay in 747 nephropathy cases and 557 control subjects. Eight single nucleotide polymorphisms within the ACE gene were significantly associated with diabetic nephropathy (P < 0.05), including five single nucleotide polymorphisms in almost complete linkage disequilibrium to the I/D polymorphism on the 16th intron (P = 0.01, odds ratio = 1.34, 95% confidence interval = 1.07 - 1.69) [197]. Subjects with the DD genotype showed less beneficial effects from treatment with RAS blockers [198,199]. A combination of 3 polymorphisms within the RAS components, ACE (I/D), AGT (M235T), and AT1 receptor (A(1166)->C) was very effective in predicting susceptibility to diabetic nephropathy [197,200]. These findings have implications for the management of diabetic nephropathy and support the rationale for treatment with RAS blockers.

7) Clinical Outcomes for RAS Blockade in Diabetic Nephropathy

As mentioned, there is growing evidence that RAS inhibition exerts a major impact on the progression of renal dysfunction in both diabetic and non-diabetic renal disease. Both ARBs and ACE inhibitors retard the development and progression of renal dysfunction [201-204]. In the BENEDICT (BErgamo NEphrologic DIabetes Complications Trial) [205], diabetic patients with no history of microalbuminuria were randomized to trandolapril vs placebo over median of 3.6 years follow up. Trandolapril resulted in a significant decrease in the development of microalbuminuria and limited the progression of renal dysfunction. This reduction was still significant even after adjusting for blood pressure reduction by trandolapril. In the AASK (African American Study of Kidney disease and hypertension) trial [206], the reduction of microalbuminuria by ACE inhibitors was also shown in the non-diabetic renal population in which patients were randomized to ramipril vs amlodipine. The benefit of ARB therapy in patients with diabetic nephropathy has been studied in 2 large trials. In the RENAAL [14] and the IDNT [207], evaluating patients with type 2 diabetes with nephropathy, the addition of ARB to standard therapy resulted in improvements in all cause mortality, progression to end stage renal disease, and doubling of serum creatinine. In the first direct comparison of ARB with an ACE inhibitor, the DETAIL trail [208] evaluated type 2 diabetic patients randomized to either enalapril or telmisartan. Telmisartan was not inferior to enalapril in the primary end point of change in baseline estimated GFR. More recently, the ONTARGET group [209] published the results of the analysis of renal outcomes. The primary renal outcome was a composite of dialysis, doubling of serum creatinine, and death. Both ARBs and ACE inhibitors were equally effective in improving outcome and the number of events for the composite primary outcome was similar for telmisartan (N = 1,147 [13.4%]) and ramipril (N = 1,150 [13.5%]; hazard ratio = 1.00, 95% confidence interval = 0.92 - 1.09). In the dual therapy group, even though there was a significant reduction in proteinuria, there was an increase in side effects and worsening renal outcomes (N = 1,233 [14.5%]; hazard ratio = 1.09, 95% confidence interval = 1.01 - 1.18, P = 0.037). The ONTARGET trial was not specifically carried out in renal patients, but with 3,500 renal events, it represents one of the largest studies on renal outcomes and dual RAS therapy. The authors noted that the only subset of patients with possible benefit of dual therapy were the patients with diabetic nephropathy. Needs for dialysis were with acute dialysis in patients with no history of renal dysfunction suggesting the potential blood pressure-lowering effects of the combination could account for the increased morbidity with dual therapy. What is missing, however, is an actual marker to test for the efficacy of treatment. If indeed, the major factor initiating the diabetic nephropathy is an inappropriate increase in intrarenal RAS, then it would seem particularly worthwhile to have a direct means of evaluating the status of the intrarenal RAS in patients and the efficacy of treatment in reducing or arresting RAS activation in the kidneys.

8) Urinary AGT as a New Biomarker of Intrarenal RAS Status in Diabetes

Microalbuminuria is the most commonly used early marker of diabetic nephropathy [210], and diabetic nephropathy is thought to be a unidirectional process from microalbuminuria to end-stage renal failure [8]. However, recent studies in type 1 diabetic patients demonstrate that a large proportion of diabetic nephropathy patients reverts to normoalbuminuria and that one-third of them exhibit reduced renal function even in the microalbuminuria stage [211]. It is claimed that urinary inflammatory markers are high in microalbuminuric type 1 diabetes having diminished renal function, but not in microalbuminuric type 1 patients with stable renal function. However, no single marker has been sufficient to represent the whole panel [169]. Therefore, a more sensitive and more specific marker for diabetic nephropathy would be highly advantageous.

AGT is the only known substrate for renin, which is the rate-limiting enzyme of the RAS. Because the level of AGT is close to the Michaelis-Menten constant for renin, not only renin levels but also AGT levels can control the activity of the RAS, and upregulation of AGT levels may lead to elevated angiotensin peptide levels [212,213]. Recent studies on experimental animal models and transgenic mice have documented the involvement of AGT in the activation of the RAS [214-222]. Genetic manipulations that lead to overexpression of the AGT gene have consistently been shown to cause hypertension [223,224]. In human genetic studies, a linkage has been established between the AGT gene and hypertension [225-228]. Enhanced intrarenal AGT mRNA and/or protein levels have also been observed in multiple experimental models of hypertension and diabetes including angiotensin II-dependent hypertensive rats [67,229-233], Dahl salt-sensitive hypertensive rats [189,190], and spontaneously hypertensive rats [234] as well as in kidney diseases including diabetic nephropathy [47,90,92,93,235,236], IgA nephropathy [237,238], and radiation nephropathy [239]. In addition, models of type 2 diabetes and metabolic syndrome also exhibit increases in intrarenal AGT and urinary AGT excretion [90-93]. Thus, AGT plays an important role in the development and progression of hypertension and kidney diseases and may be particularly useful as a predictor of developing kidney disease[18,52].

In rodents, urinary excretion rates of AGT provide a specific index of intrarenal RAS status and are correlated with kidney angiotensin II levels in angiotensin II-dependent hypertensive rats (Figure 2) [67,230-233]. Because of its potential importance, a direct quantitative method to measure urinary AGT using human AGT ELISA was recently developed [240]. Using this system, urinary excretion rates of AGT have been used as an index of intrarenal RAS status in patients with chronic kidney disease [241,242] and in patients with hypertension [243]. Recently, 2 clinical studies were performed to determine if urinary AGT levels can be used as a novel biomarker of the intrarenal RAS status in diabetes mellitus patients [244,245].

To demonstrate that the administration of an ARB interferes with the vicious cycle of high glucose-ROS-AGT-angiotensin II-AT1 receptor-ROS by suppressing ROS and inflammation, 13 hypertensive diabetic nephropathy patients who received ARBs were recruited and evaluated before and at 16 weeks after treatment [244]. Urinary AGT, albumin, 8-hydroxydeoxyguanosine, 8-epi-prostaglandin F2 alpha, monocyte chemoattractant protein-1, interleukin-6, and interleukin-10 were assessed. ARB treatment reduced the blood pressure and urinary levels of AGT, albumin, 8-hydroxydeoxyguanosine, 8-epi-prostaglandin F2 alpha, monocyte chemoattractant protein-1, and interleukin-6; while increasing urinary interleukin-10 levels. The reduction of urinary AGT correlated with the reduction of blood pressure and urinary levels of albumin, 8-hydroxydeoxyguanosine, 8-epi-prostaglandin F2 alpha, monocyte chemoattractant protein-1, and interleukin-6 and the increased urinary interleukin-10 levels. These results suggest that the mechanisms by which ARBs exert their renoprotective effect may involve the suppression of intrarenal AGT levels in association with reduced anti-inflammatory and antioxidant effects in patients with type 2 diabetes (Figure 7) [244].

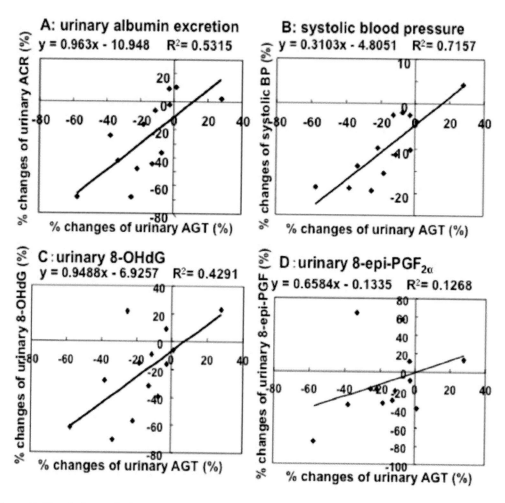

Figure 7. Correlations of urinary angiotensinogen with the reduction rates of blood pressure (B) and urinary levels of albumin (A), 8-hydroxy-deoxyguanosine (C), and 8-epi-prostaglandin F2 alpha (D) by treatment with angiotensin II type 1 receptor blocker (ARB) in type 2 diabetic patients.

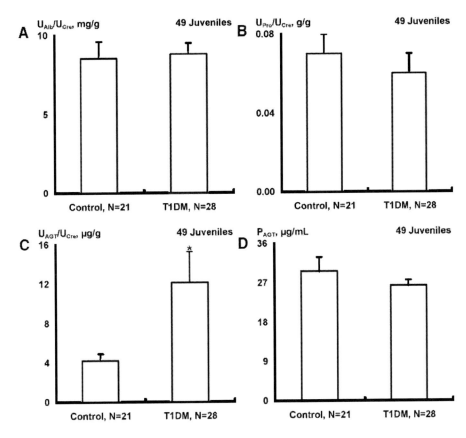

Figure 8. Urinary albumin-creatinine ratio (A) or urinary protein-creatinine ratio (B) were not increased in these type 1 diabetic patients compared to control subjects, suggesting that these patients were in their pre-microalbuminuric phase of diabetic nephropathy. However, UAGT/UCre was significantly increased in these patients compared to control subjects (C). Importantly, the AGT increase was not observed in plasma (D).

To determine if urinary AGT levels can be dissociated from urinary albumin or protein excretion rates in type 1 diabetic juveniles, early phase studies were performed in control and diabetic juveniles [245]. Of the 55 juveniles recruited, 34 were type 1 diabetic patients and 21 were gender- and age-matched control subjects. Since the primary focus of the study was comparison between characteristics of normoalbuminuric patients with type 1 diabetes and those of control subjects, 6 microalbuminuric patients with type 1 diabetes (urinary albumin-creatinine ratio> 30 mg/g) were excluded. Consequently, 49 urine and plasma samples were analyzed. None of them received treatment with RAS blockade. Neither urinary albumin-creatinine ratios or urinary protein-creatinine ratios were significantly increased in these type 1 diabetic patients compared to control subjects (urinary albumin-creatinine ratio: 8.8 +/- 0.7 mg/g vs 8.5 +/- 1.1 mg/g, P = 0.8450; urinary protein-creatinine ratio: 0.060 +/- 0.010 g/g vs 0.070 +/- 0.010 g/g, P = 0.3231), suggesting that these patients were in their pre-microalbuminuric phase of diabetic nephropathy. However, urinary AGT-creatinine ratios were significantly increased in these patients compared to control subjects (12.1 +/- 3.2 µg/g vs 4.2 +/-0.7 µg/g, P =0.0454). Importantly, the AGT increase was not observed in plasma (26.3 +/- 1.3 µg/ml vs 29.5 +/- 3.3 µg/ml, P = 0.3 148) (Figure 8). These data indicate that urinary AGT levels are increased in type 1 diabetic subjects and that increased urinary AGT levels precede the increased urinary albumin levels, suggesting a possibility that urinary AGT levels serve as a very sensitive early marker of intrarenal RAS activation and may be one of the earliest predictors of diabetic nephropathy in diabetic patients [245].

Conclusion

The complicated and pleiotropic roles of an activated RAS in pathogenesis of diabetic nephropathy continue to receive recognition from emerging and ongoing studies. Clearly, the use of ARBs and ACE inhibitors has become common practice in treating patients with diabetes. Since RAS activation plays such a central role in the development and progression of diabetic nephropathy, there has been extensive interest in the potential hope for reduction in morbidity and mortality by using agents that block one of more steps in the RAS. Accordingly, the assessment of urinary AGT as an early biomarker of the status of the intrarenal RAS may be of substantial importance. It may be particularly helpful in serving as a means to determine efficacy of the treatment to reduce intrarenal angiotensin II levels.

Acknowledgments

The authors acknowledge the assistance provided by Ms. Debbie M. Olavarrieta in preparing the manuscript.

Sources of Funding

The authors' laboratories are supported by grants from the National Institute of Diabetes and Digestive and Kidney Diseases (R01DK072408, R01DK062003), the National Center for Research Resources (P20RR017659, P20RR018766), the National Heart, Lung, and Blood Institute (R01HL026371), and by American Heart Association Grant-in-Aid (GRNT2250875, GRNT3020018).

Conflicts of Interest/Disclosures

None

References

[1] Joss N, Paterson KR, Deighan CJ, Simpson K, Boulton-Jones JM: Diabetic nephropathy: How effective is treatment in clinical practice? *QJM* 95: 41-49, 2002

[2] Mokdad AH, Ford ES, Bowman BA, Dietz WH, Vinicor F, Bales VS, Marks JS: Prevalence of obesity, diabetes, and obesity-related health risk factors, 2001. *JAMA* 289: 76-79, 2003

[3] Bays HE, Bazata DD, Clark NG, Gavin JR, 3rd, Green AJ, Lewis SJ, Reed ML, Stewart W, Chapman RH, Fox KM, Grandy S: Prevalence of self-reported diagnosis of diabetes mellitus and associated risk factors in a national survey in the US population: SHIELD (study to help improve early evaluation and management of risk factors leading to diabetes). *BMC Public Health* 7: 277, 2007

[4] National diabetes information clearinghouse: A service of the NIDDK, NIH. In; 2007.

[5] Ford ES, Giles WH, Dietz WH: Prevalence of the metabolic syndrome among US adults: Findings from the third national health and nutrition examination survey. *JAMA* 287: 356-359, 2002

[6] Wolf G, Sharma K, Ziyadeh F. Pathophysiology and pathogenesis of diabetic nephropathy. In: Alpern RJ, Hebert SC, eds. *Seldin and giebisch's the kidney physiology and pathophysiology*. 4th ed. Burlington: Elsevier; 2008:2215-2233.

[7] American Society of Nephrology, http://www.Asn-online.Org/facts_and_statistics. In; 2007.

[8] The effect of intensive treatment of diabetes on the development and progression of long-term complications in insulin-dependent diabetes mellitus. The diabetes control and complications trial research group. *N.Engl. J.Med.* 329: 977-986, 1993

[9] Intensive blood-glucose control with sulphonylureas or insulin compared with conventional treatment and risk of complications in patients with type 2 diabetes (UKPDS 33). UK prospective diabetes study (UKPDS) group. *Lancet* 352: 837-853, 1998

[10] Schrijvers BF, De Vriese AS, Flyvbjerg A: From hyperglycemia to diabetic kidney disease: The role of metabolic, hemodynamic, intracellular factors and growth factors/cytokines. *Endocr. Rev.* 25: 971-1010, 2004

[11] Jaimes EA, Hua P, Tian RX, Raij L: Human glomerular endothelium: Interplay among glucose, free fatty acids angiotensin II and oxidative stress in hyperglycemia. *Am. J. Physiol. Renal. Physiol.* 10.11 52/ajprenal .00248.02009, 2009

[12] Taguma Y, Kitamoto Y, Futaki G, Ueda H, Monma H, Ishizaki M, Takahashi H, Sekino H, Sasaki Y: Effect of captopril on heavy proteinuria in azotemic diabetics. *N. Engl. J. Med.* 313: 1617-1620, 1985

[13] Lewis EJ, Hunsicker LG, Bain KP, Rhode RD: The effect of angiotensin-converting-enzyme inhibition on diabetic nephropathy. *N. Engl. J. Med.* 329: 1456-1462, 1993

[14] Brenner BM, Cooper ME, de Zeeuw D, Keane WF, Mitch WE, Parving HH, Remuzzi G, Snapinn SM, Zhang Z, Shahinfar S: Effects of losartan on renal and cardiovascular outcomes in patients with type 2 diabetes and nephropathy. *N. Engl. J.Med.* 345: 861-869, 2001

[15] Jacobsen P, Andersen S, Rossing K, Jensen BR, Parving HH: Dual blockade of the renin-angiotensin system versus maximal recommended dose of ACE inhibition in diabetic nephropathy. *Kidney Int.* 63: 1874-1880, 2003

[16] Mogensen CE, Neldam S, Tikkanen I, Oren S, Viskoper R, Watts RW, Cooper ME: Randomised controlled trial of dual blockade of renin-angiotensin system in patients with

hypertension, microalbuminuria, and non-insulin dependent diabetes: The candesartan and lisinopril microalbuminuria (CALM) study. *BMJ* 321: 1440-1444, 2000

[17] Huang XR, Chen WY, Truong LD, Lan HY: Chymase is upregulated in diabetic nephropathy: Implications for an alternative pathway of angiotensin II-mediated diabetic renal and vascular disease. *J. Am. Soc. Nephrol.* 14: 1738-1747, 2003

[18] Navar LG, Harrison-Bernard LM, Nishiyama A, Kobori H: Regulation of intrarenal angiotensin II in hypertension. *Hypertension* 39: 3 16-322, 2002

[19] Mauer M, Zinman B, Gardiner R, Suissa S, Sinaiko A, Strand T, Drummond K, Donnelly S, Goodyer P, Gubler MC, Klein R: Renal and retinal effects of enalapril and losartan in type 1 diabetes. *N. Engl J Med* 361: 40-51, 2009

[20] Tamsma JT: Renal and retinal effects of enalapril and losartan in type 1 diabetes. *N Engl J Med* 361: 1410; author reply 1411, 2009

[21] Sowers JR, Epstein M, Frohlich ED: Diabetes, hypertension, and cardiovascular disease: An update. *Hypertension* 37: 1053-1059, 2001

[22] Hostetter TH: Diabetic nephropathy. Metabolic versus hemodynamic considerations. *Diabetes Care* 15: 1205-1215, 1992

[23] Vallon V, Richter K, Blantz RC, Thomson S, Osswald H: Glomerular hyperfiltration in experimental diabetes mellitus: Potential role of tubular reabsorption. *J. Am. Soc. Nephrol.* 10: 2569-2576, 1999

[24] Zatz R, Meyer TW, Rennke HG, Brenner BM: Predominance of hemodynamic rather than metabolic factors in the pathogenesis of diabetic glomerulopathy. *Proc. Natl. Acad. Sci. USA* 82: 5963-5967, 1985

[25] Gurley SB, Clare SE, Snow KP, Hu A, Meyer TW, Coffman TM: Impact of genetic background on nephropathy in diabetic mice. *Am. J. Physiol. Renal. Physiol.* 290: F214-222, 2006

[26] Carmines PK, Ohishi K, Ikenaga H: Functional impairment of renal afferent arteriolar voltage-gated calcium channels in rats with diabetes mellitus. *J Glin Invest* 98: 2564-2571, 1996

[27] Thomson SC, Vallon V, Blantz RC: Kidney function in early diabetes: The tubular hypothesis of glomerular filtration. *Am. J. Physiol. Renal. Physiol.* 286: F8-15, 2004

[28] Ohishi K, Okwueze MI, Vari RC, Carmines PK: Juxtamedullary microvascular dysfunction during the hyperfiltration stage of diabetes mellitus. *Am. J. Physiol.* 267: F99-105, 1994

[29] Ikenaga H, Bast JP, Fallet RW, Carmines PK: Exaggerated impact of ATP-sensitive K(+) channels on afferent arteriolar diameter in diabetes mellitus. *J. Am. Soc. Nephrol.* 11: 1199-1207, 2000

[30] Bank N, Aynedjian HS: Role of EDRF (nitric oxide) in diabetic renal hyperfiltration. *Kidney Int.* 43: 1306-1312, 1993

[31] Komers R, Anderson S: Paradoxes of nitric oxide in the diabetic kidney. *Am. J. Physiol. Renal. Physiol.* 284: F1121-1137, 2003

[32] Sugimoto H, Shikata K, Matsuda M, Kushiro M, Hayashi Y, Hiragushi K, Wada J, Makino H: Increased expression of endothelial cell nitric oxide synthase (ecnos) in afferent and glomerular endothelial cells is involved in glomerular hyperfiltration of diabetic nephropathy. *Diabetologia* 41: 1426-1434, 1998

[33] Veelken R, Hilgers KF, HartnerA, Haas A, Bohmer KP, Sterzel RB: Nitric oxide synthase isoforms and glomerular hyperfiltration in early diabetic nephropathy. *J. Am. Soc. Nephrol.* 11: 71-79, 2000

[34] Tolins JP, Shultz PJ, Raij L, Brown DM, Mauer SM: Abnormal renal hemodynamic response to reduced renal perfusion pressure in diabetic rats: Role of no. *Am. J. Physiol.* 265: F886-895, 1993

[35] Levine DZ, Iacovitti M, Robertson SJ, Mokhtar GA: Modulation of single-nephron GFR in the db/db mouse model of type 2 diabetes mellitus. *Am. J. Physiol. Regul. Integr. Comp. Physiol*.290: R975-981, 2006

[36] Bell TD, DiBona GF, Biemiller R, Brands MW: Continuously measured renal blood flow does not increase in diabetes if nitric oxide synthesis is blocked. *Am. J. Physiol. Renal. Physiol.* 295: F1449-1456, 2008

[37] Brands MW, Bell TD, Gibson B: Nitric oxide may prevent hypertension early in diabetes by counteracting renal actions of superoxide. *Hypertension* 43: 57-63, 2004

[38] Ishii N, Patel KP, Lane PH, Taylor T, Bian K, Murad F, Pollock JS, Carmines PK: Nitric oxide synthesis and oxidative stress in the renal cortex of rats with diabetes mellitus. *J.Am. Soc. Nephrol.* 12: 1630-1639, 2001

[39] Komers R, Oyama TT, Chapman JG, Allison KM, Anderson S: Effects of systemic inhibition of neuronal nitric oxide synthase in diabetic rats. *Hypertension* 35: 655-661, 2000

[40] Prabhakar SS: Role of nitric oxide in diabetic nephropathy. *Semin Nephrol* 24: 333-344, 2004

[41] Ohishi K, Carmines PK: Superoxide dismutase restores the influence of nitric oxide on renal arterioles in diabetes mellitus. *J.Am. Soc. Nephrol.* 5: 1559-1566, 1995

[42] PfluegerAC, Larson TS, Hagl S, Knox FG: Role of nitric oxide in intrarenal hemodynamics in experimental diabetes mellitus in rats. *Am. J. Physiol.* 277: R725-733, 1999

[43] Keynan S, Hirshberg B, Levin-Iaina N, Wexler ID, Dahan R, Reinhartz E, Ovadia H, Wollman Y, Chernihovskey T, Iaina A, Raz I: Renal nitric oxide production during the early phase of experimental diabetes mellitus. *Kidney Int.* 58: 740-747, 2000

[44] Schoonmaker GC, Fallet RW, Carmines PK: Superoxide anion curbs nitric oxide modulation of afferent arteriolar ANG II responsiveness in diabetes mellitus. *Am. J. Physiol. Renal. Physiol.* 278: F302-309, 2000

[45] Zhao HJ, Wang S, Cheng H, Zhang MZ, Takahashi T, Fogo AB, Breyer MD, Harris RC: Endothelial nitric oxide synthase deficiency produces accelerated nephropathy in diabetic mice. *J. Am. Soc. Nephrol.* 17: 2664-2669,2006

[46] Sochett EB, Cherney DZ, Curtis JR, Dekker MG, Scholey JW, Miller JA: Impact of renin angiotensin system modulation on the hyperfiltration state in type 1 diabetes. *J.Am. Soc. Nephrol.* 17: 1703-1709, 2006

[47] Anderson S, Jung FF, Ingelfinger JR: Renal renin-angiotensin system in diabetes: Functional, immunohistochemical, and molecular biological correlations. *Am. J. Physiol.* 265: F477-486, 1993

[48] Andersen S, Tarnow L, Rossing P, Hansen BV, Parving HH: Renoprotective effects of angiotensin II receptor blockade in type 1 diabetic patients with diabetic nephropathy. *Kidney Int.* 57: 601-606, 2000

[49] Hollenberg NK, Price DA, Fisher ND, Lansang MC, Perkins B, Gordon MS, Williams GH, Laffel LM: Glomerular hemodynamics and the renin-angiotensin system in patients with type 1 diabetes mellitus. *Kidney Int.* 63: 172-178, 2003

[50] Giunti S, Barit D, Cooper ME: Mechanisms of diabetic nephropathy: Role of hypertension. *Hypertension* 48: 5 19-526, 2006

[51] Mitchell KD, Navar LG. Intrarenal actions of angiotensin II in the pathogenesis of experimental hypertension. In: Laragh JH, Brenner BM, eds. *Hypertension: Pathophysiology, diagnosis and management.* 2nd ed. New York, NY: Raven Press; 1995:1437-1450.

[52] Kobori H, Nangaku M, Navar LG, Nishiyama A: The intrarenal renin-angiotensin system: From physiology to the pathobiology of hypertension and kidney disease. *Pharmacol. Rev.* 59: 25 1-287, 2007

[53] Carey RM, Siragy HM: The intrarenal renin-angiotensin system and diabetic nephropathy. *Trends Endocrinol. Metab.* 14: 274-281, 2003

[54] Santos RA, Simoes e Silva AC, Maric C, Silva DM, Machado RP, de Buhr I, Heringer-Walther S, Pinheiro SV, Lopes MT, Bader M, Mendes EP, Lemos VS, Campagnole-Santos MJ, Schultheiss HP, Speth R, Walther T: Angiotensin-(1-7) is an endogenous ligand for the G protein-coupled receptor mas. *Proc. Natl. Acad. Sci. USA* 100: 8258-8263, 2003

[55] Navar LG, Prieto-Carrasquero MC, Kobori H. Chapter 1: Molecular aspects of the renal renin-angiotensin system. In: Re RN, DiPette DJ, Schiffrin EL, Sowers JR, eds. *Molecular mechanisms in hypertension.* 1st ed. Oxfordshire, UK: Taylor and Francis Medical; 2006:3-14.

[56] Dzau VJ, Re R: Tissue angiotensin system in cardiovascular medicine. A paradigm shift? *Circulation* 89: 493-498, 1994

[57] Baltatu O, Silva JA, Jr., Ganten D, Bader M: The brain renin-angiotensin system modulates angiotensin II-induced hypertension and cardiac hypertrophy. *Hypertension* 35: 409-4 12, 2000

[58] Dell'Italia LJ, Meng QC, Balcells E, Wei CC, Palmer R, Hageman GR, Durand J, Hankes GH, Oparil S: Compartmentalization of angiotensin II generation in the dog heart evidence for independent mechanisms in intravascular and interstitial spaces. *J. Clin. Invest.* 100: 253-258, 1997

[59] Mazzocchi G, Malendowicz LK, Markowska A, Albertin G, Nussdorfer GG: Role of adrenal renin-angiotensin system in the control of aldosterone secretion in sodium-restricted rats. *Am. J. Physiol. Endocrinol. Metab.* 278: E1027-1030, 2000

[60] Danser AH, Admiraal PJ, Derkx FH, Schalekamp MA: Angiotensin I-to-II conversion in the human renal vascular bed. *J. Hypertens.* 16: 205 1-2056, 1998

[61] Griendling KK, Minieri CA, Ollerenshaw JD, Alexander RW: Angiotensin II stimulates nadh and NADPH oxidase activity in cultured vascular smooth muscle cells. *Circ. Res.* 74: 1141-1148, 1994

[62] Ingelfinger JR, Zuo WM, Fon EA, Ellison KE, Dzau VJ: In situ hybridization evidence for angiotensinogen messenger RNA in the rat proximal tubule. An hypothesis for the intrarenal renin angiotensin system. *J. Clin. Invest.* 85: 417-423, 1990

[63] Terada Y, Tomita K, Nonoguchi H, Marumo F: PCR localization of angiotensin II receptor and angiotensinogen mRNAs in rat kidney. *Kidney Int.* 43: 125 1-1259, 1993

[64] Richoux JP, Cordonnier JL, Bouhnik J, Clauser E, Corvol P, Menard J, Grignon G: Immunocytochemical localization of angiotensinogen in rat liver and kidney. *Cell Tissue Res.* 233: 439-451, 1983

[65] Darby IA, Congiu M, Fernley RT, Sernia C, Coghlan JP: Cellular and ultrastructural location of angiotensinogen in rat and sheep kidney. *Kidney Int.* 46: 1557-1560, 1994

[66] Darby IA, Sernia C: In situ hybridization and immunohistochemistry of renal angiotensinogen in neonatal and adult rat kidneys. *Cell Tissue Res.* 281: 197-206, 1995

[67] Kobori H, Harrison-Bernard LM, Navar LG: Expression of angiotensinogen mRNA and protein in angiotensin II-dependent hypertension. *J. Am. Soc. Nephrol.* 12: 43 1-439, 2001

[68] Leyssac PP: Changes in single nephron renin release are mediated by tubular fluid flow rate. *Kidney Int.* 30: 332-339, 1986

[69] Yanagawa N, Capparelli AW, Jo OD, Friedal A, Barrett JD, Eggena P: Production of angiotensinogen and renin-like activity by rabbit proximal tubular cells in culture. *Kidney Int.* 39: 938-941, 1991

[70] Henrich WL, McAllister EA, Eskue A, Miller T, Moe OW: Renin regulation in cultured proximal tubular cells. *Hypertension* 27: 1337-1340, 1996

[71] Moe OW, Ujiie K, Star RA, Miller RT, Widell J, Alpern RJ, Henrich WL: Renin expression in renal proximal tubule. *J. Glin. Invest.* 91: 774-779, 1993

[72] Sibony M, Gasc JM, Soubrier F, Alhenc-Gelas F, Corvol P: Gene expression and tissue localization of the two isoforms of angiotensin I converting enzyme. *Hypertension* 21: 827-835, 1993

[73] Schulz WW, Hagler HK, Buja LM, Erdos EG: Ultrastructural localization of angiotensin I-converting enzyme (EC 3.4.15.1) and neutral metalloendopeptidase (EC 3.4.24.11) in the proximal tubule of the human kidney. *Lab. Invest.* 59: 789-797, 1988

[74] Vio CP, Jeanneret VA: Local induction of angiotensin-converting enzyme in the kidney as a mechanism of progressive renal diseases. *Kidney Int. Suppl.* S57-63, 2003

[75] Casarini DE, Boim MA, Stella RC, Krieger-Azzolini MH, Krieger JE, Schor N: Angiotensin I-converting enzyme activity in tubular fluid along the rat nephron. *Am. J. Physiol.* 272: F405-409, 1997

[76] Kang JJ, Toma I, Sipos A, Meer EJ, Vargas SL, Peti-Peterdi J: The collecting duct is the major source of prorenin in diabetes. *Hypertension* 51: 1597-1604, 2008

[77] Prieto-Carrasquero MC, Botros FT, Pagan J, Kobori H, Seth DM, Casarini DE, Navar LG: Collecting duct renin is upregulated in both kidneys of 2-kidney, 1-clip goldblatt hypertensive rats. *Hypertension* 51: 1590-1596, 2008

[78] Prieto-Carrasquero MC, Kobori H, Ozawa Y, Gutierrez A, Seth D, Navar LG: AT1 receptor-mediated enhancement of collecting duct renin in angiotensin II-dependent hypertensive rats. *Am. J. Physiol. Renal. Physiol.* 289: F632-637, 2005

[79] Rohrwasser A, Morgan T, Dillon HF, Zhao L, Callaway CW, Hillas E, Zhang S, Cheng T, Inagami T, Ward K, Terreros DA, Lalouel JM: Elements of a paracrine tubular renin-angiotensin system along the entire nephron. *Hypertension* 34: 1265-1274, 1999

[80] Nguyen G, Delarue F, Burckle C, Bouzhir L, Giller T, Sraer JD: Pivotal role of the renin/prorenin receptor in angiotensin II production and cellular responses to renin. *J. Glin. Invest.* 109: 1417-1427, 2002

[81] Advani A, Kelly DJ, Cox AJ, White KE, Advani SL, Thai K, Connelly KA, Yuen D, Trogadis J, Herzenberg AM, Kuliszewski MA, Leong-Poi H, Gilbert RE: The (pro)renin

receptor: Site-specific and functional linkage to the vacuolar H+-atpase in the kidney. *Hypertension* 54: 261-269, 2009

[82] Wang ZQ, Millatt LJ, Heiderstadt NT, Siragy HM, Johns RA, Carey RM: Differential regulation of renal angiotensin subtype AT1A and AT2 receptor protein in rats with angiotensin-dependent hypertension. *Hypertension* 33: 96-101, 1999

[83] Miyata N, Park F, Li XF, Cowley AW, Jr.: Distribution of angiotensin AT1 and AT2 receptor subtypes in the rat kidney. *Am. J. Physiol.* 277: F437-446, 1999

[84] Bouby N, Hus-Citharel A, Marchetti J, Bankir L, Corvol P, Llorens-Cortes C: Expression of type 1 angiotensin II receptor subtypes and angiotensin II-induced calcium mobilization along the rat nephron. *J. Am. Soc. Nephrol.* 8: 1658-1667, 1997

[85] Harrison-Bernard LM, Navar LG, Ho MM, Vinson GP, El-Dahr SS: Immunohistochemical localization of ANG II AT1 receptor in adult rat kidney using a monoclonal antibody. *Am. J. Physiol.* 273: F170-F177, 1997

[86] Anderson S: Physiologic actions and molecular expression of the renin-angiotensin system in the diabetic rat. *Miner Electrolyte Metab.* 24: 406-411, 1998

[87] Harrison-Bernard LM, Imig JD, Carmines PK: Renal AT1 receptor protein expression during the early stage of diabetes mellitus. *Int. J. Exp. Diabetes Res.* 3: 97-108, 2002

[88] Zimpelmann J, Kumar D, Levine DZ, Wehbi G, Imig JD, Navar LG, Burns KD: Early diabetes mellitus stimulates proximal tubule renin mRNA expression in the rat. *Kidney Int.* 58: 2320-2330, 2000

[89] Wehbi GJ, Zimpelmann J, Carey RM, Levine DZ, Burns KD: Early streptozotocin-diabetes mellitus downregulates rat kidney AT2 receptors. *Am. J. Physiol. Renal. Physiol.* 280: F254-265, 2001

[90] Nagai Y, Yao L, Kobori H, Miyata K, Ozawa Y, Miyatake A, Yukimura T, Shokoji T, Kimura S, Kiyomoto H, Kohno M, Abe Y, Nishiyama A: Temporary angiotensin II blockade at the prediabetic stage attenuates the development of renal injury in type 2 diabetic rats. *J. Am. Soc. Nephrol.* 16: 703-711, 2005

[91] Nishiyama A, Nakagawa T, Kobori H, Nagai Y, Okada N, Konishi Y, Morikawa T, Okumura M, MedaI, Kiyomoto H, Hosomi N, Mori T, Ito S, Imanishi M: Strict angiotensin blockade prevents the augmentation of intrarenal angiotensin II and podocyte abnormalities in type 2 diabetic rats with microalbuminuria. *J. Hypertens.* 26: 1849-1859, 2008

[92] Suzaki Y, Ozawa Y, Kobori H: Intrarenal oxidative stress and augmented angiotensinogen are precedent to renal injury in Zucker diabetic fatty rats. *Int. J. Biol. Sci.* 3: 40-46, 2007

[93] Miyata K, Ohashi N, Suzaki Y, KatsuradaA, Kobori H: Sequential activation of the reactive oxygen species/angiotensinogen/renin-angiotensin system axis in renal injury of type 2 diabetic rats. *Clin. Exp. Pharmacol. Physiol.* 35: 922-927, 2008

[94] Ichihara A, Hayashi M, Kaneshiro Y, Suzuki F, Nakagawa T, Tada Y, Koura Y, Nishiyama A, Okada H, Uddin MN, Nabi AH, Ishida Y, Inagami T, Saruta T: Inhibition of diabetic nephropathy by a decoy peptide corresponding to the "Handle" Region for nonproteolytic activation of prorenin. *J. Glin. Invest.* 114: 1128-1135, 2004

[95] Feldman DL, Jin L, Xuan H, Contrepas A, Zhou Y, Webb RL, Mueller DN, Feldt S, Cumin F, Maniara W, Persohn E, Schuetz H, Jan Danser AH, Nguyen G: Effects of aliskiren on blood pressure, albuminuria, and (pro)renin receptor expression in diabetic tg(mren-2)27 rats. *Hypertension* 52: 130-136, 2008

[96] Takahashi H, Ichihara A, Kaneshiro Y, Inomata K, Sakoda M, Takemitsu T, Nishiyama A, Itoh H: Regression of nephropathy developed in diabetes by (pro)renin receptor blockade. *J. Am. Soc. Nephrol.* 18: 2054-2061, 2007

[97] Ichihara A, Sakoda M, Kurauchi-Mito A, Nishiyama A, Itoh H: Involvement of receptor-bound prorenin in development of nephropathy in diabetic db/db mice. *J. Am. Soc. Hypertens* 2: 332-340, 2008

[98] IchiharaA, Suzuki F, Nakagawa T, Kaneshiro Y, Takemitsu T, Sakoda M, Nabi AH, Nishiyama A, Sugaya T, Hayashi M, Inagami T: Prorenin receptor blockade inhibits development of glomerulosclerosis in diabetic angiotensin II type 1 a receptor-deficient mice. *J. Am. Soc. Nephrol.* 17: 1950-1961, 2006

[99] Batenburg WW, Jan Danser AH: The (pro)renin receptor: A new addition to the renin-angiotensin system? *Eur. J. Pharmacol.* 585: 320-324, 2008

[100] Wolf G, Ritz E: Combination therapy with ACE inhibitors and angiotensin II receptor blockers to halt progression of chronic renal disease: Pathophysiology and indications. *Kidney Int.* 67: 799-812, 2005

[101] Yamamoto T, Nakamura T, Noble NA, Ruoslahti E, Border WA: Expression of transforming growth factor beta is elevated in human and experimental diabetic nephropathy. *Proc. Natl. Acad. Sci. USA* 90: 1814-1818, 1993

[102] Teles F, Machado FG, Ventura BH, Malheiros DM, Fujihara CK, Silva LF, Zatz R: Regression of glomerular injury by losartan in experimental diabetic nephropathy. *Kidney Int.* 75: 72-79, 2009

[103] Azizi M, Chatellier G, Guyene TT, Murieta-Geoffroy D, Menard J: Additive effects of combined angiotensin-converting enzyme inhibition and angiotensin II antagonism on blood pressure and renin release in sodium-depleted normotensives. *Circulation* 92: 825-834, 1995

[104] Menard J, Campbell DJ, Azizi M, Gonzales MF: Synergistic effects of ACE inhibition and Ang II antagonism on blood pressure, cardiac weight, and renin in spontaneously hypertensive rats. *Circulation* 96: 3072-3078, 1997

[105] Cohen DL, Townsend RR: Is there added value to adding ARB to ACE inhibitors in the management of CKD? *J.Am. Soc. Nephrol.* 20: 1666-1668, 2009

[106] Skeggs LT, Jr., Kahn JR, Shumway NP: The preparation and function of the hypertensin-converting enzyme. *J.Exp. Med.* 103: 295-299, 1956

[107] Donoghue M, Hsieh F, Baronas E, Godbout K, Gosselin M, Stagliano N, Donovan M, Woolf B, Robison K, Jeyaseelan R, Breitbart RE, Acton S: A novel angiotensin-converting enzyme-related carboxypeptidase (ACE2) converts angiotensin I to angiotensin 1-9. *Circ. Res.* 87: E1-9, 2000

[108] Crackower MA, Sarao R, Oudit GY, Yagil C, Kozieradzki I, Scanga SE, Oliveira-dosSantos AJ, da Costa J, Zhang L, Pei Y, Scholey J, Ferrario CM, Manoukian AS, Chappell MC, Backx PH, Yagil Y, Penninger JM: Angiotensin-converting enzyme 2 is an essential regulator of heart function. *Nature* 417: 822-828, 2002

[109] Ferrario CM, Chappell MC, Tallant EA, Brosnihan KB, Diz DI: Counterregulatory actions of angiotensin-(1-7). *Hypertension* 30: 535-541, 1997

[110] Vickers C, Hales P, Kaushik V, Dick L, Gavin J, Tang J, Godbout K, Parsons T, Baronas E, Hsieh F, Acton S, Patane M, Nichols A, Tummino P: Hydrolysis of biological peptides by human angiotensin-converting enzyme-related carboxypeptidase. *J. Biol. Chem.* 277: 14838-14843, 2002

[111] Oudit GY, Herzenberg AM, Kassiri Z, Wong D, Reich H, Khokha R, Crackower MA, Backx PH, Penninger JM, Scholey JW: Loss of angiotensin-converting enzyme-2 leads to the late development of angiotensin II-dependent glomerulosclerosis. *Am. J. Pathol.* 168: 1808-1820, 2006

[112] Wong DW, Oudit GY, Reich H, Kassiri Z, Zhou J, Liu QC, Backx PH, Penninger JM, Herzenberg AM, Scholey JW: Loss of angiotensin-converting enzyme-2 (ace2) accelerates diabetic kidney injury. *Am. J. Pathol.* 171: 438-451, 2007

[113] Wysocki J, Ye M, Soler MJ, Gurley SB, Xiao HD, Bernstein KE, Coffman TM, Chen S, Batlle D: ACE and ACE2 activity in diabetic mice. *Diabetes* 55: 2132-2139, 2006

[114] Soler MJ, Wysocki J, Ye M, Lloveras J, Kanwar Y, Batlle D: ACE2 inhibition worsens glomerular injury in association with increased ACE expression in streptozotocin-induced diabetic mice. *Kidney Int.* 72: 614-623, 2007

[115] Ye M, Wysocki J, Naaz P, Salabat MR, LaPointe MS, Batlle D: Increased ACE 2 and decreased ACE protein in renal tubules from diabetic mice: A renoprotective combination? *Hypertension* 43: 1120-1125, 2004

[116] Park S, Bivona BJ, Kobori H, Seth DM, Chappell MC, Lazartigues E, Harrison-Bernard LM: Major role for ACE-independent intrarenal ANGII formation in type II diabetes. *Am. J. Physiol. Renal. Physiol.* 298:F37-F48, 2010

[117] Lazartigues E, Feng Y, Lavoie JL: The two faces of the tissue renin-angiotensin systems: Implication in cardiovascular diseases. *Curr. Pharm. Des.* 13: 1231-1245, 2007

[118] Navar LG, Inscho EW, Majid SA, Imig JD, Harrison-Bernard LM, Mitchell KD: Paracrine regulation of the renal microcirculation. *Physiol. Rev.* 76: 425-536, 1996

[119] Navar LG, Imig JD, Zou L, Wang CT: Intrarenal production of angiotensin II. *Sem. Nephrol.* 17: 412-422, 1997

[120] IchiharaA, Kobori H, Nishiyama A, Navar LG: Renal renin-angiotensin system. *Contrib. Nephrol.* 143: 117-130, 2004

[121] Burrell LM, Johnston CI, Tikellis C, Cooper ME: ACE2, a new regulator of the renin-angiotensin system. *Trends Endocrinol. Metab.* 15: 166-169, 2004

[122] Danilczyk U, Penninger JM: Angiotensin-converting enzyme II in the heart and the kidney. *Circ Res* 98: 463-471, 2006

[123] Danilczyk U, Eriksson U, Oudit GY, Penninger JM: Physiological roles of angiotensin-converting enzyme 2. *Cell Mol. Life Sci.* 61: 2714-2719, 2004

[124] Shaltout HA, Westwood B, Averill DB, Ferrario CM, Figueroa J, Diz DI, Rose JC, Chappell MC: Angiotensin metabolism in renal proximal tubules, urine and serum of sheep: Evidence for ACE2-dependent processing of angiotensin II. *Am. J. Physiol. Renal. Physiol.* 2006

[125] Stegbauer J, Vonend O, Oberhauser V, Rump LC: Effects of angiotensin-(1-7) and other bioactive components of the renin-angiotensin system on vascular resistance and noradrenaline release in rat kidney. *J.Hypertens* 21: 1391-1399, 2003

[126] Modrall JG, Sadjadi J, Brosnihan KB, Gallagher PE, Yu CH, Kramer GL, Bernstein KE, Chappell MC: Depletion of tissue angiotensin-converting enzyme differentially influences the intrarenal and urinary expression of angiotensin peptides. *Hypertension* 43: 849-853, 2004

[127] Zhong JC, Huang DY, Yang YM, Li YF, Liu GF, Song XH, Du K: Upregulation of angiotensin-converting enzyme 2 by all-trans retinoic acid in spontaneously hypertensive rats. *Hypertension* 44: 907-912, 2004

[128] Tikellis C, Johnston CI, Forbes JM, Burns WC, Burrell LM, Risvanis J, Cooper ME: Characterization of renal angiotensin-converting enzyme 2 in diabetic nephropathy. *Hypertension* 41: 392-397, 2003

[129] Belova LA: Angiotensin II-generating enzymes. *Biochemistry (Mosc)* 65: 1337-1345, 2000

[130] Urata H, Boehm KD, Philip A, Kinoshita A, Gabrovsek J, Bumpus FM, Husain A: Cellular localization and regional distribution of an angiotensin II-forming chymase in the heart. *J. Clin. Invest.* 91: 1269-1281, 1993

[131] Miyazaki M, Takai S: Local angiotensin II-generating system in vascular tissues: The roles of chymase. *Hypertens. Res.* 24: 189-193, 2001

[132] Miyazaki M, Takai S: Role of chymase on vascular proliferation. *J. Renin. Angiotensin Aldosterone Syst.* 1: 23-26, 2000

[133] McEuenAR, Sharma B, Walls AF: Regulation of the activity of human chymase during storage and release from mast cells: The contributions of inorganic cations, ph, heparin and histamine. *Biochim. Biophys. Acta* 1267: 115-121, 1995

[134] Takai S, Shiota N, Yamamoto D, Okunishi H, Miyazaki M: Purification and characterization of angiotensin II-generating chymase from hamster cheek pouch. *Life Sci.* 58: 59 1-597, 1996

[135] Nakano K, Takaishi K, KodamaA, Mammoto A, Shiozaki H, Monden M, Takai Y: Distinct actions and cooperative roles of ROCK and mdia in Rho small G protein-induced reorganization of the actin cytoskeleton in madin-darby canine kidney cells. *Mol. Biol. Cell* 10: 2481-2491, 1999 .

[136] Guo C, Ju H, Leung D, Massaeli H, Shi M, Rabinovitch M: A novel vascular smooth muscle chymase is upregulated in hypertensive rats. *J. Clin. Invest.* 107: 703-7 15, 2001

[137] Ju H, Gros R, You X, Tsang S, Husain M, Rabinovitch M: Conditional and targeted overexpression of vascular chymase causes hypertension in transgenic mice. *Proc. Natl. Acad. Sci. USA* 98: 7469-7474, 2001

[138] Akasu M, Urata H, Kinoshita A, Sasaguri M, Ideishi M, Arakawa K: Differences in tissue angiotensin II-forming pathways by species and organs in vitro. *Hypertension* 32: 5 14-520, 1998

[139] Kishi K, Jin D, Takai S, Muramatsu M, Katayama H, Tamai H, Miyazaki M: Role of chymase-dependent angiotensin II formation in monocrotaline-induced pulmonary hypertensive rats. *Pediatr. Res.* 60: 77-82, 2006

[140] Petrie MC, Padmanabhan N, McDonald JE, Hillier C, Connell JM, McMurray JJ: Angiotensin converting enzyme (ACE) and non-ACE dependent angiotensin II generation in resistance arteries from patients with heart failure and coronary heart disease. *J. Am. Coll Cardiol.* 37: 1056-1061, 2001

[141] Wei CC, Tian B, Perry G, Meng QC, Chen YF, Oparil S, Dell'Italia LJ: Differential ANG II generation in plasma and tissue of mice with decreased expression of the ACE gene. *Am. J. Physiol. Heart Circ. Physiol.* 282: H2254-2258, 2002

[142] Murakami M, Matsuda H, Kubota E, Wakino S, Honda M, Hayashi K, Saruta T: Role of angiotensin II generated by angiotensin converting enzyme-independent pathways in canine kidney. *Kidney Int. Suppl.* 63: S132-135, 1997

[143] Tokuyama H, Hayashi K, Matsuda H, Kubota E, Honda M, Okubo K, Takamatsu I, Tatematsu S, Ozawa Y, Wakino S, Saruta T: Differential regulation of elevated renal angiotensin II in chronic renal ischemia. *Hypertension* 40: 34-40, 2002

[144] Sadjadi J, Kramer GL, Yu CH, Burress Welborn M, 3rd, Chappell MC, Gregory Modrall J: Angiotensin converting enzyme-independent angiotensin ii production by chymase is up-regulated in the ischemic kidney in renovascular hypertension. *J. Surg. Res.* 127: 65-69, 2005

[145] Yamada M, Ueda M, Naruko T, Tanabe S, Han YS, Ikura Y, Ogami M, Takai S, Miyazaki M: Mast cell chymase expression and mast cell phenotypes in human rejected kidneys. *Kidney Int.* 59: 1374-1381, 2001

[146] Morikawa T, Imanishi M, Suzuki H, Okada N, Okumura M, Konishi Y, Yoshioka K, Takai S, Miyazaki M: Mast cell chymase in the ischemic kidney of severe unilateral renovascular hypertension. *Am. J. Kidney Dis.* 45: e45-50, 2005

[147] Koka V, Wang W, Huang XR, Kim-Mitsuyama S, Truong LD, Lan HY: Advanced glycation end products activate a chymase-dependent angiotensin II-generating pathway in diabetic complications. *Circulation* 113: 1353-1360, 2006

[148] Ritz E: Chymase: A potential culprit in diabetic nephropathy? *J Am Soc Nephrol* 14: 1952-1954, 2003

[149] Haneda M, Koya D, Kikkawa R: Cellular mechanisms in the development and progression of diabetic nephropathy: Activation of the DAG-PKC-ERK pathway. *Am. J. Kidney Dis.* 38: S178-181, 2001

[150] Kikkawa R, Koya D, Haneda M: Progression of diabetic nephropathy. *Am. J. Kidney Di.s* 41: S19-21, 2003

[151] Park JY, Ha SW, King GL: The role of protein kinase C activation in the pathogenesis of diabetic vascular complications. *Perit Dial Int* 19 Suppl 2: S222-227, 1999

[152] Shah SV: Light emission by isolated rat glomeruli in response to phorbol myristate acetate. *J LabClin Med* 98: 46-57, 1981

[153] Miyanoshita A, Takahashi T, Endou H: Inhibitory effect of cyclic amp on phorbol ester-stimulated production of reactive oxygen metabolites in rat glomeruli. *Biochem. Biophys. Res. Commun.* 165: 519-525, 1989

[154] Ha H, Endou H: Lipid peroxidation in isolated rat nephron segments. *Am. J. Physiol.* 263: F201-207, 1992

[155] Ha H, Lee HB: Reactive oxygen species as glucose signaling molecules in mesangial cells cultured under high glucose. *Kidney Int. Suppl.* 77: S 19-25, 2000

[156] Hsieh TJ, Zhang SL, Filep JG, Tang SS, Ingelfinger JR, Chan JS: High glucose stimulates angiotensinogen gene expression via reactive oxygen species generation in rat kidney proximal tubular cells. *Endocrinology* 143: 2975-2985, 2002

[157] Tomlinson DR: Mitogen-activated protein kinases as glucose transducers for diabetic complications. *Diabetologia* 42: 1271-1281, 1999

[158] Berk BC: Redox signals that regulate the vascular response to injury. *Thromb Haemost.* 82: 810-817, 1999

[159] Zhou G, Bao ZQ, Dixon JE: Components of a new human protein kinase signal transduction pathway. *J. Biol. Chem.* 270: 12665-12669, 1995

[160] Strawn WB: Pathophysiological and clinical implications of AT(1) and AT(2) angiotensin II receptors in metabolic disorders: Hypercholesterolaemia and diabetes. *Drugs* 62: 31-41, 2002

[161] Davi G, Chiarelli F, Santilli F, Pomilio M, Vigneri S, Falco A, Basili S, Ciabattoni G, Patrono C: Enhanced lipid peroxidation and platelet activation in the early phase of type 1

diabetes mellitus: Role of interleukin-6 and disease duration. *Circulation* 107: 3 199-3203, 2003

[162] McFarlane SI, Kumar A, Sowers JR: Mechanisms by which angiotensin-converting enzyme inhibitors prevent diabetes and cardiovascular disease. *Am. J. Cardiol.* 91: 30H-37H, 2003

[163] Mezzano S, Droguett A, Burgos ME, Ardiles LG, Flores CA, Aros CA, Caorsi I, Vio CP, Ruiz-Ortega M, Egido J: Renin-angiotensin system activation and interstitial inflammation in human diabetic nephropathy. *Kidney Int.* 64: Suppl 86 S64-70, 2003

[164] Utimura R, Fujihara CK, Mattar AL, Malheiros DM, Noronha IL, Zatz R: Mycophenolate mofetil prevents the development of glomerular injury in experimental diabetes. *Kidney Int.* 63: 209-216, 2003

[165] Yozai K, Shikata K, Sasaki M, ToneA, Ohga S, Usui H, Okada S, Wada J, Nagase R, Ogawa D, Shikata Y, Makino H: Methotrexate prevents renal injury in experimental diabetic rats via anti-inflammatory actions. *J. Am. Soc. Nephrol.* 16: 3326-3338, 2005

[166] Ogawa S, Mori T, Nako K, Kato T, Takeuchi K, Ito S: Angiotensin II type 1 receptor blockers reduce urinary oxidative stress markers in hypertensive diabetic nephropathy. *Hypertension* 47: 699-705, 2006

[167] de Vinuesa SG, Goicoechea M, Kanter J, Puerta M, Cachofeiro V, Lahera V, Gomez-Campdera F, Luno J: Insulin resistance, inflammatory biomarkers, and adipokines in patients with chronic kidney disease: Effects of angiotensin II blockade. *J. Am. Soc. Nephrol.* 17: S206-212, 2006

[168] Egido J, Ruiz-Ortega M: Anti-inflammatory actions of quinapril. *Cardiovasc. Drugs Ther.* 2007

[169] Wolkow PP, Niewczas MA, Perkins B, Ficociello LH, Lipinski B, Warram JH, Krolewski AS: Association of urinary inflammatory markers and renal decline in microalbuminuric type 1 diabetics. *J.Am. Soc. Nephrol.* 19: 789-797, 2008

[170] Kagami S, Border WA, Miller DE, Noble NA: Angiotensin II stimulates extracellular matrix protein synthesis through induction of transforming growth factor-beta expression in rat glomerular mesangial cells. *J. Cuin. Invest.* 93: 2431-2437, 1994

[171] Border WA, Noble NA: Cytokines in kidney disease: The role of transforming growth factor-beta. *Am. J. Kidney Dis* 22: 105-113, 1993

[172] Rao GN: Hydrogen peroxide induces complex formation of shc-grb2-sos with receptor tyrosine kinase and activates ras and extracellular signal-regulated protein kinases group of mitogen-activated protein kinases. *Oncogene* 13: 713-719, 1996

[173] Yoshizumi M, Abe J, Haendeler J, Huang Q, Berk BC: Src and cas mediate JNK activation but not ERK1/2 and p38 kinases by reactive oxygen species. *J.Biou. Chem.* 275: 11706-11712, 2000

[174] Suzaki Y, Yoshizumi M, Kagami S, Koyama AH, Taketani Y, Houchi H, Tsuchiya K, Takeda E, Tamaki T: Hydrogen peroxide stimulates c-src-mediated big mitogen-activated protein kinase 1 (BMK1) and the MEF2C signaling pathway in PC12 cells: Potential role in cell survival following oxidative insults. *J. Biou. Chem.* 277: 9614-9621, 2002

[175] Suzaki Y, Yoshizumi M, Kagami S, NishiyamaA, Ozawa Y, Kyaw M, Izawa Y, Kanematsu Y, Tsuchiya K, Tamaki T: BMK1 is activated in glomeruli of diabetic rats and in mesangial cells by high glucose conditions. *Kidney Int.* 65: 1749-1760, 2004

[176] Schreck R, Rieber P, Baeuerle PA: Reactive oxygen intermediates as apparently widely used messengers in the activation of the NF-kappa B transcription factor and HIV-1. *EMBO J.* 10: 2247-2258, 1991

[177] Perona R, Montaner S, Saniger L, Sanchez-Perez I, Bravo R, Lacal JC: Activation of the nuclear factor-kappaB by Rho, CDC42, and Rac-1 proteins. *Genes. Dev.* 11: 463-475, 1997

[178] Zhang SL, Tang SS, Chen X, Filep JG, Ingelfinger JR, Chan JS: High levels of glucose stimulate angiotensinogen gene expression via the p38 mitogen-activated protein kinase pathway in rat kidney proximal tubular cells. *Endocrinology* 141: 4637-4646, 2000

[179] Li J, Brasier AR: Angiotensinogen gene activation by angiotensin II is mediated by the rel A (nuclear factor-kappaB p65) transcription factor: One mechanism for the renin angiotensin system positive feedback loop in hepatocytes. *Mol. Endocrinol.* 10: 252-264, 1996

[180] Brinkmann MM, Glenn M, Rainbow L, Kieser A, Henke-Gendo C, Schulz TF: Activation of mitogen-activated protein kinase and NF-kappaB pathways by a kaposi's sarcoma-associated herpesvirus k15 membrane protein. *J. Virol.* 77: 9346-9358, 2003

[181] Hoffmann E, Thiefes A, Buhrow D, Dittrich-Breiholz O, Schneider H, Resch K, Kracht M: Mek1-dependent delayed expression of fos-related antigen-1 counteracts c-fos and p65 NFkappaB-mediated interleukin-8 transcription in response to cytokines or growth factors. *J. Biol. Chem.* 280: 9706-97 18, 2005

[182] Zhang SL, Filep JG, Hohman TC, Tang SS, Ingelfinger JR, Chan JS: Molecular mechanisms of glucose action on angiotensinogen gene expression in rat proximal tubular cells. *Kidney Int.* 55: 454-464, 1999

[183] Zhang SL, To C, Chen X, Filep JG, Tang SS, Ingelfinger JR, Chan JS: Essential role(s) of the intrarenal renin-angiotensin system in transforming growth factor-beta 1 gene expression and induction of hypertrophy of rat kidney proximal tubular cells in high glucose. *J.Am. Soc. Nephrol.* 13: 302-312, 2002

[184] Zhang SL, Chen X, Hsieh TJ, Leclerc M, Henley N, Allidina A, Halle JP, Brunette MG, Filep JG, Tang SS, Ingelfinger JR, Chan JS: Hyperglycemia induces insulin resistance on angiotensinogen gene expression in diabetic rat kidney proximal tubular cells. *J. Endocrinol.* 172: 333-344, 2002

[185] Zhang SL, Chen X, Wei CC, Filep JG, Tang SS, Ingelfinger JR, Chan JS: Insulin inhibits dexamethasone effect on angiotensinogen gene expression and induction of hypertrophy in rat kidney proximal tubular cells in high glucose. *Endocrinology* 143: 4627-4635, 2002

[186] Hsieh TJ, Fustier P, Zhang SL, Filep JG, Tang SS, Ingelfinger JR, Fantus IG, Hamet P, Chan JS: High glucose stimulates angiotensinogen gene expression and cell hypertrophy via activation of the hexosamine biosynthesis pathway in rat kidney proximal tubular cells. *Endocrinology* 144: 4338-4349, 2003

[187] Chen X, Zhang SL, Pang L, Filep JG, Tang SS, Ingelfinger JR, Chan JS: Characterization of a putative insulin-responsive element and its binding protein(s) in rat angiotensinogen gene promoter: Regulation by glucose and insulin. *Endocrinology* 142: 2577-2585, 2001

[188] Hsieh TJ, Fustier P, Wei CC, Zhang SL, Filep JG, Tang SS, Ingelfinger JR, Fantus IG, Hamet P, Chan JS: Reactive oxygen species blockade and action of insulin on expression of angiotensinogen gene in proximal tubular cells. *J.Endocrinol.* 183: 535-550, 2004

[189] Kobori H, Nishiyama A, Abe Y, Navar LG: Enhancement of intrarenal angiotensinogen in Dahl salt-sensitive rats on high salt diet. *Hypertension* 41: 592-597, 2003

[190] Kobori H, Nishiyama A: Effects of tempol on renal angiotensinogen production in Dahl salt-sensitive rats. *Biochem. Biophys. Res. Commu.n* 315: 746-750, 2004

[191] Rigat B, Hubert C, Alhenc-Gelas F, Cambien F, Corvol P, Soubrier F: An insertion/deletion polymorphism in the angiotensin I-converting enzyme gene accounting for half the variance of serum enzyme levels. *J. Clin. Invest.* 86: 1343-1346, 1990

[192] Mizuiri S, Hemmi H, Kumanomidou H, Iwamoto M, Miyagi M, Sakai K, Aikawa A, Ohara T, Yamada K, Shimatake H, Hasegawa A: Angiotensin-converting enzyme (ACE) I/d genotype and renal ACE gene expression. *Kidney Int.* 60: 1124-1130, 2001

[193] Marre M, Jeunemaitre X, Gallois Y, Rodier M, Chatellier G, Sert C, Dusselier L, Kahal Z, Chaillous L, Halimi S, Muller A, Sackmann H, Bauduceau B, Bled F, Passa P, Alhenc-Gelas F: Contribution of genetic polymorphism in the renin-angiotensin system to the development of renal complications in insulin-dependent diabetes: Genetique de la nephropathie diabetique (GENEDIAB) study group. *J. Clin. Invest.* 99: 1585-1595, 1997

[194] Hadjadj S, Belloum R, Bouhanick B, Gallois Y, Guilloteau G, Chatellier G, Alhenc-Gelas F, Marre M: Prognostic value of angiotensin-I converting enzyme I/d polymorphism for nephropathy in type 1 diabetes mellitus: A prospective study. *J.Am. Soc. Nephrol.* 12: 54 1-549, 2001

[195] Parving HH, Tarnow L, Rossing P: Genetics of diabetic nephropathy. *J.Am. Soc. Nephrol.* 7: 2509-2517, 1996

[196] Ng DP, Tai BC, Koh D, Tan KW, Chia KS: Angiotensin-I converting enzyme insertion/deletion polymorphism and its association with diabetic nephropathy: A meta-analysis of studies reported between 1994 and 2004 and comprising 14,727 subjects. *Diabetologia* 48: 1008-1016, 2005

[197] Osawa N, Koya D, Araki S, Uzu T, Tsunoda T, Kashiwagi A, Nakamura Y, Maeda S: Combinational effect of genes for the renin-angiotensin system in conferring susceptibility to diabetic nephropathy. *J.Hum. Genet.* 52: 143-151, 2007

[198] So WY, Ma RC, Ozaki R, Tong PC, Ng MC, Ho CS, Lam CW, Chow CC, Chan WB, Kong AP, Chan JC: Angiotensin-converting enzyme (ACE) inhibition in type 2, diabetic patients--interaction with ACE insertion/deletion polymorphism. *Kidney Int.* 69: 1438-1443, 2006

[199] Jacobsen PK, Tarnow L, Parving HH: Time to consider ACE insertion/deletion genotypes and individual renoprotective treatment in diabetic nephropathy? *Kidney Int.* 69: 1293-1295, 2006

[200] Jacobsen P, Tarnow L, Carstensen B, Hovind P, Poirier O, Parving HH: Genetic variation in the renin-angiotensin system and progression of diabetic nephropathy. *J.Am. Soc. Nephrol.* 14: 2843-2850, 2003

[201] Hansson L, Lindholm LH, Niskanen L, Lanke J, Hedner T, Niklason A, Luomanmaki K, Dahlof B, de Faire U, Morlin C, Karlberg BE, Wester PO, Bjorck JE: Effect of angiotensin-converting-enzyme inhibition compared with conventional therapy on cardiovascular morbidity and mortality in hypertension: The captopril prevention project (CAPPP) randomised trial. *Lancet* 353: 611-616, 1999

[202] Efficacy of atenolol and captopril in reducing risk of macrovascular and microvascular complications in type 2 diabetes: UKPDS 39. UK prospective diabetes study group. *BMJ* 317: 713-720, 1998

[203] Schmieder RE: Endothelial dysfunction: How can one intervene at the beginning of the cardiovascular continuum? *J.Hypertens. Suppl.* 24: S31-35, 2006

[204] Parving HH, Lehnert H, Brochner-Mortensen J, Gomis R, Andersen S, Arner P, Irbesartan in Patients with Type 2 Diabetes and Microalbuminuria Study G: The effect of irbesartan on the development of diabetic nephropathy in patients with type 2 diabetes. *N. Engl. J. Med.* 345: 870-878, 2001

[205] Ruggenenti P, Fassi A, IlievaAP, Bruno S, Iliev IP, Brusegan V, Rubis N, Gherardi G, Arnoldi F, Ganeva M, Ene-Iordache B, Gaspari F, Perna A, Bossi A, Trevisan R, Dodesini AR, Remuzzi G, Bergamo Nephrologic Diabetes Complications Trial I: Preventing microalbuminuria in type 2 diabetes. *N. Engl. J. Med.* 351: 1941-1951, 2004

[206] Agodoa LY, Appel L, Bakris GL, Beck G, Bourgoignie J, Briggs JP, Charleston J, Cheek D, Cleveland W, Douglas JG, Douglas M, Dowie D, Faulkner M, Gabriel A, Gassman J, Greene T, Hall Y, Hebert L, Hiremath L, Jamerson K, Johnson CJ, Kopple J, Kusek J, Lash J, Lea J, Lewis JB, Lipkowitz M, Massry S, Middleton J, Miller ER, 3rd, Norris K, O'Connor D, Ojo A, Phillips RA, Pogue V, Rahman M, Randall OS, Rostand S, Schulman G, Smith W, ThornleyBrown D, Tisher CC, Toto RD, Wright JT, Jr., Xu S,African American Study of Kidney Disease and Hypertension Study G: Effect of ramipril vs amlodipine on renal outcomes in hypertensive nephrosclerosis: A randomized controlled trial. *JAMA* 285: 27 19-2728, 2001

[207] Lewis EJ, Hunsicker LG, Clarke WR, Berl T, Pohl MA, Lewis JB, Ritz E,Atkins RC, Rohde R, Raz I: Renoprotective effect of the angiotensin-receptor antagonist irbesartan in patients with nephropathy due to type 2 diabetes. *N.Eng.l J. Med.* 345: 85 1-860, 2001

[208] Barnett AH, Bain SC, Bouter P, Karlberg B, Madsbad S, Jervell J, Mustonen J: Angiotensin-receptor blockade versus converting-enzyme inhibition in type 2 diabetes and nephropathy. *N. Engl.J.Med.* 351: 1952-1961, 2004

[209] Mann JF, Schmieder RE, McQueen M, Dyal L, Schumacher H, Pogue J, Wang X, Maggioni A, Budaj A, Chaithiraphan S, Dickstein K, Keltai M, Metsarinne K, Oto A, Parkhomenko A, Piegas LS, Svendsen TL, Teo KK, Yusuf S, investigators O: Renal outcomes with telmisartan, ramipril, or both, in people at high vascular risk (the ONTARGET study): A multicentre, randomised, double-blind, controlled trial. *Lancet* 372: 547-553, 2008

[210] Coresh J, Selvin E, Stevens LA, Manzi J, Kusek JW, Eggers P, Van Lente F, Levey AS: Prevalence of chronic kidney disease in the United States. *JAMA* 298: 2038-2047,2007

[211] Perkins BA, Ficociello LH, Silva KH, Finkelstein DM, Warram JH, Krolewski AS: Regression of microalbuminuria in type 1 diabetes. *NEngl. J.Med.* 348: 2285-2293,2003

[212] Gould AB, Green D: Kinetics of the human renin and human substrate reaction. *Cardiovasc. Res.* 5: 86-89, 1971

[213] Brasier AR, Li J: Mechanisms for inducible control of angiotensinogen gene transcription. *Hypertension* 27: 465-475, 1996

[214] Ding Y, Davisson RL, Hardy DO, Zhu LJ, Merrill DC, Catterall JF, Sigmund CD: The kidney androgen-regulated protein promoter confers renal proximal tubule cell-specific

and highly androgen-responsive expression on the human angiotensinogen gene in transgenic mice. *JBiou Chem.* 272: 28142-28148, 1997

[215] Kimura S, Mullins JJ, Bunnemann B, Metzger R, Hilgenfeldt U, Zimmermann F, Jacob H, Fuxe K, Ganten D, Kaling M: High blood pressure in transgenic mice carrying the rat angiotensinogen gene. *EMBO J.* 11: 821-827, 1992

[216] Fukamizu A, Sugimura K, Takimoto E, Sugiyama F, Seo MS, Takahashi S, Hatae T, Kajiwara N, Yagami K, Murakami K: Chimeric renin-angiotensin system demonstrates sustained increase in blood pressure of transgenic mice carrying both human renin and human angiotensinogen genes. *J. Biou. Chem.* 268: 11617-11621, 1993

[217] Bohlender J, Menard J, Ganten D, Luft FC: Angiotensinogen concentrations and renin clearance: Implications for blood pressure regulation. *Hypertension* 35: 780-786, 2000

[218] Smithies O: Theodore cooper memorial lecture. A mouse view of hypertension. *Hypertension* 30: 1318-1324, 1997

[219] Merrill DC, Thompson MW, Carney CL, Granwehr BP, Schlager G, Robillard JE, Sigmund CD: Chronic hypertension and altered baroreflex responses in transgenic mice containing the human renin and human angiotensinogen genes. *J. Cuin. Invest.* 97: 1047-1055, 1996

[220] Kobori H, Ozawa Y, Satou R, Katsurada A, Miyata K, Ohashi N, Hase N, Suzaki Y, Sigmund CD, Navar LG: Kidney-specific enhancement of ANG II stimulates endogenous intrarenal angiotensinogen in gene-targeted mice. *Am J Physiol Renal Physiol* 293: F938-F945, 2007

[221] Sachetelli S, Liu Q, Zhang SL, Liu F, Hsieh TJ, Brezniceanu ML, Guo DF, Filep JG, Ingelfinger JR, Sigmund CD, Hamet P, Chan JS: RAS blockade decreases blood pressure and proteinuria in transgenic mice overexpressing rat angiotensinogen gene in the kidney. *Kidney Int.* 69: 1016-1023, 2006

[222] Lavoie JL, Lake-Bruse KD, Sigmund CD: Increased blood pressure in transgenic mice expressing both human renin and angiotensinogen in the renal proximal tubule. *Am. J. Physiol. Renal. Physiol.* 286: F965-971, 2004

[223] Smithies O, Kim HS: Targeted gene duplication and disruption for analyzing quantitative genetic traits in mice. *Proc. Natl. Acad. Sci. U S A* 91: 3612-3615, 1994

[224] Kim HS, Krege JH, Kluckman KD, Hagaman JR, Hodgin JB, Best CF, Jennette JC, Coffman TM, Maeda N, Smithies O: Genetic control of blood pressure and the angiotensinogen locus. *Proc. Natl. Acad. Sci. U S A* 92: 2735-2739, 1995

[225] Inoue I, Nakajima T, Williams CS, Quackenbush J, Puryear R, Powers M, Cheng T, Ludwig EH, Sharma AM, Hata A, Jeunemaitre X, Lalouel JM: A nucleotide substitution in the promoter of human angiotensinogen is associated with essential hypertension and affects basal transcription in vitro. *J. Clin. Invest.* 99: 1786-1797, 1997

[226] Jeunemaitre X, Soubrier F, Kotelevtsev YV, Lifton RP, Williams CS, Charru A, Hunt SC, Hopkins PN, Williams RR, Lalouel JM: Molecular basis of human hypertension: Role of angiotensinogen. *Cell* 71: 169-180, 1992

[227] Zhao YY, Zhou J, Narayanan CS, Cui Y, Kumar A: Role of C/A polymorphism at -20 on the expression of human angiotensinogen gene. *Hypertension* 33: 108-115, 1999

[228] Ishigami T, Umemura S, Tamura K, Hibi K, Nyui N, Kihara M, Yabana M, Watanabe Y, Sumida Y, Nagahara T, Ochiai H, Ishii M: Essential hypertension and 5' upstream core promoter region of human angiotensinogen gene. *Hypertension* 30: 1325-1330, 1997

[229] Schunkert H, Ingelfinger JR, Jacob H, Jackson B, Bouyounes B, Dzau VJ: Reciprocal feedback regulation of kidney angiotensinogen and renin mRNA expressions by angiotensin II. *Am. J. Physiol.* 263: E863-E869, 1992

[230] Kobori H, Prieto-Carrasquero MC, Ozawa Y, Navar LG: AT1 receptor mediated augmentation of intrarenal angiotensinogen in angiotensin II-dependent hypertension. *Hypertension* 43: 1126-1132, 2004

[231] Kobori H, Nishiyama A, Harrison-Bernard LM, Navar LG: Urinary angiotensinogen as an indicator of intrarenal angiotensin status in hypertension. *Hypertension* 41: 42-49, 2003

[232] Kobori H, Harrison-Bernard LM, Navar LG: Urinary excretion of angiotensinogen reflects intrarenal angiotensinogen production. *Kidney Int.* 61: 579-585, 2002

[233] Kobori H, Harrison-Bernard LM, Navar LG: Enhancement of angiotensinogen expression in angiotensin II-dependent hypertension. *Hypertension* 37: 1329-1335, 2001

[234] Kobori H, Ozawa Y, Suzaki Y, Nishiyama A: Enhanced intrarenal angiotensinogen contributes to early renal injury in spontaneously hypertensive rats. *J Am Soc Nephrol* 16: 2073-2080, 2005

[235] Singh R, Singh AK, Leehey DJ: A novel mechanism for angiotensin II formation in streptozotocin-diabetic rat glomeruli. *Am. J. Physiol. Renal. Physiol.* 288: F1183-1190, 2005

[236] Leehey DJ, Singh AK, Bast JP, Sethupathi P, Singh R: Glomerular renin angiotensin system in streptozotocin diabetic and Zucker diabetic fatty rats. *Transl. Res.* 151: 208-216, 2008

[237] Kobori H, Katsurada A, Ozawa Y, Satou R, Miyata K, Hase N, Suzuki Y, Shoji T: Enhanced intrarenal oxidative stress and angiotensinogen in IgA nephropathy patients. *Biochem Biophys. Res. Commun.* 358: 156-163, 2007

[238] Takamatsu M, Urushihara M, Kondo S, Shimizu M, Morioka T, Oite T, Kobori H, Kagami S: Glomerular angiotensinogen protein is enhanced in pediatric IgA nephropathy. *Pediat. Nephrol.* 23: 1257-1267, 2008

[239] Kobori H, Ozawa Y, Suzaki Y, Prieto-Carrasquero MC, NishiyamaA, Shoji T, Cohen EP, Navar LG: Young scholars award lecture: Intratubular angiotensinogen in hypertension and kidney diseases. *Am. J. Hypertens.* 19: 541-550, 2006

[240] Katsurada A, Hagiwara Y, Miyashita K, Satou R, Miyata K, Ohashi N, Navar LG, Kobori H: Novel sandwich ELISA for human angiotensinogen. *Am. J. Physiol. Renal Physiol.* 293: F956-F960, 2007

[241] Yamamoto T, Nakagawa T, Suzuki H, Ohashi N, Fukasawa H, Fujigaki Y, Kato A, Nakamura Y, Suzuki F, Hishida A: Urinary angiotensinogen as a marker of intrarenal angiotensin II activity associated with deterioration of renal function in patients with chronic kidney disease. *Jam. Soc. Nephrol.* 18: 1558-1565, 2007

[242] Kobori H, Ohashi N, Katsurada A, Miyata K, Satou R, Saito T, Yamamoto T: Urinary angiotensinogen as a potential biomarker of severity of chronic kidney diseases. *Jam. Soc. Hypertens* 2: 349-354, 2008

[243] Kobori H, Alper AB, Shenava R, Katsurada A, Saito T, Ohashi N, Urushihara M, Miyata K, Satou R, Hamm LL, Navar LG: Urinary angiotensinogen as a novel biomarker of the intrarenal renin-angiotensin system status in hypertensive patients. *Hypertension* 53: 344-350, 2009

[244] Ogawa S, Kobori H, Ohashi N, Urushihara M, Nishiyama A, Mori T, Ishizuka T, Nako K, Ito S: Angiotensin II type 1 receptor blockers reduce urinary angiotensinogen excretion and the levels of urinary markers of oxidative stress and inflammation in patients with type 2 diabetic nephropathy. *Biomark Insights* 4: 97-102, 2009

[245] Saito T, Urushihara M, Kotani Y, Kagami S, Kobori H: Increased urinary angiotensinogen is precedent to increased urinary albumin in patients with type 1 diabetes. *Am. J. Med. Sci.* 338: 478-480, 2009

In: Advances in Pathogenesis of Diabetic Nephropathy
Editor: Sharma S. Prabhakar

ISBN: 978-1-61122-134-3
© 2012 Nova Science Publishers, Inc.

Chapter IX

Role of Oxidative Stress in Diabetic Nephropathy

Josephine M. Forbes[1,2,*], Melinda T. Coughlan[1] and Mark E. Cooper[1,2]

[1]JDRF Einstein Centre for Diabetes Complications, Division of Diabetes Complications, Baker IDI Heart and Diabetes Institute, Melbourne, Australia
[2]Departments of Medicine and Immunology, Monash University, AMREP Precinct, Melbourne, Australia

Abstract

Oxidative stress, occurs primarily as the result of normal metabolism but is facilitated by the conditions present in a number of chronic disorders, including diabetic nephropathy (DN). It is postulated, that oxidative stress is an early link between hyperglycaemia and renal disease but also likely occurs as a consequence of other primary pathogenic mechanisms seen in diabetes. There are a number of pathways which generate reactive oxygen species (ROS) in the kidney such as glycolysis, specific defects in the polyol pathway, uncoupling of nitric oxide synthase, xanthine oxidase, NAD(P)H oxidase and advanced glycation which have each been identified as potentially major contributors to the pathogenesis of diabetic kidney disease. In addition, mitochondrial production of ROS in response to chronic hyperglycaemia may also be a key contributor to each of these pathogenic pathways.

To date, it is unclear as to why antioxidants *per se* have demonstrated such poor renoprotection in humans, despite exciting positive preclinical research findings, however, it seems evident that therapies such as vitamins may not be the ideal antioxidant strategy in human diabetic nephropathy. More recent data have suggested that combined strategies involving a more targeted antioxidant approach, using agents which penetrate specific cellular compartments, may be the elusive additive therapy required to optimise renoprotection in diabetes.

---

[*] Corresponding Author: A/Professor Josephine Forbes, Head, JDRF Einstein Centre, Division of Diabetes Complications, Baker IDI Heart & Diabetes Institute, Postal Address: PO Box 6492, St Kilda Rd Central, Melbourne, Vic 8008, Australia, Courier address: 75 Commercial Rd, Melbourne, Vic, 3004. Australia, Ph: 61 3 8532 1456, Fax: 61 3 8532 1480, josephine.forbes@bakeridi.edu.au.

Keywords: mitochondrial dysfunction, reactive oxygen species, NADPH oxidase, diabetes complications, mitochondria

Introduction

Diabetes and its complications are the most rapidly growing epidemic of the 21st century, with some 25-40% of patients developing renal impairment. Diabetic renal disease is characterised by functional as well as structural abnormalities [1]. Structural changes include thickening of basement membranes, mesangial expansion, hypertrophy and glomerular epithelial cell (podocyte) loss within glomeruli. Concomitantly, the tubulointerstitial compartment demonstrates expansion of tubular basement membranes, tubular atrophy, interstitial fibrosis and arteriosclerosis.

Many large clinical trials (DCCT/UKPDS/ACCORD/ADVANCE) have established that the most important, and yet obvious, risk factor for diabetic microvascular disease, in particular nephropathy, is poor metabolic control, resulting in hyperglycaemia [2-4]. To date, aside from strict metabolic control, the most effective treatments for progressive diabetic nephropathy appear to be anti-hypertensive agents, particularly those that target the renin-angiotensin system (RAS), such as angiotensin converting enzyme inhibitors, angiotensin receptor-1 antagonists or their combination [5-7]. Although these treatments retard the relentless progression to end stage renal disease that occurs in diabetic patients susceptible to nephropathy, these agents do not prevent this disorder.

Defining "Oxidative Stress"

Oxidative stress (or oxidant-derived tissue injury) represents an imbalance among production of pro-oxidants or reactive oxygen species (ROS) which exceeds local antioxidant capacity. When this occurs, there is oxidation of important macromolecules including proteins, lipids and carbohydrates. Many experimental animal studies have demonstrated that potent inhibition of oxidative stress with certain antioxidants [8, 9] provides end organ protection in experimental diabetes. Sadly, human studies with various antioxidants including α-tocopherol [10] have in general, been disappointing. Thus, there is a general view that conventional antioxidant therapy is not likely to have particular benefit as part of the strategy to reduce diabetic complications including nephropathy. In this chapter, we focus on the diverse sources of ROS generation in a diabetic milieu and postulate that more targeted, rationally designed antioxidant approaches may ultimately be worth considering as part of the therapeutic strategy to optimise renoprotection in diabetes.

Within the diabetic kidney, there are a number of enzymatic and non-enzymatic sources of ROS. These include autooxidation of glucose, transition metal catalysed Fenton reactions, advanced glycation, polyol pathway flux, mitochondrial respiratory chain deficiencies, xanthine oxidase activity, peroxidases, nitric oxide synthase (NOS) and nicotinamide adenine dinucleotide phosphate (NAD(P)H) oxidase (11). Reactive oxygen species liberated within the kidney include free radicals such as superoxide ($^{\bullet}O_2^-$), hydroxyl ($^{\bullet}OH$), peroxyl ($^{\bullet}RO_2$) as well as non-radical species such as hydrogen peroxide (H_2O_2) and hypoochlorous acid

(HOCl) [12]. There are also reactive nitrogen species produced from similar pathways, which include the radicals nitric oxide (•NO) and nitrogen dioxide (•NO$_2^-$) as well as the non-radical peroxynitrite (ONOO$^-$), nitrous oxide (HNO$_2$) and alkyl peroxynitrates (RONOO) (12). Of these, •O$_2^-$, •NO, H$_2$O$_2$ and ONOO$^-$ have been the most widely investigated in the diabetic kidney and hence these sources are the focus of this chapter.

Antioxidants and their Role in Detoxifying ROS

Mammals have evolved numerous antioxidant systems in response to excess ROS production as a consequence of respiration and metabolism during homeostasis. Arguably, the most important of these antioxidant enzymes is superoxide dismutase which exists in three major cellular forms, copper zinc superoxide dismutase, (CuZnSOD, *SOD1*), manganese SOD (MnSOD, *SOD2*) and extracellular SOD (*SOD3*). These enzymes are responsible for the detoxification of superoxide radicals to hydrogen peroxide and water in different cellular compartments. Glutathione peroxidase (GPx) and catalase are other antioxidant enzymes, which catalyse the conversion of hydrogen peroxide to water.

Decreases in expression and in some instances the activity of each of these antioxidant enzymes has been previously reported in diabetic microvascular disease [13]. Indeed, the over-expression of CuZnSOD protects against end organ damage in experimental models of type 2 diabetic nephropathy [14]. More recently, multiple CuZnSOD gene variants have shown associations with the development of diabetic nephropathy in humans [15]. Other studies in mice with genetic deletions of various antioxidant enzymes have also provided insight into the relative contribution of MnSOD [16] to the development of diabetic complications. MnSOD mimetics such as MnTBAP have also shown efficacy in preventing ROS induced injury *in vitro* [17] although the utility *in vivo* of such drugs is likely to be limited [18]. Further strengthening a potential role for the antioxidant MnSOD, specific polymorphisms of the MnSOD gene are associated with the development of diabetic nephropathy in humans [19].

Interestingly, GPx-1 deficient mice have no increased risk for microvascular disease, in particular diabetic nephropathy [20], which may be due to redundancy with respect to other renal GPx isoforms, in particular including GPx-3. However, podocyte specific knockout of selenoproteins does not exacerbate nephropathy in experimental models of diabetes suggesting that functional GPx may not be important for protection against the development and progression of nephropathy [21]. Over-expression of catalase in experimental models of type 2 diabetic nephropathy appears to be protective [22]. However, in contrast to both CuZnSOD and MnSOD, catalase gene polymorphisms which interfere with its cellular expression are not associated with increased incidence of nephropathy in type 2 diabetic patients [23].

Lipoic acid is an organosulfur compound, which is an essential cofactor for many enzyme complexes, termed "lipoate" in physiological systems. It is essential for aerobic life and is a common and sometimes controversial dietary supplement. There have been a number of studies demonstrating the benefits of treatment with α-lipoic acid in both experimental models [24] and in human clinical studies of patients with diabetic nephropathy [25] often above those seen with vitamin C or E [24].

There are numerous other antioxidants present within cells, such as the vitamins benfotiamine and thiamine [26], metallothionein [27], thioredoxin [28] and amino acids such as taurine [29], which may also play a role in protection against diabetic nephropathy, although these are not discussed in detail within this chapter.

Glucose Uptake in Renal Cells

It is not surprising that the most important factor in the excessive intracellular generation of ROS by hyperglycaemia, is the ability of individual cell types to process glucose. Renal cells must be able to modulate the transport of glucose across the plasma membrane into the cytosol, in order to maintain intracellular glucose homeostasis. It is well understood that certain cell populations including the retinal capillary endothelial cells, mesangial cells in the renal glomeruli, and neuronal and Schwann cells in peripheral nerves, do not have the ability to control glucose transport rates in order to prevent excessive changes in intracellular glucose concentrations during hyperglycaemia [30]. Indeed, enhanced glucose uptake has been identified in many of the cell populations within the diabetic kidney, including glomerular epithelial cells [31], mesangial cells [32] and proximal tubular epithelial cells [33]. Thus, these specific cell populations may be particularly susceptible to the changing milieu of diabetes, since they are unable to prevent fluctuations in intracellular glucose concentrations in the setting of altered systemic glucose concentrations. It is not hard to see why intensive glycaemic control is the most desirable method to prevent progressive diabetic renal disease, particularly as an early intervention to limit cellular ROS generation by enabling these specific susceptible cell populations to decrease glucose uptake in hyperglycaemic environments. This is substantiated by studies in experimental diabetic nephropathy with interventions to prevent membrane localisation of glucose transporters, in particular GLUT-1 [30, 34].

Auto-oxidation of glucose in the presence of transition metals is also thought to generate ROS in diabetes, although this theoretical pathway, which has been shown *in vitro*, has never been substantiated *in vivo*. Since both high glucose concentrations and the non-metabolizable glucose analogue 3-O-methylglucopyranose (3-OMG) cause equivocal increases in $^\bullet O_2^-$, it is hypothesized that the metabolism of glucose is not necessary for the production of ROS [35]. Therefore, it is predicted that auto-oxidation of glucose may occur within the circulation, extracellular spaces or within cells. Furthermore, this process is not inhibited by blockade of enzymatic sources of ROS, but only with metal chelators such as diethylenetriamine penta-acetic acid or EDTA [36]. However, the contribution of this process to the development of diabetic renal disease remains to be determined.

Cytosolic Sources of Reactive Oxygen Species

Glycolysis

Following its transport into the cell, glucose is converted via glycolysis to glucose-6-phosphate, which is then sequentially processed to pyruvate. Cellular glycolysis has many paradoxes relating to the production of excess ROS. On one hand, in diabetic complications it is intuitive that restricting cellular glucose uptake in order to maintain intracellular glucose homeostasis is likely a critical protection mechanism in susceptible cell populations to minimise cellular damage and ROS generation. On the other hand there is evidence, suggesting that restriction of cellular glucose uptake causes production of small quantities of cellular ROS, which improve cell survival [37]. This finding is further supported by data in *C.elegans* which demonstrate that antioxidant therapies impair cellular survival, by restoring glucose uptake [37]. Theoretically, it is thought that exposure to low grade stress and associated elevations in ROS, primes cells against pathological injury when vast changes occur in cellular glycolysis. Not surprising in this context is that either caloric restriction [38] or intermittent feeding patterns [39], protect against diabetic renal disease in rodent models of diabetes. In reality, long term compliance to such a dietary oriented regimen is unlikely and therefore caloric restriction mimetics are currently being tested in ageing [40] where declining renal function also occurs. Although the effects of these mimetics are unknown, disruption of glycolysis can ultimately facilitate the excessive generation of ROS by a number of pathways as reviewed below.

Glucose-6-Phosphate Dehydrogenase

Glucose-6-phosphate dehydrogenase (G6PDH) is a rate limiting enzyme involved in the pentose phosphate pathway and therefore ultimately responsible for ribose synthesis, which is the main source of NAD(P)H, glutathione (GSH) reductase and aldose reductase. A number of studies have identified that altered activity of G6PDH results in cellular oxidative stress [41]. Indeed, deficiencies in the activity of G6PDH are common human enzymopathies, resulting in increased ROS generation and decreases in antioxidants such as GSH [42]. Interestingly, the activity of G6PDH is increased in kidneys from rodents with experimental diabetic nephropathy [43]. This pathway as a potential source of ROS in diabetic nephropathy warrants further investigation.

Flux through the Sorbitol Pathway

Sorbitol/polyol pathway flux was documented more than forty years ago in the hyper-glycaemic setting [44]. The cytosolic enzyme aldose reductase converts high intracellular glucose concentrations to sorbitol using NAD(P)H derived from the pentose phosphate pathway as a cofactor. It is likely that during hyperglycaemia, consumption of NAD(P)H by this reaction inhibits replenishment of reduced glutathione which is required to maintain glutathione peroxidase activity. This would ultimately decrease cellular antioxidant activity. Subsequently, sorbitol is oxidized to fructose via sorbitol dehydrogenase, with NAD+ reduced to NADH, providing increased substrate to complex I of the mitochondrial respiratory chain. Since the mitochondrial respiratory chain is thought to be a major source of excess ROS in diabetes, provision of additional electrons for transfer to oxygen forming superoxide would augment mitochondrial ROS production. In addition, since sorbitol does not cross cell membranes, its intracellular accumulation results in osmotic stress. Osmotic stress *per se* increases cellular cytosolic generation of H_2O_2 [Beffagna, 2005 #647].

Therefore, not surprisingly, administration of osmotic diuretics protects proximal tubular cells from ROS mediated apoptosis [45].

Inhibition of sorbitol accumulation with aldose reductase blockade has been shown to delay, prevent, and at early stages, to reverse diabetic complications, particularly experimental diabetic neuropathy [46]. Clinical trials, have in general been disappointing, despite decades of investigation and have been marred by limited tissue penetration and a range of side effects from most of these agents. Despite this, two aldose reductase inhibitors, zenarestat and fidarestat, have demonstrated improvements in neural function and fibre density [47, 48] in humans. Currently, however, the clinical utility of aldose reductase inhibitors remains uncertain.

Advanced Glycation

Non-enzymatic glycation of free amino groups on proteins and amino acids begins with covalent attachment of sugar moieties at a rate determined by a number of factors including intracellular glucose concentrations, pH and time in a biochemical "Maillard reaction" [49]. Physiologically, this is thought to be an evolutionary pathway for labelling of senescent cellular proteins for their recognition and ultimate turnover. In both major forms of diabetes, persistent hyperglycaemia and oxidative stress act to hasten the formation of advanced glycation end products (AGEs) [50], causing long-lived proteins to become more heavily altered, in addition to modifying shorter-lived molecules [51, 52]. Furthermore, elevated intracellular glucose degradation products such as glyoxal resulting from glycolysis and the tricarboxylic acid (TCA) cycle, initiate the glycation of intracellular proteins far more rapidly than glucose itself [53]. These advanced glycation end products (AGEs) can be generated from intracellular auto-oxidation of glucose to glyoxal [54], decomposition of early glycation (Amadori) products to 3-deoxyglucosone, and fragmentation of metabolites of the pentose phosphate pathway such as glyceraldehyde-3-phosphate and dihydroxyacetone phosphate to the reactive carbonyl methylglyoxal [55]. Excess ROS are generated during the formation of AGEs causing a self-perpetuating cycle of ROS/AGE formation in diseases such as diabetes. The proposed sources of ROS in the Maillard reaction are many and include the autoxidation of glucose (Wolff pathway), Schiff bases (Namiki pathway) and Amadori adducts (Hodge pathway), as well as AGE modified proteins themselves [50].

Since the ultimate fate of most AGEs within the body is renal clearance, AGEs can also interact with a number of renal cellular binding sites, which mediate many of their biological effects. Perhaps the most important of these binding sites is the immunoglobulin superfamily protein, the receptor for advanced glycation end products (RAGE) [56]. RAGE is a multi ligand pattern recognition receptor that is involved in the amplification of immune and inflammatory responses [57]. *In vitro* studies have shown cytosolic generation of ROS through activation of the RAGE receptor in both proximal tubular and mesangial cells, most likely through NAD(P)H oxidase [58] This further supports the interaction of AGEs with full-length cellular RAGE and subsequent cytosolic ROS generation as a major player in the development of nephropathy. AGE-RAGE interactions leading to ROS generation have also been suggested as pathogenic pathways in complementary *in vivo* studies in diabetic nephropathy [59].

While there are a number of antioxidant systems in place to limit tissue damage initiated by the Maillard reaction including detoxification systems such as the glyoxalase pathway, aldose reductases, aldehyde dehydrogenases and the chelation of metal ions [60, 61], the ultimate development of tissue injury depends on the balance between the rate of formation of AGE modified proteins, protection by these various systems, in addition to renal clearance. Of particular interest, is that AGE modifications can occur on antioxidant enzymes such as CuZnSOD and MnSOD in diabetes [62], which would alter the activity of these enzymes, ultimately further contributing to excess cellular ROS accumulation.

In models of experimentaldiabetic nephropathy, there are clear benefits associated with a variety of AGE inhibitors [63-66], which act in disparate ways in the context of improvements in cellular ROS generation. In experimental diabetic nephropathy, alagebrium chloride decreases renal mitochondrial ROS generation, which is not seen with RAS blockade [67]. Indeed, the utility of alagebrium chloride is currently being investigated in type 1 diabetic patients with microalbuminuria, treated with concomitant ACE inhibition (PHASE IIb, http://www.alteon.com). In addition, benfotiamine has also shown efficacy in the treatment of patients with painful diabetic neuropathy, but to date has not been studied in clinical diabetic nephropathy [68]. However, another study has demonstrated a lack of effect of benfotiamine on complication causing pathways in type 1 diabetic patients [69].

Blockade of RAGE signal transduction [58, 70] may also be a useful strategy to improve diabetic renal disease, although amelioration of renal ROS generation with this approach has not been documented to date. Furthermore, the clinical utility of such agents targeting AGEs and/or RAGE in preventing or retarding diabetic nephropathy is yet to be determined but is an area of active preclinical and clinical investigation.

NAD(P)H Oxidase

The best characterised NAD(P)H oxidase is a cytosolic enzyme complex which was initially discovered in neutrophils where it plays a critical role in "oxidative burst" in non-specific host-pathogen defence, producing millimolar quantities of $^\bullet O_2^-$ by electron transport [71]. This enzyme complex is composed of five subunits comprising a membrane-associated $p22^{phox}$ and a $gp91^{phox}$ subunit and at least four cytosolic subunits, $p47^{phox}$, $p67^{phox}$, $p40^{phox}$, and GTPase $rac1$ or $rac2$ [71]. The gp91phox subunit has other renal homologues namely Nox-3 and Nox-4, which have been identified in foetal kidney and renal cortical tissues respectively [72]. In addition to residing in phagocytic cells, NAD(P)H oxidase is present in non-phagocytic renal cell types such as mesangial and proximal tubular cells, vascular smooth muscle cells, endothelial cells and fibroblasts. In these cell types, however, $^\bullet O_2^-$ production is proportionally lower than in activated neutrophils and hence, the intrinsic function of this enzyme in non-phagocytic cells is likely different to that seen in phagocytic and other white cell populations since. Indeed, ROS generated in this context in the intracellular compartment by NAD(P)H oxidase most likely act as second messengers. Indeed, binding of several cytokines and hormones such as tumour necrosis factor-α (TNF-α), platelet derived growth factor (PDGF) and angiotensin II to their cognate receptors rapidly activates NAD(P)H oxidase followed by intracellular $^\bullet O_2^-$ and H_2O_2 generation [73]. This is evident from studies using pharmacological inhibition of NAD(P)H oxidase, mice with deletions of the various NAD(P)H oxidase subunits, or treatment with anti-sense oligonucleotides [73].

Non-phagocytic NAD(P)H oxidase can also generate excessive ROS production, contributing to cellular oxidative stress. This has been shown in renal pathological states such as diabetic nephropathy [74], hypertension, inflammation and ischemia-reperfusion injury [75, 76]. Within the kidney, various subunits of NAD(P)H oxidase are increased in experimental diabetic nephropathy [77]. In addition, pharmacological inhibition of NAD(P)H oxidase with apocynin prevents up-regulation of $p47^{phox}$ and $gp91^{phox}$ over-expression seen in experimental diabetic nephropathy [74, 78]. Furthermore, a more specific therapeutic approach using anti-sense oligonucleotides to Nox-4, the renal $gp91^{phox}$ homologue, inhibited NAD(P)H-dependent ROS generation in renal cortical and glomerular homogenates resulting in attenuation of renal hypertrophy [79]. These data highlight the importance of NAD(P)H oxidase as a potential pathogenic mediator of hyperglycaemia induced ROS production.

Xanthine Oxidase

Xanthine oxidase is the enzyme which catalyzes the oxidation of hypoxanthine to uric acid using molecular oxygen as the electron acceptor. Consequently, this liberates a number of ROS including $^{\bullet}O_2^-$, $^{\bullet}OH$ and H_2O_2. Under normal physiological conditions, levels of xanthine oxidase activity are unmeasurable in most cell types, although sensitive electron spin technologies have confirmed xanthine oxidase as an important source of vascular superoxide generation in experimental models of type 1 diabetes [80]. Indeed the xanthine oxidase inhibitor allopurinol has shown therapeutic benefit in experimental diabetic rodent models of neuropathy and vascular dysfunction [81]. Despite these data, there is no direct evidence of abnormalities in this pathway within renal tissues in experimental or human diabetes and thus the contribution of this enzyme to the pathogenesis of diabetic nephropathy remains to be elucidated.

Uncoupling of Nitric Oxide Synthase

There are three major isoforms of nitric oxide synthase (NOS), inducible (iNOS), neuronal (nNOS) and endothelial (eNOS). Each of these isoforms requires five cofactors/prosthetics such as flavinmononucleotide (FMN), bihydrobiopterin (BH4), calmodulin and flavin adenine dinucleotide (FAD) to produce $^{\bullet}NO$ [82]. In diabetes, uncoupling of NOS due to restricted substrate (L-arginine) availability or the absence of cofactors, is thought to generate $^{\bullet}O_2^-$ in preference to $^{\bullet}NO$ [82]. Indeed, one study in experimental diabetic nephropathy has suggested that uncoupling of NOS, in addition to NADPH oxidase are two major sources of glomerular superoxide [83]. In that study, restoration of physiological levels of BH4 attenuated ROS production and improved renal function.

There are however, numerous paradoxical roles for $^{\bullet}NO$ seen in diabetic nephropathy. Based on current findings, it is reasonable to suggest that early nephropathy in diabetes is associated with increased intrarenal $^{\bullet}NO$ production [84] mediated primarily by constitutively released $^{\bullet}NO$ (endothelial nitric oxide synthase, eNOS and neuronal nitric oxide synthase, nNOS) [83]. Indeed, enhanced •NO production may contribute to the hyperfiltration and other haemodynamic changes that characterize early diabetic nephropathy [85]. This is supported by studies in early diabetic nephropathy where L-NAME reversed haemodynamic changes and renal damage [86].

On the other hand, the majority of the studies in advanced diabetic renal disease indicate that severe proteinuria, declining renal function, and hypertension are associated with a state of progressive •NO deficiency [87]. Advanced renal changes attributed to •NO are thought to be mediated through multiple mechanisms such as glucose and AGE quenching, and inhibition and/or post-translational modification of NOS, which changes the activity of both endothelial and inducible isoforms. Indeed, some authors have reported no effect [88] or aggravation of renal damage by chronic NO inhibition in models of type 1 and type 2 diabetic nephropathy respectively [89]. Furthermore, mice with a genetic deficiency in eNOS have exacerbated renal disease in the context of diabetes [90].

Genetic polymorphisms of the NOS enzyme may also play a role in the •NO abnormalities that contribute to the development and progression of diabetic nephropathy [87]. Owing to the different temporal changes in •NO production during the pathogenesis of diabetic nephropathy, there is much controversy as to the utility of approaches, which inhibit NOS activity for clinical application.

Therefore, owing to the complex temporal changes in •NO production during the evolution of diabetic nephropathy, there is ongoing controversy as to the clinical applicability of approaches which directly inhibit NOS activity.

Mitochondrial Sources of ROS

Oxidative Phosphorylation

Most glucose which enters the cell is sequentially processed to become fuel for oxidative phosphorylation by the mitochondrial respiratory chain. Once transported intracellularly, glucose is converted to pyruvate and eventually nicotinamide adenine dinucleotide (NADH; reduced form) in addition to reduced flavin adenine dinucleotide ($FADH_2$) by the glycolytic pathway. NADH and $FADH_2$ are then transported into the mitochondria via either the malate-aspartate or the glycerol phosphate shuttle systems. NADH is the main electron donor to the mitochondrial respiratory chain and it is hypothesized that hyperglycaemia increases the NADH/NAD+ ratio in complication prone cell populations [91], although this has not been shown in vivo [92]. Therefore, therapies which would partially lower chronic glycolysis present in cells exposed to hyperglycaemia may be of therapeutic benefit in diabetic complication prone tissues [93], by decreasing the fuel availability to the mitochondrial electron transport chain. Mitochondria can also utilise free fatty acids (FFA), where β-oxidation and oxidation of FFA in the TCA cycle generate the same electron donors for oxidative phosphorylation (NADH and $FADH_2$). Therefore excess FFA can replicate hyperglycaemia induced mitochondrial defects. It is likely that in the context of established renal disease, control of dietary fat intake and circulating LDL cholesterol and triglycerides with HMG-CoA reductase inhibitors, should further protect the mitochondria from FFA induced oxidative damage as has been shown in some studies [94].

The generation of ROS, specifically $^\bullet O_2^-$, by damaged or dysfunctional mitochondria, has previously been postulated as the primary initiating event in the development of diabetic complications [17], although this is now controversial. Despite this, decreasing mitochondrial ROS generation is still considered a relevant aim in ameliorating the burden of diabetic renal disease. Oxidative phosphorylation consumes 90% of all oxygen in humans, and is the process whereby electrons from glucose and other fuels are transferred to molecular oxygen, involving complexes I to IV and finally adenosine triphosphate (ATP) synthase. Protons are pumped across the mitochondrial membrane creating a voltage gradient, which is collapsed to generate ATP. This series of reactions is tightly regulated, however, it is estimated that up to 1% of oxygen is only partially reduced to $^\bullet O_2^-$, instead of fully to water under physiological conditions. The two major sites of electron leakage are at NADH dehydrogenase (Complex I) and at the interface between Coenzyme Q (CoQ) and complex III [95]. Therefore, in diabetes where there is an excess of fuels supplied as a result of chronic hyperglycaemia feeding into the respiratory chain, it has been hypothesized, based primarily on *in vitro* studies [17], that excess production of $^\bullet O_2^-$ is via the premature collapse of the mitochondrial membrane potential, which rather than driving ATP production, leaks electrons to oxygen to form $^\bullet O_2^-$. While these findings are exciting, these predominantly tissue culture studies [96] remain to be fully substantiated *in vivo*, particularly with respect to nephropathy although there is now some suggestion that this may occur *in vivo* [62, 92].

Specifically, dysfunction of the mitochondrial respiratory chain has been postulated to contribute to various disease pathologies, including not only diabetes complications but also a number of other diseases such as Parkinson's disease, Huntington's disease and Alzheimer's disease as well as being implicated in the pathophysiology of aging. Furthermore, patients with genetic defects that decrease the activity of complex I have vastly elevated rates of mitochondrial $^\bullet O_2^-$ production [97]. Additional evidence for mitochondrial oxidative phosphorylation as a candidate in the pathogenesis of diabetic complications comes from the disease Friedreich Ataxia, a genetic disorder due to frataxin mutations causing excessive mitochondrial ROS generation in association with down-regulation of mitochondrial complex I [98]. Indeed, in addition to the well-characterised cardiac dysfunction seen in this disorder, some individuals with Friedreich Ataxia develop renal disease . A role for mitochondria in the development of diabetic kidney disease is further strengthened by the recent observation that up to 50% of children with mitochondrial diseases have renal impairment [99]. Furthermore, some of these subjects with mitochondrial respiratory chain defects have demonstrated renal disease as their primary pathology, including a newly described mitochondriopathy involving a deficiency in coenzyme Q10 which also has primary renal involvement [100]. This suggests that investigation into specific mitochondrial defects and their contribution to diabetic kidney disease are warranted and should be highlighted as a research priority.

Intramitochondrial $^\bullet O_2^-$ production initiates a range of damaging reactions through the production of H_2O_2, ferrous iron, $^\bullet OH$ and $ONOO^-$, which can then damage lipids, proteins and nucleic acids. A number of functional enzymes within the mitochondria are particularly susceptible to ROS mediated damage, leading to altered ATP synthesis, cellular calcium dysregulation and induction of mitochondrial permeability transition, all of which predispose the cell to necrosis or apoptosis. Indeed, localised swelling of mitochondria via induction of mitochondrial pore transition has been previously shown to induce a decrease in the activity of complex I (98). Indeed, localised swelling of mitochondria via induction of mitochondrial pore transition has been previously shown to induce a decrease in the activity of complex I

[101] and which has been postulated as a contributing factor in experimental models of diabetic nephropathy [92].

Idebenone is a new generation mitochondrial antioxidant, which has a high uptake into organs such as the kidney, where one third of its intracellular content is localised within the mitochondria. Studies in humans with Friedreich Ataxia suggest that this antioxidant is a safe and highly efficient way to protect mitochondrial function from oxidative damage [102]. Interestingly, unlike traditional antioxidants such as α-tocopherol, idebenone has been shown to reduce cardiomyopathy in these subjects [102]. It remains to be determined if such an agent may have renoprotective effects in a setting such as diabetes. Mito Q is another new generation antioxidant with selective uptake into mitochondria. This is due to covalent attachment of its antioxidant moiety to the lipophilic triphenylphosphonium cation, which is being tested in patients with Alzheimer's disease (http://www.antipodeanpharma.com). This molecule accumulates 5-10 fold in mitochondria but changes in the membrane potential can increase its uptake by between 100-500 fold [103]. The efficacy of these relatively selective mitochondrial antioxidants in diabetic nephropathy remains to be determined, however, their targeted specificity for mitochondria suggests that intensive preclinical and subsequently clinical investigation is warranted for these agents.

Uncoupling of the Respiratory Chain – Dissipating Energy as Heat

The collapse of the mitochondrial membrane potential can occur via uncoupling of the respiratory chain, dissipating electrons as heat rather than for ATP synthesis. Indeed, chronic uncoupling decreases ATP synthesis and increases the leakage of electrons to oxygen to form $^{\bullet}O_2^-$. There are three major isoforms of uncoupling proteins, UCP-1 to 3 [104], which bind to the respiratory chain at the location of ATP synthase. Studies in diabetic neural tissues [105] and retinal endothelial cells [106] have suggested that chronic over-expression of uncoupling proteins is responsible for the "back up" of electrons in the respiratory chain and their subsequent leakage to $^{\bullet}O_2^-$, although this phenomenon is unsubstantiated *in vivo* in renal tissues [105]. Therefore therapeutic agents lowering mitochondrial superoxide generation by modulating the levels of these proteins may lead to a novel treatment strategy for diabetic renal disease. Indeed, this has been used successfully in other experimental models of disease including those studying beta cell death [107]. Paradoxically, however, low levels of artificial uncouplers may be useful in disorders such as obesity. Thus, the challenge is to create an agent which sufficiently attenuates mitochondrial ROS production without significantly compromising ATP generation.

Interactions among Prominent Pathogenic Pathways in Diabetic Nephropathy and ROS Generation

Given the evidence presented within this chapter, it is likely that changes in cellular function resulting in oxidative stress play a key role in the development and progression of diabetic nephropathy. Early points for therapeutic intervention to reduce ROS generation would include decreasing the cellular uptake and processing of glucose and restricting the feeding of glucose derived metabolites into cellular respiration. It is however, increasingly considered, that normalisation of mitochondrial function including maintenance of oxidative phosphorylation is a key strategy to reduce the progression of diabetic nephropathy. Further to this, a "unifying hypothesis" [17], suggests that the initiator of hyperglycaemia-induced damage in the diabetic kidney is excess generation of mitochondrial $^{\bullet}O_2^-$ which then leads to activation of four major biochemical pathways. These include increased advanced glycation end product (AGE) formation, increased flux through the polyol and hexosamine pathways and activation of protein kinase C (PKC) isoforms [17]. In addition, each of these pathways can initiate and perpetuate intracellular ROS generation. Inhibition of other cellular pathways including NADPH oxidase or reversing the uncoupling of eNOS may also warrant further investigation to assess their relative importance in progressive renal disease in particular, their role in human disease. Another important area of investigation is the role of depletion of specific cellular antioxidants in the development and progression of diabetic renal disease.

As outlined above, current strategies to treat, prevent or reverse diabetic nephropathy rely on widespread use of agents that interrupt the RAS. As such, it is important to appreciate that angiotensin II itself can produce ROS, primarily via NADPH oxidase [108] and it is therefore likely that strategies which interrupt the RAS have the capacity to significantly lower cellular ROS generation. However, RAS blockade may not fully suppress ROS generation, particularly from other sources such as mitochondria [67], which could explain the persistent progression of disease, albeit at a slower rate, seen in subjects with diabetic nephropathy concomitantly treated with agents that interrupt the RAS. Therefore, novel therapeutic targets that could lead to new treatments that confer synergistic effects with those seen with RAS blockade are of paramount importance for maximal renoprotection in this disorder.

Conclusion

Although a single cellular source of ROS as the initiator of diabetic nephropathy is an attractive prospect and potentially simplifies therapeutic targets, it is unlikely that this fully explains what occurs in the kidney, which has marked heterogeneity in resident cell populations. Therefore therapeutic *in vitro* studies in individual renal cell types are essential, however, one must be cautious in their interpretation. Indeed, these must be performed in association with appropriate *in vivo* models of diabetic nephropathy, although these also have obvious limitations related to their translatability to the clinical context. Overall, it is clear from the evidence presented within this chapter, that more than one source of ROS in diabetic nephropathy may be pathogenic. Therefore, the goal of designing new generation antioxidant therapies is to identify agents which are potentially effective and penetrative of specific cell compartments, providing superior renoprotection upon their combination with RAS blockade.

Acknowledgments

The work of the authors was completed with support from the Juvenile Diabetes Research Foundation (JDRF), the National Health and Medical Research Council of Australia (NHMRC) and National Institutes of Health (United States of America). Josephine Forbes is a JDRF Career Development Fellow.

References

[1] Cooper ME. Pathogenesis, prevention, and treatment of diabetic nephropathy. *Lancet.* 1998 Jul 18;352(9123):213-9.
[2] Effect of intensive therapy on the microvascular complications of type 1 diabetes mellitus. *Jama.* 2002 May 15;287(19):2563-9.
[3] Dluhy RG, McMahon GT. Intensive glycemic control in the ACCORD and ADVANCE trials. *N. Engl. J. Med.* 2008 Jun 12;358(24):2630-3.
[4] UK Prospective Diabetes Study (UKPDS) Group. Intensive blood-glucose control with sulphonylureas or insulin compared with conventional treatment and risk of complications in patients with type 2 diabetes (UKPDS 33). *Lancet.* 1998;352(9131):837-53.
[5] Brenner BM, Cooper ME, de Zeeuw D, Keane WF, Mitch WE, Parving HH, et al. Effects of losartan on renal and cardiovascular outcomes in patients with type 2 diabetes and nephropathy. *N. Engl. J. Med.* 2001;345(12):861-9.
[6] Lewis EJ, Hunsicker LG, Bain RP, Rohde RD. The effect of angiotensin-converting-enzyme inhibition on diabetic nephropathy. The Collaborative Study Group. *N. Engl. J. Med.* 1993;329(20):1456-62.
[7] Mogensen CE, Neldam S, Tikkanen I, Oren S, Viskoper R, Watts RW, et al. Randomised controlled trial of dual blockade of renin-angiotensin system in patients with hypertension, microalbuminuria, and non-insulin dependent diabetes: the candesartan and lisinopril microalbuminuria (CALM) study. *Bmj.* 2000 Dec 9;321(7274):1440-4.
[8] Koya D, Haneda M, Nakagawa H, Isshiki K, Sato H, Maeda S, et al. Amelioration of accelerated diabetic mesangial expansion by treatment with a PKC beta inhibitor in diabetic db/db mice, a rodent model for type 2 diabetes. *FASEB J.* 2000 Mar;14(3):439-47.
[9] Koya D, Lee IK, Ishii H, Kanoh H, King GL. Prevention of glomerular dysfunction in diabetic rats by treatment with d-alpha-tocopherol. *J. Am. Soc. Nephrol.* 1997 Mar;8(3):426-35.
[10] Heart Outcomes Prevention Evaluation Study Investigators. Effects of ramipril on cardiovascular and microvascular outcomes in people with diabetes mellitus: results of the HOPE study and MICRO-HOPE substudy. *Lancet.* 2000;355(9200):253-9.

[11] Baynes JW, Thorpe SR. Role of oxidative stress in diabetic complications: a new perspective on an old paradigm. *Diabetes.* 1999 Jan;48(1):1-9.

[12] Evans JL, Goldfine ID, Maddux BA, Grodsky GM. Oxidative stress and stress-activated signaling pathways: a unifying hypothesis of type 2 diabetes. *Endocr. Rev.* 2002 Oct;23(5):599-622.

[13] Ceriello A, Morocutti A, Mercuri F, Quagliaro L, Moro M, Damante G, et al. Defective intracellular antioxidant enzyme production in type 1 diabetic patients with nephropathy. *Diabetes.* 2000 Dec;49(12):2170-7.

[14] DeRubertis FR, Craven PA, Melhem MF. Acceleration of diabetic renal injury in the superoxide dismutase knockout mouse: effects of tempol. *Metabolism.* 2007 Sep;56(9):1256-64.

[15] Al-Kateb H, Boright AP, Mirea L, Xie X, Sutradhar R, Mowjoodi A, et al. Multiple superoxide dismutase 1/splicing factor serine alanine 15 variants are associated with the development and progression of diabetic nephropathy: the Diabetes Control and Complications Trial/Epidemiology of Diabetes Interventions and Complications Genetics study. *Diabetes.* 2008 Jan;57(1):218-28.

[16] Hinerfeld D, Traini MD, Weinberger RP, Cochran B, Doctrow SR, Harry J, et al. Endogenous mitochondrial oxidative stress: neurodegeneration, proteomic analysis, specific respiratory chain defects, and efficacious antioxidant therapy in superoxide dismutase 2 null mice. *J. Neurochem.* 2004 Feb;88(3):657-67.

[17] Nishikawa T, Edelstein D, Du XL, Yamagishi S, Matsumura T, Kaneda Y, et al. Normalizing mitochondrial superoxide production blocks three pathways of hyperglycaemic damage. *Nature.* 2000;404(6779):787-90.

[18] Asaba K, Tojo A, Onozato ML, Goto A, Fujita T. Double-edged action of SOD mimetic in diabetic nephropathy. *J. Cardiovasc. Pharmacol.* 2007 Jan;49(1):13-9.

[19] Mollsten A, Marklund SL, Wessman M, Svensson M, Forsblom C, Parkkonen M, et al. A functional polymorphism in the manganese superoxide dismutase gene and diabetic nephropathy. *Diabetes.* 2007 Jan;56(1):265-9.

[20] de Haan JB, Stefanovic N, Nikolic-Paterson D, Scurr LL, Croft KD, Mori TA, et al. Kidney expression of glutathione peroxidase-1 is not protective against streptozotocin-induced diabetic nephropathy. *Am. J. Physiol. Renal. Physiol.* 2005 Sep;289(3):F544-51.

[21] Blauwkamp MN, Yu J, Schin MA, Burke KA, Berry MJ, Carlson BA, et al. Podocyte specific knock out of selenoproteins does not enhance nephropathy in streptozotocin diabetic C57BL/6 mice. *BMC Nephrol.* 2008;9:7.

[22] Brezniceanu ML, Liu F, Wei CC, Tran S, Sachetelli S, Zhang SL, et al. Catalase overexpression attenuates angiotensinogen expression and apoptosis in diabetic mice. *Kidney Int.* 2007 May;71(9):912-23.

[23] dos Santos KG, Canani LH, Gross JL, Tschiedel B, Souto KE, Roisenberg I. The catalase -262C/T promoter polymorphism and diabetic complications in Caucasians with type 2 diabetes. Dis Markers. 2006;22(5-6):355-9.

[24] Melhem MF, Craven PA, Derubertis FR. Effects of dietary supplementation of alpha-lipoic acid on early glomerular injury in diabetes mellitus. *J. Am. Soc. Nephrol.* 2001 Jan;12(1):124-33.

[25] Borcea V, Nourooz-Zadeh J, Wolff SP, Klevesath M, Hofmann M, Urich H, et al. alpha-Lipoic acid decreases oxidative stress even in diabetic patients with poor

glycemic control and albuminuria. *Free Radic. Biol. Med.* 1999 Jun;26(11-12):1495-500.

[26] Babaei-Jadidi R, Karachalias N, Ahmed N, Battah S, Thornalley PJ. Prevention of incipient diabetic nephropathy by high-dose thiamine and benfotiamine. *Diabetes.* 2003 Aug;52(8):2110-20.

[27] Zheng S, Carlson EC, Yang L, Kralik PM, Huang Y, Epstein PN. Podocyte-specific overexpression of the antioxidant metallothionein reduces diabetic nephropathy. *J. Am. Soc. Nephrol.* 2008 Nov;19(11):2077-85.

[28] Hamada Y, Miyata S, Nii-Kono T, Kitazawa R, Kitazawa S, Higo S, et al. Overexpression of thioredoxin1 in transgenic mice suppresses development of diabetic nephropathy. *Nephrol. Dial. Transplant.* 2007 Jun;22(6):1547-57.

[29] Winiarska K, Szymanski K, Gorniak P, Dudziak M, Bryla J. Hypoglycaemic, antioxidative and nephroprotective effects of taurine in alloxan diabetic rabbits. *Biochimie.* 2009 Feb;91(2):261-70.

[30] Heilig CW, Concepcion LA, Riser BL, Freytag SO, Zhu M, Cortes P. Overexpression of glucose transporters in rat mesangial cells cultured in a normal glucose milieu mimics the diabetic phenotype. *J. Clin. Invest.* 1995 Oct;96(4):1802-14.

[31] Coward RJ, Welsh GI, Yang J, Tasman C, Lennon R, Koziell A, et al. The human glomerular podocyte is a novel target for insulin action. *Diabetes.* 2005 Nov;54(11):3095-102.

[32] Han DC, Isono M, Chen S, Casaretto A, Hong SW, Wolf G, et al. Leptin stimulates type I collagen production in db/db mesangial cells: glucose uptake and TGF-beta type II receptor expression. *Kidney Int.* 2001;59(4):1315-23.

[33] Rahmoune H, Thompson PW, Ward JM, Smith CD, Hong G, Brown J. Glucose transporters in human renal proximal tubular cells isolated from the urine of patients with non-insulin-dependent diabetes. *Diabetes.* 2005 Dec;54(12):3427-34.

[34] Asada T, Ogawa T, Iwai M, Shimomura K, Kobayashi M. Recombinant insulin-like growth factor I normalizes expression of renal glucose transporters in diabetic rats. *Am. J. Physiol.* 1997 Jul;273(1 Pt 2):F27-37.

[35] Graier WF, Simecek S, Kukovetz WR, Kostner GM. High D-glucose-induced changes in endothelial Ca2+/EDRF signaling are due to generation of superoxide anions. *Diabetes.* 1996 Oct;45(10):1386-95.

[36] Graier WF, Simecek S, Hoebel BG, Wascher TC, Dittrich P, Kostner GM. Antioxidants prevent high-D-glucose-enhanced endothelial Ca2+/cGMP response by scavenging superoxide anions. *Eur. J. Pharmacol.* 1997 Mar 12;322(1):113-22.

[37] Schulz TJ, Zarse K, Voigt A, Urban N, Birringer M, Ristow M. Glucose restriction extends Caenorhabditis elegans life span by inducing mitochondrial respiration and increasing oxidative stress. *Cell Metab.* 2007 Oct;6(4):280-93.

[38] Nangaku M, Izuhara Y, Usuda N, Inagi R, Shibata T, Sugiyama S, et al. In a type 2 diabetic nephropathy rat model, the improvement of obesity by a low calorie diet reduces oxidative/carbonyl stress and prevents diabetic nephropathy. *Nephrol. Dial. Transplant.* 2005 Dec;20(12):2661-9.

[39] Tikoo K, Tripathi DN, Kabra DG, Sharma V, Gaikwad AB. Intermittent fasting prevents the progression of type I diabetic nephropathy in rats and changes the expression of Sir2 and p53. *FEBS Lett.* 2007 Mar 6;581(5):1071-8.

[40] Ingram DK, Zhu M, Mamczarz J, Zou S, Lane MA, Roth GS, et al. Calorie restriction mimetics: an emerging research field. *Aging Cell.* 2006 Apr;5(2):97-108.

[41] Zhang Z, Apse K, Pang J, Stanton RC. High glucose inhibits glucose-6-phosphate dehydrogenase via cAMP in aortic endothelial cells. *J. Biol. Chem.* 2000 Dec 22;275(51):40042-7.

[42] Pandolfi PP, Sonati F, Rivi R, Mason P, Grosveld F, Luzzatto L. Targeted disruption of the housekeeping gene encoding glucose 6-phosphate dehydrogenase (G6PD): G6PD is dispensable for pentose synthesis but essential for defense against oxidative stress. *Embo. J.* 1995 Nov 1;14(21):5209-15.

[43] Kunjara S, Sochor M, Ali M, Bennett M, Greenbaum AL, McLean P. Uridine and cytidine nucleotide synthesis in renal hypertrophy: biochemical differences in response to the growth stimulus of diabetes and unilateral nephrectomy. *Biochem. Med. Metab. Biol.* 1992 Apr;47(2):168-80.

[44] Morrison AD, Clements RS, Jr., Winegrad AI. Effects of elevated glucose concentrations on the metabolism of the aortic wall. *J. Clin. Invest.* 1972 Dec;51(12):3114-23.

[45] Pingle SC, Mishra S, Marcuzzi A, Bhat SG, Sekino Y, Rybak LP, et al. Osmotic diuretics induce adenosine A1 receptor expression and protect renal proximal tubular epithelial cells against cisplatin-mediated apoptosis. *J. Biol. Chem.* 2004 Oct 8;279(41):43157-67.

[46] Kaiser N, Sasson S, Feener EP, Boukobza-Vardi N, Higashi S, Moller DE, et al. Differential regulation of glucose transport and transporters by glucose in vascular endothelial and smooth muscle cells. *Diabetes.* 1993 Jan;42(1):80-9.

[47] Greene DA, Arezzo JC, Brown MB. Effect of aldose reductase inhibition on nerve conduction and morphometry in diabetic neuropathy. Zenarestat Study Group. *Neurology.* 1999 Aug 11;53(3):580-91.

[48] Hotta N, Toyota T, Matsuoka K, Shigeta Y, Kikkawa R, Kaneko T, et al. Clinical efficacy of fidarestat, a novel aldose reductase inhibitor, for diabetic peripheral neuropathy: a 52-week multicenter placebo-controlled double-blind parallel group study. *Diabetes Care.* 2001 Oct;24(10):1776-82.

[49] Maillard L. Action des acides amines sur les sucres: formation des melanoidines par voie methodique. CR *Acad. Sci.* 1912;154:66-8.

[50] Fu MX, Wells-Knecht KJ, Blackledge JA, Lyons TJ, Thorpe SR, Baynes JW. Glycation, glycoxidation, and cross-linking of collagen by glucose. Kinetics, mechanisms, and inhibition of late stages of the Maillard reaction. *Diabetes.* 1994;43(5):676-83.

[51] Vlassara H. The AGE-receptor in the pathogenesis of diabetic complications. *Diabetes Metab. Res. Rev.* 2001 Nov-Dec;17(6):436-43.

[52] Brownlee M. Biochemistry and molecular cell biology of diabetic complications. *Nature.* 2001 Dec 13;414(6865):813-20.

[53] Hamada Y, Araki N, Koh N, Nakamura J, Horiuchi S, Hotta N. Rapid formation of advanced glycation end products by intermediate metabolites of glycolytic pathway and polyol pathway. *Biochem. Biophys. Res. Commun.* 1996 Nov 12;228(2):539-43.

[54] Wells-Knecht KJ, Zyzak DV, Litchfield JE, Thorpe SR, Baynes JW. Mechanism of autoxidative glycosylation: identification of glyoxal and arabinose as intermediates in

the autoxidative modification of proteins by glucose. *Biochemistry.* 1995 Mar 21;34(11):3702-9.
[55] Thornalley PJ, Langborg A, Minhas HS. Formation of glyoxal, methylglyoxal and 3-deoxyglucosone in the glycation of proteins by glucose. *Biochem. J.* 1999 Nov 15;344 Pt 1:109-16.
[56] Neeper M, Schmidt AM, Brett J, Yan SD, Wang F, Pan YC, et al. Cloning and expression of a cell surface receptor for advanced glycosylation end products of proteins. *J. Biol. Chem.* 1992 Jul 25;267(21):14998-5004.
[57] Schmidt AM, Hori O, Chen JX, Li JF, Crandall J, Zhang J, et al. Advanced glycation endproducts interacting with their endothelial receptor induce expression of vascular cell adhesion molecule-1 (VCAM-1) in cultured human endothelial cells and in mice. A potential mechanism for the accelerated vasculopathy of diabetes. *J. Clin. Invest.* 1995 Sep;96(3):1395-403.
[58] Wendt TM, Tanji N, Guo J, Kislinger TR, Qu W, Lu Y, et al. RAGE drives the development of glomerulosclerosis and implicates podocyte activation in the pathogenesis of diabetic nephropathy. *Am. J. Pathol.* 2003 Apr;162(4):1123-37.
[59] Inagi R, Yamamoto Y, Nangaku M, Usuda N, Okamato H, Kurokawa K, et al. A severe diabetic nephropathy model with early development of nodule-like lesions induced by megsin overexpression in RAGE/iNOS transgenic mice. *Diabetes.* 2006 Feb;55(2):356-66.
[60] Shinohara M, Thornalley PJ, Giardino I, Beisswenger P, Thorpe SR, Onorato J, et al. Overexpression of glyoxalase-I in bovine endothelial cells inhibits intracellular advanced glycation endproduct formation and prevents hyperglycemia-induced increases in macromolecular endocytosis. *J. Clin. Invest.* 1998 Mar 1;101(5):1142-7.
[61] Thornalley PJ. Glutathione-dependent detoxification of alpha-oxoaldehydes by the glyoxalase system: involvement in disease mechanisms and antiproliferative activity of glyoxalase I inhibitors. *Chem. Biol. Interact.* 1998 Apr 24;111-112:137-51.
[62] Rosca MG, Mustata TG, Kinter MT, Ozdemir AM, Kern TS, Szweda LI, et al. Glycation of mitochondrial proteins from diabetic rat kidney is associated with excess superoxide formation. *Am. J. Physiol. Renal. Physiol.* 2005 Aug;289(2):F420-30.
[63] Degenhardt TP, Alderson NL, Arrington DD, Beattie RJ, Basgen JM, Steffes MW, et al. Pyridoxamine inhibits early renal disease and dyslipidemia in the streptozotocin-diabetic rat. *Kidney Int.* 2002 Mar;61(3):939-50.
[64] Forbes JM, Thallas V, Thomas MC, Founds HW, Burns WC, Jerums G, et al. The breakdown of preexisting advanced glycation end products is associated with reduced renal fibrosis in experimental diabetes. *Faseb. J.* 2003 Sep;17(12):1762-4.
[65] Nakamura S, Makita Z, Ishikawa S, Yasumura K, Fujii W, Yanagisawa K, et al. Progression of nephropathy in spontaneous diabetic rats is prevented by OPB-9195, a novel inhibitor of advanced glycation. *Diabetes.* 1997 May;46(5):895-9.
[66] Soulis-Liparota T, Cooper M, Papazoglou D, Clarke B, Jerums G. Retardation by aminoguanidine of development of albuminuria, mesangial expansion, and tissue fluorescence in streptozocin-induced diabetic rat. *Diabetes.* 1991;40(10):1328-34.
[67] Coughlan MT, Thallas-Bonke V, Pete J, Long DM, Gasser A, Tong DC, et al. Combination therapy with the advanced glycation end product cross-link breaker, alagebrium, and angiotensin converting enzyme inhibitors in diabetes: synergy or redundancy? *Endocrinology.* 2007 Feb;148(2):886-95.

[68] Stracke H, Lindemann A, Federlin K. A benfotiamine-vitamin B combination in treatment of diabetic polyneuropathy. *Exp. Clin. Endocrinol. Diabetes.* 1996;104(4):311-6.

[69] Du X, Edelstein D, Brownlee M. Oral benfotiamine plus alpha-lipoic acid normalises complication-causing pathways in type 1 diabetes. *Diabetologia.* 2008 Oct;51(10):1930-2.

[70] Flyvbjerg A, Denner L, Schrijvers BF, Tilton RG, Mogensen TH, Paludan SR, et al. Long-term renal effects of a neutralizing RAGE antibody in obese type 2 diabetic mice. *Diabetes.* 2004 Jan;53(1):166-72.

[71] Babior BM, Lambeth JD, Nauseef W. The neutrophil NADPH oxidase. *Arch. Biochem. Biophys.* 2002 Jan 15;397(2):342-4.

[72] Gill PS, Wilcox CS. NADPH oxidases in the kidney. *Antioxid Redox. Signal.* 2006 Sep-Oct;8(9-10):1597-607.

[73] Li JM, Shah AM. ROS generation by nonphagocytic NADPH oxidase: potential relevance in diabetic nephropathy. *J. Am. Soc. Nephrol.* 2003 Aug;14(8 Suppl 3):S221-6.

[74] Thallas-Bonke V, Thorpe SR, Coughlan MT, Fukami K, Yap FY, Sourris K, et al. Inhibition of NADPH oxidase prevents AGE mediated damage in diabetic nephropathy through a protein kinase C-{alpha} dependent pathway. *Diabetes.* 2007 Oct 24.

[75] Griendling KK, Sorescu D, Ushio-Fukai M. NAD(P)H oxidase: role in cardiovascular biology and disease. *Circ Res.* 2000 Mar 17;86(5):494-501.

[76] Zalba G, San Jose G, Moreno MU, Fortuno MA, Fortuno A, Beaumont FJ, et al. Oxidative stress in arterial hypertension: role of NAD(P)H oxidase. *Hypertension.* 2001 Dec 1;38(6):1395-9.

[77] Onozato ML, Tojo A, Goto A, Fujita T, Wilcox CS. Oxidative stress and nitric oxide synthase in rat diabetic nephropathy: effects of ACEI and ARB. *Kidney Int.* 2002;61(1):186-94.

[78] Asaba K, Tojo A, Onozato ML, Goto A, Quinn MT, Fujita T, et al. Effects of NADPH oxidase inhibitor in diabetic nephropathy. *Kidney Int.* 2005 May;67(5):1890-8.

[79] Gorin Y, Block K, Hernandez J, Bhandari B, Wagner B, Barnes JL, et al. Nox4 NAD(P)H oxidase mediates hypertrophy and fibronectin expression in the diabetic kidney. *J. Biol. Chem.* 2005 Nov 25;280(47):39616-26.

[80] Matsumoto S, Koshiishi I, Inoguchi T, Nawata H, Utsumi H. Confirmation of superoxide generation via xanthine oxidase in streptozotocin-induced diabetic mice. *Free Radic. Res.* 2003 Jul;37(7):767-72.

[81] Inkster ME, Cotter MA, Cameron NE. Treatment with the xanthine oxidase inhibitor, allopurinol, improves nerve and vascular function in diabetic rats. *Eur. J. Pharmacol.* 2007 Apr 30;561(1-3):63-71.

[82] Guzik TJ, Mussa S, Gastaldi D, Sadowski J, Ratnatunga C, Pillai R, et al. Mechanisms of increased vascular superoxide production in human diabetes mellitus: role of NAD(P)H oxidase and endothelial nitric oxide synthase. *Circulation.* 2002 Apr 9;105(14):1656-62.

[83] Satoh M, Fujimoto S, Haruna Y, Arakawa S, Horike H, Komai N, et al. NAD(P)H oxidase and uncoupled nitric oxide synthase are major sources of glomerular superoxide in rats with experimental diabetic nephropathy. *Am. J. Physiol. Renal. Physiol.* 2005 Jun;288(6):F1144-52.

[84] Komers R, Allen TJ, Cooper ME. Role of endothelium-derived nitric oxide in the pathogenesis of the renal hemodynamic changes of experimental diabetes. *Diabetes.* 1994 Oct;43(10):1190-7.

[85] Komers R, Lindsley JN, Oyama TT, Allison KM, Anderson S. Role of neuronal nitric oxide synthase (NOS1) in the pathogenesis of renal hemodynamic changes in diabetes. *Am. J. Physiol. Renal. Physiol.* 2000 Sep;279(3):F573-83.

[86] Choi KC, Lee SC, Kim SW, Kim NH, Lee JU, Kang YJ. Role of nitric oxide in the pathogenesis of diabetic nephropathy in streptozotocin-induced diabetic rats. *Korean J. Intern. Med.* 1999 Jan;14(1):32-41.

[87] Prabhakar SS. Role of nitric oxide in diabetic nephropathy. *Semin. Nephrol.* 2004 Jul;24(4):333-44.

[88] Soulis T, Cooper ME, Sastra S, Thallas V, Panagiotopoulos S, Bjerrum OJ, et al. Relative Contributions of Advanced Glycation and Nitric Oxide Synthase Inhibition to Aminoguanidine-Mediated Renoprotection in Diabetic Rats. *Diabetologia.* 1997;40(10):1141-51.

[89] Kamijo H, Higuchi M, Hora K. Chronic inhibition of nitric oxide production aggravates diabetic nephropathy in Otsuka Long-Evans Tokushima Fatty rats. *Nephron. Physiol.* 2006;104(1):p12-22.

[90] Nakagawa T, Sato W, Glushakova O, Heinig M, Clarke T, Campbell-Thompson M, et al. Diabetic endothelial nitric oxide synthase knockout mice develop advanced diabetic nephropathy. *J. Am. Soc. Nephrol.* 2007 Feb;18(2):539-50.

[91] Kabat A, Ponicke K, Salameh A, Mohr FW, Dhein S. Effect of a beta 2-adrenoceptor stimulation on hyperglycemia-induced endothelial dysfunction. *J. Pharmacol. Exp. Ther.* 2004 Feb;308(2):564-73.

[92] Coughlan MT, Thorburn DR, Penfold SA, Laskowski A, Harcourt BE, Sourris KC, et al. RAGE-Induced Cytosolic ROS Promote Mitochondrial Superoxide Generation in Diabetes. *J. Am. Soc. Nephrol.* 2009 Apr;20(4):742-52.

[93] Hipkiss AR. Does chronic glycolysis accelerate aging? Could this explain how dietary restriction works? *Ann. N Y Acad. Sci.* 2006 May;1067:361-8.

[94] Tonolo G, Ciccarese M, Brizzi P, Puddu L, Secchi G, Calvia P, et al. Reduction of albumin excretion rate in normotensive microalbuminuric type 2 diabetic patients during long-term simvastatin treatment. *Diabetes Care.* 1997 Dec;20(12):1891-5.

[95] Turrens JF, Boveris A. Generation of superoxide anion by the NADH dehydrogenase of bovine heart mitochondria. *Biochem. J.* 1980 Nov 1;191(2):421-7.

[96] Kiritoshi S, Nishikawa T, Sonoda K, Kukidome D, Senokuchi T, Matsuo T, et al. Reactive oxygen species from mitochondria induce cyclooxygenase-2 gene expression in human mesangial cells: potential role in diabetic nephropathy. *Diabetes.* 2003 Oct;52(10):2570-7.

[97] Verkaart S, Koopman WJ, van Emst-de Vries SE, Nijtmans LG, van den Heuvel LW, Smeitink JA, et al. Superoxide production is inversely related to complex I activity in inherited complex I deficiency. *Biochim. Biophys. Acta.* 2007 Jan 4.

[98] Rotig A, de Lonlay P, Chretien D, Foury F, Koenig M, Sidi D, et al. Aconitase and mitochondrial iron-sulphur protein deficiency in Friedreich ataxia. *Nat. Genet.* 1997 Oct;17(2):215-7.

[99] Martin-Hernandez E, Garcia-Silva MT, Vara J, Campos Y, Cabello A, Muley R, et al. Renal pathology in children with mitochondrial diseases. *Pediatr. Nephrol.* 2005 Sep;20(9):1299-305.

[100] Diomedi-Camassei F, Di Giandomenico S, Santorelli FM, Caridi G, Piemonte F, Montini G, et al. COQ2 nephropathy: a newly described inherited mitochondriopathy with primary renal involvement. *J. Am. Soc. Nephrol.* 2007 Oct;18(10):2773-80.

[101] Batandier C, Leverve X, Fontaine E. Opening of the mitochondrial permeability transition pore induces reactive oxygen species production at the level of the respiratory chain complex I. *J. Biol. Chem.* 2004 Apr 23;279(17):17197-204.

[102] Hausse AO, Aggoun Y, Bonnet D, Sidi D, Munnich A, Rotig A, et al. Idebenone and reduced cardiac hypertrophy in Friedreich's ataxia. *Heart.* 2002 Apr;87(4):346-9.

[103] Green K, Brand MD, Murphy MP. Prevention of mitochondrial oxidative damage as a therapeutic strategy in diabetes. *Diabetes.* 2004 Feb;53 Suppl 1:S110-8.

[104] Boss O, Samec S, Paoloni-Giacobino A, Rossier C, Dulloo A, Seydoux J, et al. Uncoupling protein-3: a new member of the mitochondrial carrier family with tissue-specific expression. *FEBS Lett.* 1997 May 12;408(1):39-42.

[105] Rudofsky G, Jr., Schroedter A, Schlotterer A, Voron'ko OE, Schlimme M, Tafel J, et al. Functional polymorphisms of UCP2 and UCP3 are associated with a reduced prevalence of diabetic neuropathy in patients with type 1 diabetes. *Diabetes Care.* 2006 Jan;29(1):89-94.

[106] Cui Y, Xu X, Bi H, Zhu Q, Wu J, Xia X, et al. Expression modification of uncoupling proteins and MnSOD in retinal endothelial cells and pericytes induced by high glucose: the role of reactive oxygen species in diabetic retinopathy. *Exp. Eye Res.* 2006 Oct;83(4):807-16.

[107] Krauss S, Zhang CY, Scorrano L, Dalgaard LT, St-Pierre J, Grey ST, et al. Superoxide-mediated activation of uncoupling protein 2 causes pancreatic beta cell dysfunction. *J. Clin. Invest.* 2003 Dec;112(12):1831-42.

[108] Griendling KK, Minieri CA, Ollerenshaw JD, Alexander RW. Angiotensin II stimulates NADH and NADPH oxidase activity in cultured vascular smooth muscle cells. *Circ. Res.* 1994;74(6):1141-8.

In: Advances in Pathogenesis of Diabetic Nephropathy
Editor: Sharma S. Prabhakar

ISBN: 978-1-61122-134-3
© 2012 Nova Science Publishers, Inc.

Chapter X

Role of Vaso-Active Factors in Diabetic Nephropathy

Sharma S. Prabhakar[*]
Department of Medicine, Texas Tech University Health Sciences Center, Lubbock, TX 79430, US

Abstract

The pathogenesis of diabetic nephropathy remains incompletely understood. The conventional pathogenic factors do not account for the development of nephropathy in diabetes. The last few decades has witnessed tremendous research examining novel pathogenic mechanisms causing or contributing to diabetic nephropathy. These include growth factors such as TGF beta, VEGF, IGF, and other vasodilatory mediators such as nitric oxide, prostaglandins, endothelin, angiotensin etc. This chapter focuses on a review of published literature that such supports the role of the vasodilatory mediators in the mediation of renal injury in diabetes. Specifically, the role of nitric oxide in contributing to the progression of diabetic nephropathy has been much debated while the evidence for role of endothelins and prostaglandins is continuing to build. In addition the in vitro and in vivo evidence directly incriminating these factors in diabetic nephropathy, experimental data from transgenic knockout models and studies examining genetic polymorphisms of factors such as eNOS and angiotensin etc. have strengthened the etio-pathogenic role of such factors. There is a separate chapter that discusses renin angiotensin system activation in diabetic nephropathy and another that deals with all growth factors so as such those subjects will not be described in this review.

---

[*] Address for correspondence: Sharma S Prabhakar MD MBA FACP FASN, Professor and Chief, Division of Nephrology and Hypertension, Vice-Chairman, Department of Medicine, Texas Tech University Health Sciences Center, Lubbock, TX 79430, T (806)743-3155 ext 252, F (806)743-3148).

Introduction

Diabetic nephropathy is a major microvascular complication of diabetes and the most common cause of kidney failure needing renal replacement therapy. The treatment options used currently to manage DN are suboptimal since the pathogenesis remains unclear. Since the well established conventional risk factors do not adequately account for the pathogenesis, investigators have shifted the focus of investigation in the past two decades to the role of growth factors, cytokines and second messengers. The development of an optimal animal model to study the pathogenesis of DN has been the focus of the Animal Models of Diabetic Complications Consortium (AMDCC), created by the National Institutes of Health [1]. Emerging information from such studies has substantially contributed to our current understanding of the disease. In addition, a sizable volume of scientific evidence has developed recently to incriminate endothelial dysfunction in microvascular complications of diabetes and consequently such research has expanded to examine the role of vasoactive peptides such as endothelins, nitric oxide, prostaglandins and others [2,3]. Hemodynamic alterations occur very early in the course of human and experimental DN [4] and it is therefore logical to incriminate these vasoactive factors in the pathogenesis of diabetic complications [5]. Furthermore, the non-hemodynamic effects of these factors have received a lot of attention in the recent past so that the pathophysiologic significance of perturbations of these factors became even more crucial in the pathogenesis of DN [6]. However these studies often yielded data that is often conflicting and complex contributing the confusion relating to the role of these factors. Furthermore current evidence suggests that most of these vasoactive factors as well as others such as AGEs may target their effects in the kidney through mesangial cells [7,8] and podocytes [8,9,10]. The objective of this review is to present a balanced view of the current knowledge and controversies relating to this field.

Nitric Oxide and Diabetic Nephropathy

Nitric Oxide- Significance in Human Physiology

Nitric oxide is a simple gas that exists as an inert gas and as a pollutant in atmosphere and in biological solutions in the form of it's end products namely nitrites and nitrates. The physiological significance of nitric oxide was uncovered only about two decades ago when it was the recognized that the putative humoral factor elaborated by endothelium-hethereto known as endothelial derived relaxing factor or EDRF was indeed nitric oxide. Since that discovery, the scientific interest in NO resulted in thousands of publications encompassing its role in human physiology and pathophysiology and yielded the much coveted Nobel prize in 1998 to its original discoverers Louis Ignarro, Robert Furchgart and Ferid Murad. Nitric oxide is synthesized from its sole precursor, L-arginine through the action of NO synthase (NOS), of which there are three isoforms. The constitutively expressed isoforms include neuronal NOS (NOS I)- expressed in neurons, and macula densa of the kidney and endothelial NOS (NOS III) expressed in endothelium while the inducible NOS (NOS II) is induced by cytokines and is expressed in cells of mesenchymal origin including mesangial cells and macrophages.

The physiological significance of nitric oxide has expanded exponentially since its original discovery. The initial focus of functional role of NO was on the vasodilatory and hemodynamic effects. However with the broader understanding of the biosynthesis and regulation, it became clear the functions depend also on the source of NO generation ie. the isoforms mediating the synthesis and cell source of NO generation. Thus NO generated from NOS I plays a major role in neuronal and cell signaling while NO from NOS II is involved in immune regulation and inflammatory responses. Finally NO derived from NOS III is important in vasodilatation and hemodynamic responses. In diabetes and its vascular complications, the role of all isoforms of NOS have been investigated but the significance of eNOS or NOS III in particular in mediating the structural and functional alterations of diabetic nephropathy has received by far the greatest attention [11]. The prominent role of NOS III was documented not only in animal models of DN but alos in human DN [12]. While neuronal NOS (NOS I) has been implicated widely in the early DN particularly in mediating hyperfiltration, other studies suggested that chronic NOS I inhibition had no impact some animal models of nephropathy of diabetes [13].

eNOS knockout studies: The strong evidence in support of the role of eNOS and its polymorphisms in DN has stimulated a strong interest in developing a eNOS knockout animal model. One of the most well quoted model was reported recently by Nakagawa et al. [14]. These mice developed not only early but also advanced lesions of DN including glomerulosclerosis. These mice were characterized by activation of RAAS and unusually high plasma aldosterone levels. Thus the response to inhibitors of RAAS such as enalapril and telmisartan tried in this model was less impressive both in terms of blood pressure and renal injury compared to wild type diabetic mice underscoring the endothelial dysfunction that characterizes this model. Furthermore, an impressive prevention of renal injury and blood pressure control with spironolactone in this study emphasized the role of aldosterone in mediating nephropathy of diabetes [15]. These authors further noted that there is an uncoupling of VEGF with NO leading to endothelial cell proliferation smooth muscle cell activation and vascular injury leading to advanced nephropathy. The VEGF-NO uncoupling is discussed in detail in the sections that follow. Another diabetic mouse model reported recently by Mohan et al. [16] from University of Texas San Antonio involved lepr db/db mice in which eNOS expression was genetically disrupted. The double knockout (eNOS-/-lepr db/db) mice developed hyperglycemia, hypertension and hyperinsulinemia. The renal disease per authors was very similar to human diabetic nephropathy despite lower fasting plasma glucose levels compared to lepr db/db mice where eNOS was preserved. The authors note that the eNOS disruption specifically led to enhanced microvascular as opposed to macrovascular injury in these mice.

eNOS polymorphism and DN: Nitric oxide is important in vascular tone and regulation of tissue hemodynamics. The susceptibility to nephropathy and vascular disease may depend to some extent on genetic factors. Several recent studies underscored the significance of several genetic polymorphisms in the development and progression of diabetic nephropathy. Most studies focused on eNOS since NO derived from endothelium is a major determinant of endothelial function and endothelial dysfunction is the hallmark of most vascular complications of diabetes. Most studies examined the Glu298Asp mutation at exon [17] and a 27bp variable number tandem repeat in intron 4 insertion/deletion polymorphism of the eNOS gene. While some studies reported strong association, others found none. Thaha et al. [18] found the association between the Glu298Asp mutation and end stage renal disease from diabetes. Ezzidi et al. [18] compared 515 diabetic nephropathy patients with 402 diabetics with no nephropathy and 748 healthy subjects and found that Asp 298 polymorphisms (especially Asp 298/4a/-786T haplotype) were significantly associated with nephropathy. A recent study by Mollsten et al. [19] reported that in a study of 458 cases with diabetic nephropathy were compared to 319 controls (long standing diabetics with no nephropathy). These were type I patients from the Steno Diabetes center. A significant association was noted between rs743507 TT- genotype and diabetic nephropathy and the authors concluded that NOS3 gene polymorphisms may be involved in the development of diabetic nephropathy. Another group [20] described that G894T polymorphism of the NOS gene has no impact on the basal NO generation in renal circulation. However the T allele is associated with increased oxidative stress and susceptibility to nephropathy in diabetes. In a study of 384 type II diabetics and 190 controls from West Africa, Chen et al. [21] reported that G894T polymorphism of eNOS gene was not associated with diabetic nephropathy. Finally a recent meta-analysis by Zintzaras [22] examining the association of eNOS polymorphisms (G894T, 4b/a and T786C) reported that the associations are inconclusive. G894T is more strongly associated with diabetic nephropathy than the other alleles while 4b/a polymorphisms were associated with DN in only East Asians. Thus more studies need to be performed to better understand the role of polymorphisms and susceptibility association with DN. A more detailed discussion of this topic is presented n the chapter on genetic determinants of diabetic nephropathy.

Nitric oxide – role in diabetes. The significance of renal nitric oxide generation in regulation of regional blood flow and hemodynamics in the kidney had been established by several investigators [23]. Several experimental observations have supported the role of nitric oxide in regulating the insulin secretion and release from pancreas. In turn insulin regulates nitric oxide generation in many tissues including the kidneys. These interactions between insulin and nitric oxide are the subject of many investigations in vitro and in vivo. Furthermore ambient glucose concentrations have been shown to affect the synthesis of nitric oxide in may tissues including endothelium, renal mesangium and vascular smooth muscle. We have recently shown that angiotensin inhibitors used commonly in diabetes increase insulin secretion in cultured pancreatic islet B cells, a phenomenon mediated by enhanced local nitric oxide synthesis [24]. This effect was observed in cultured hamster pancreatic islet B cells exposed to either ACE inhibitors and ARBs. Insulin secretion was assayed by commercial insulin ELISA kit using a guinea pig anti-insulin antibody and measuring absorbance at 492 nm. Co-incubation with NOS inhibitor L-NMMA abolished the increase in insulin secretion seen with ACEi and ARBs. These data suggest that angiotensin inhibition enhances insulin secretion and release from pancreatic islets by a NO –dependent mechanism and this effect may contribute to improved glycemic control seen with clinical usage of RAAS blockade.

Nitric oxide and hyperglycemia In general high glucose upregulates endothelial nitric oxide synthesis through eNOS while inhibiting the iNOS mediated NO generation, Our in vitro experiments in renal mesangial cells support these observations. We demonstrated that high ambient glucose inhibited nitric oxide synthesis mediated by iNOS in renal mesangial cells through a mechanism that was post translational and involved stability of tetrahydrobiopterin, a co-factor needed for nitric oxide synthase [25]. We also demonstrated that despite this effect of high glucose on iNOS, the eNOS derived NO is upregulated by ambient glucose in vitro and and is contributed in vivo by the activation of angiotensin and

VEGF that occurs early in the course of diabetic nephropathy [26]. High glucose induces oxidative and nitrosative stress in many cell types causing generation of superoxide, NO and peroxynitrite, which induce apoptosis and contribute to progression of DN [27]. Furthermore glucose and glucose transporter-1 (GLUT-1) have been suggested as links between glomerular hyperfiltration and cascade of events that injure the kidney in diabetes [28], thus forming the bridge between the metabolic and hemodynamic pathways leading DN. Recently Nordquist et al. [29] have discussed the role of sustained hyperglycemia leading to low oxygen tension and a high degree of non-oxygen dependent metabolism leads to medullary ischemia and consequent generation of reactive oxygen species. The role of hepatic arginine metabolism [30] and renal NO generation in mediating renal medullary hypoxia has been the subject many critical reviews [31]. The critical role of oxidative stress as a consequence of chronic hyperglycemia induced superoxide generation in decreasing NO synthesis and/or bioavailability has been underscored by Haidara et al. [32]. The ability of glucose to scavenge nitric oxide is proposed as an initiating event in the endothelial dysfunction and inhibition of NOS by AGE and PAI-1 are additional factors instrumental in contributing to NO deficiency in advanced DN [33]. Finally several investigators attempted to develop a unifying pathogenic basis for DN stemming from consequences of hyperglycemia such as activation of RAAS, endothelins, abnormal NO synthesis, activation of multiple growth factors and formation of AGE all leading to endothelial dysfunction and tissue injury in diabetes [34].

Nitric oxide and angiotensin interactions: Experiments from our laboratory have clearly demonstrated that angiotensin stimulated nitric oxide generation from cultured endothelial cells and in the kidneys of intact Sprague-Dawley rats [24]. Adult SD rats (20 weeks) were anesthetized and angiotensin II (10^{-8} M) infused intravenously for 4 hours after which the rats were sacrificed and kidneys harvested. As compared to controls (5mM glucose infusion) eNOS expression and activity was increased and iNOS expression was inhibited by angiotensin treatment. This was associated with increased urinary excretion of NO metabolites suggesting that the angiotensin stimulatory effects on the eNOS superseded the iNOS inhibition in terms of the effect on overall NO generation in the kidney.

As mentioned earlier, high glucose inhibited NO generation mediated by iNOS in Mesangial cells. However the effect of high glucose in the diabetic kidney depends on the composite effects of changes in all NOS isoforms in the kidney. Furthermore such effects are additionally modified by other factors concomitantly altered in the diabetic kidney such as the angiotensin Therefore we examined the effects of administration of glucose (20 mM) and angiotensin II separately and simultaneously for 4 hours intravenously in adult SD rats on the expression and activity of NOS isoforms in the kidney. We observed that despite high glucose inhibition of eNOS, intra renal eNOS activity, expression and overall NO generation as reflected by NO metabolites remained higher with concomitant angiotensin administration [24]. Thus the effects of angiotensin II on eNOS are stronger than the high glucose effects.

Renin angiotensin system plays a vital role in the hemodynamic, humoral and metabolic pathways in the pathophysiology of renal disease in diabetes and hypertension [35] and it is suggested that a balance between nitric oxide and angiotensin is a key determinant of whether renal injury or protection ensues under given circumstances.

Dual Role of Nitric Oxide in DN

It has been established for a long time that the principal risk factors that affect the development and progression of diabetic nephropathy includes uncontrolled hyperglycemia, hypertension (systemic and glomerular) and activation of RAAS. All these three factors have been shown to modulate intra renal NO generation either directly or through signaling pathways. The role of NO in affecting the renal structure and function is very complicated and depends on several factors including the stage of diabetic renal disease, isoforms of NOS involved, structures in the kidney, and influence of other factors in diabetic milieu [36]. The complex metabolic milieu in diabetes triggers several pathophysiological mechanisms that simultaneously stimulate and suppress intrarenal NO production [37]. The net effect on renal NO levels depends on the mechanisms that prevail in a given stage of the disease process.

The currently available evidence enables us to reasonably conclude that early diabetic nephropathy is associated with increased renal NO production mediated primarily by constitutively released NO through eNOS or NOS III activation. There is some contribution to this augmented NO production through nNOS (NOS I) derived enhanced synthesis, particularly from macula densa region of the kidney. Together the increased intrarenal NO generation contributes to the development of glomerular hyperfiltration and microalbuminuria that characterize early diabetic nephropathy [38]. Serum NO levels (NO2-+ NO3-) correlated with the development of diastolic hypertension and microalbuminuria in subjects with type I diabetes [39]. On the other hand, advanced diabetic nephropathy with severe proteinuria, hypertension and renal failure is associated with a state of progressive NO deficiency. As the duration of diabetic state increases, factors that suppress NO bioavailability prevail [40]. Many factors including activation of protein kinase C, activation of TGF-beta, NO quenching by advanced glycosylation end products (AGE) contribute to the NO deficient state – either directly or by inhibiting and/or by post translational modification of activity of NOS isoforms. Other inhibitors of NOS enzyme such as asymmetric dimethylarginine (ADMA) accumulate in diabetic nephropathy and may contribute to progression of DN [41] and such association has also been observed in other microvascular complications such as retinopathy [42]. Such correlations are not uniform since Yonem et al. [43] found no correlation of ADMA levels with retinopathy and Sibal et al. [44] found an association of elevated ADMA levels in plasma with endothelial dysfunction in diabetes without nephropathy but not in the presence of nephropathy. Shibata et al. [45] hypothesized that NO inhibition induced by ADMA decreases the peritubular blood flow leading to tubulointerstitial ischemia and injury, which is a major determinant of renal functional demise in DN. They argued that pharmacological manipulations to enhance the activity of dimethylarginine dimethylaminohydrolase (DDAH), an enzyme that increases the breakdown of ADMS could prove to be a novel therapeutic strategy for treatment of early DN. Complex interplay of these mechanisms results in a perturbation of the physiological properties of NO in metabolism of endothelial homeostasis such as vasodilation, anticoagulation, smooth cell proliferation etc. These changes in turn predispose to glomerular hyperfiltration, sclerosis and loss of renal function in diabetes [46]. Huang et al. [47] reported that AGE stimulates renal tubular cell hypertrophy in diabetes by a mechanism that involves oxidant injury since antioxidants prevent such hypertrophy partly by induction of NO/cGMP/PKG signaling. Inhibitors of AGE formation such as aminoguanidine have been shown to slow the progression of microvascular complications of diabetes including neuropathy and nephropathy [48]. However clinical trial of aminoguanidine to prevent progression of DN was terminated early due to safety concerns [49] and newer analogs of aminoguanidine are currently being evaluated. Furthermore oxidative stress mediated by hyperglycemia and angiotensin leads to sustained activation of NADPH as discussed by Gao et al. [50] may lead to depletion of intracellular NADPH, an intracellular co-factor for eNOS. In addition overproduction of reactive oxygen species (ROS) leads to uncoupling of eNOS, mitochondrial dysfunction, and impaired antioxidant defense mechanism. Satoh et al. [51] have shown that angiotensin receptor blockers improved the NOS uncoupling due to ROS by increasing the bioavailability of tetrahydrobiopterin, a co-factor for NOS. These findings underscore the role of angiotensin in the oxidative stress of DN and the impact of such alterations on eNOS function. Furthermore, the superoxide radical reacts with NO [52], accounting for decreased NO bioavailability along with other causes and also forming peroxynitrite, a very potent vascular and cellular toxin, contributing to the progression of diabetic nephropathy [53]. We have described similar observations in ZSF rats, an excellent rat model for diabetic nephropathy, with decreased renal NO production associated with oxidative stress [54]. Some studies have focused on the role of iNOS (as opposed to eNOS) generated peroxynitrite in the oxidative damage and glomerular lesions of the diabetic kidney [55]. Studies by Wang et al. demonstrated that the glomerular damage mediate peroxynitrite involved activation of JAK/STAT signaling pathways [56]. Neutralization of peroxynitrite or pharmacological inhibition of poly (ADP-ribose) polymerase (PARP) is a promising new approach in the therapy and prevention of diabetic vascular complications [57]. Oxidative stress has been linked to endothelial dysfunction and microvascular damage in diabetes [58]. Several models of DN, both experimental and clinical have underscored the role of oxidative stress as a pathogenic factor in DN. Recently DeRubertis et al. [59] has used a superoxide dismutase (SOD) knockout mouse to demonstrate the role of SOD1and the interaction of superoxide and NO in the pathogenesis of DN. The role of oxidative stress in DN is discussed in a separate chapter. In spite of extensive experimental evidence incriminating oxidative stress in the pathogenesis of DN, most animal and human studies using common antioxidants have yielded negative results [60]. Strategies involving a more targeted antioxidant approach using agents that penetrate specific cellular compartments may be n attractive and effective therapeutic addition to strengthen renoprotective interventions [61]. Targeting the redox-sensitive transcription factor Nfr2 may be a viable strategy to restore antioxidant activity in diabetes. In chronic diabetic kidney NO bioavailability is impaired but free radical scavenging with tempol, increased NO levels in renal tubules though a mechanism that involved PP2B dependent activation of NOS1 and NOS2 [62]. Recent studies have yielded increasing evidence that dysfunctional NO systems in the kidney may lead to impaired oxygen availability and disturbed mitochondrial respiration in the kidney [63]. Most recently Brosius et al. [64] has incriminated eNOS along with TGF-beta and bradykinins in the glomerular and interstitial fibrosis that so clearly characterizes the advanced phases of DN. Other studies have shown that therapy with antioxidants such as curcumin reverses such activation of eNOS and TGF- that occurs in diabetic nephropathy and ameliorate the renal disease [65]. Since kidney is an important site of L-arginine synthesis, it is logical to assume that arginine stores and consequently serum levels decline with progressive renal failure, Indeed, Baris et al. [66] had shown that lower L-arginine levels in the serum are an important predictor of nephropathy in diabetes. The progressive NO deficiency in advanced diabetic nephropathy is a reflection of gross endothelial dysfunction that ensues in DN and is a fore-runner of hypertension [67] and atherosclerotic vascular disease. Nacci et al. [68] have incriminated hyperinsulinemia and abnormal insulin signaling in endothelium in defective endothelial NO release and NO deficiency in diabetes. Recent studies suggest that endothelial dependent vasodilatation can be improved by using angiotensin receptor blockers [69].

Most of these changes are mediated by endothelial and partly inducible NOS in the chronic advanced stage of DN. Progressive loss of renal parenchyma also contributes partially to the NO deficiency since kidney is a major source of L-arginine, the sole precursor of NO. These changes and the factors affecting them are schematically represented in the figure below [26].

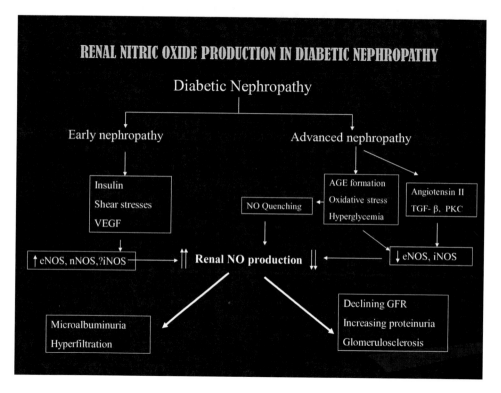

Chronic NO inhibition using NOS inhibitors in diabetic animals with nephropathy has been shown to accelerate renal structural and functional damage [26]. Some studies in human diabetic subjects suggested that people of African heritage could be more susceptible to such effects of NOS inhibition than subjects of Caucasian heritage [70]. Interestingly, modulation of testosterone by orchiectomy did not influence the effects of chronic NO inhibition on diabetic kidney [71]. Based on the findings described in the preceding section that basically underscore the NO deficient state that occurs in DN, several investigators explored the potential role of L-arginine supplementation in animal models of DN since L-arginine is the sole precursor of NO. While some reported amelioration of hyperfitration and reduction of proteinuria in diabetic rats [72] treated with L-arginine, convincing evidence of such approaches in human studies is lacking. Other investigators have reported a beneficial effect in structural and functional components of DN, by increasing dietary nitrite consumption in animal models of DN [73].

VEGF and NO Uncoupling

Vascular endothelial growth factor (VEGF) has been incriminated in the pathogenesis of DN particularly in the early phases when it contributes to hyperfiltration and increased capillary permeability leading to microalbuminuria. The role of VEGF and other growth factors is discussed in detail in another chapter in this book. One of the mechanisms of actions of VEGF involves activation of eNOS and this particular effect may be responsible for at least partially for glomerular hyperfiltration. [74,75]. VEGF normally stimulates endothelial NO production and along with NO acts as a trophic factor for the endothelium. The increased local NO levels act as inhibitory to prevent excess endothelial cell proliferation and smooth muscle cell proliferation. More recently Nakagawa et al. [76] hypothesized that the endothelial dysfunction in diabetic nephropathy induced by hyperglycemia and other factors may underlie the high VEGF state and action in DN. Under these circumstances they predicted that high VEGF and a low NO state characteristic of DN, leads to uninhibited proliferation of vascular endothelium and vascular smooth muscle cell proliferation. Nakagawa et al. [77] confirmed this hypothesis in their eNOS knout mice model of DN. Furthermore in vitro studies demonstrated that VEGF induced endothelial cell proliferation was enhanced by blocking NO with L-NAME and suppressed by exogenous NO administration whereas macrophage migration in response to VEGF was inhibited by exogenous NO suggesting that uncoupling condition could cause abnormal angiogenesis and macrophage infiltration [78]. Other investigators [79] described the role of NO in negatively regulating VEGF induced macrophage migration by inhibiting Flt-1 expression. Nakagawa et al. therefore concluded that this phenomenon of VEGF-NO uncoupling whereby a NO deficient state leads excess VEGF levels and its uninhibited action may be a key pathogenic factor in DN [80].

ANGIOTENSIN and Diabetic Nephropathy

Activation of renin angiotensin system particularly in the kidney plays an early and active role in the pathogenesis of diabetic nephropathy [81]. The mechanisms of such activation of angiotensin and the downstream events leading to renal injury and proteinuric renal failure are the sole contents of another chapter in this book and hence this aspect will not be further discussed in this chapter. For obvious reasons, the antagonists of RAAS have not only been effective in reducing proteinuria and slowing the progression of DN independent of their blood pressure effects in several animal models [82] and in humans with diabetic nephropathy, but it is also now a standard of care in the management of this condition.

ENDOTHELINS and Diabetic Nephropathy

Endothelins are vasoactive factors elaborated by endothelium and many other tissues that predominantly are vasoconstrictive. In addition to direct vasoconstrictor effects, endothelin -1 also causes endothelial dysfunction by inhibiting nitric oxide production [83]. Endothelins have also been incriminated in non hemodynamic effects such as mitosis, apoptosis and fibrosis and have been incriminated in micro and macrovascular complications of diabetes and antagonists of endothelins have been shown to prevent structural and functional changes induced by diabetes in animal models [84]. Increased circulating endothelin -1 levels have been described in microvascular complications of diabetes [3]. ET-1 has also been incriminated in development of insulin resistance [85]. Hyperinsulinemia has also been incriminated in development of CKD by stimulating the production and the renal actions of ET-1 [83]. Activation of endothelins in early diabetic nephropathy has been incriminated in the microvascular hemodynamic changes leading to functional and structural changes through intracellular second messengers and transcription factors [86].

More recently Kalani et al. [87] found not only high levels of ET-1 in plasma of patients with type II diabetes but a positive correlation between the ET-1 levels and microangioathy in such patients. The authors suggested ET-1 cause not only endothelial dysfunction directly and indirectly through inhibiting NO, but also contributed insulin resistance and accelerated development of metabolic syndrome in such patients. Not all studies found comparable results when evaluating endothelin levels in DN. For example Mukulic et al. [88] found high levels of Big endothelin and not endothelin-1 in the urine of patients with DN versus controls. Tomic et al. [89] demonstrated that in a group of diabetic subjects that included both type I and II, that higher plasma endothelin-1 levels was associated with development of systolic and diastolic hypertension.

PROSTAGLANDINS and Diabetic Nephropathy

Prostaglandins are eicosonoids generated by the action of the enzyme cyclooxegease (COX) that are vasoactive, some being vaso-constrictive and others vaso-dilatory. In addition PGs also influence the regulation of other vasoactive factors in the kidney such as the angiotensin and nitric oxide production. The kallikrein- kinin system suppresses mitochondrial respiration n nitric oxide production [90] Local production of PGs in the kidney is increased in clinical and experimental DN but the role of PGs in the pathogenesis of DN remains unclear. While the stimulus for enhanced PG synthesis remains debated, Kiritoshi et al. [91] showed in vitro studies that hyperglemia induced ROS generation may a play a role in PG synthesis. Abnormalities of excretion of PGs in the urine have been demonstrated several years ago and have been linked to hemodynamic changes of early DN [92, 93]. Umeda et al. [94] demonstrated that urinary excretion ratio of 6-keto-PGF1 alpha to TXB2 is decreased in patients with type II diabetes. Later the same authors demonstrated that Ozagrel, a TXB inhibitor improved the ratio in such patients. Other PG inhibitors such as Cilostazol and Berprost also reduced albuminuria and improved renal function. Mahadevan et al. [95] have shown at the same time that exposure in vivo or in vitro to elevated glucose increased the production of PGs by glomeruli and mesangial cells, which was linked to increased hyaluran production in the kidney. Indomethacin reduced the hyaluran production in the glomeruli linking prostaglandins to glomerular sclerosis. Hyama et al. [96] could reproduce similar findings in mesangial cells and incriminated activation of cytosolic phospholipase 2 activation and MAPK pathway in the stimulation of renal prostaglandins. Using OLETF strain of rats, Okumara et al. [97] demonstrated that urinary excretion of TXB2, PGI2 were both high in diabetic rats compared to healthy rats at 14 weeks but PGI2 normalized at 54 weeks while TXB2 remained high. Such altered renal production of PGs have been incriminated in structural and functional changes of DN. Komers et al. [98]

demonstrated an increase in COX-2 expression in diabetic rats compared to controls while administration of COX-2 inhibitor decreased the hyperfiltration in diabetic rats without changing the systemic blood pressure. While COX-I inhibition had no such benefit. The authors concluded that COX-2 as opposed to COX-1 played a role in the pathogenesis of DN. Itoh et al. [99] studied other markers of renal injury such as urinary N-acetyl –beta-D-glucosaminidase (NAG) along with ET-1 levels in the serum and kidney and found that they are all elevated in STZ diabetic rats and the levels decreased with PGI(2) derivatives implicating prostaglandins as mediators of pathogenesis through ET-1. Zuo et al. [100] showed in STZ-diabetic rats that administration of COX-2 inhibitors significantly decreased the matrix expansion and glomerular sclerosis that involved TGF-beta 1 and AT-1 receptor expression. While the observation is interesting the explanation and implications remain to be elucidated. That Beraprost, a prostacyclin analogue improved glomerular hyperfiltration and proteinuria in STZ –diabetic rats by inhibiting eNOS was shown recently by Yamashita et al. [101] and by Watanabe et al. in OLETF rats [102] while Owada et al. [92] demonstrated in clinical trials that beraprost administered for 24 months decreased proteinuria in diabetic subjects with incipient nephropathy.

Using a mouse model of diabetes (B-6 Ins2-Akita) Nasrallah et al. [103] demonstrated when ibuprofen was given from 20th to 36th week (microalbuminuric phase) that urinary excretion of PGE(2) PGEM, TXB(2) and 6 keto –PGF(1)-alpha were increased in diabetes and were reduced with administration of NSAIDs . The authors concluded that prostaglandins are involved in the functional changes of early DN and by inhibiting those changes, PG inhibitors prevent hyperfiltration, and decreased albuminuria and fibronectin deposition in the kidney. Makino et al. [104] have demonstrated an antagonist of PGE2 receptor EP1 subtype attenuated glomerular hypertrophy, mesangial expansion and proteinuria in STZ-diabetic rats by inhibiting TGF-beta expression in diabetic nephropathy. The role of thromboxanes in DN was examined by Okumura et al. [105] using diabetic rat models. They demonstrated that TXA2 excretion was increased in urine in diabetic rats and was associated with intraglomerular thrombi, both of which were decreased by OKY-046, an inhibitor of TXA2 synthesis. Cherney et al. [106] examined the hypothesis that COX2 regulated vasoreactivity in diabetic subjects in a gender dependent manner and found that COX2 inhibition hasd stronger effects in females and also that prostaglandins contributed to angiotensin II mediated gender differences in vasoreactivity, suggesting augmented female prostanoid dependence.

Summary

Nephropathy in diabetes remains a common and serious vascular complication associated with unusually high morbidity and mortality because of attendant cardiovascular risk and associated complications of advancing renal failure. Despite substantial advances in managing the obvious predisposing factors viz. hypertension, uncontrolled hyperglycemia and activated rennin angiotensin system, the treatment of this condition remains suboptimal in view of incomplete understanding of the pathogenesis. For these reasons, research in the pathogenesis of DN in the past decades has shifted towards understanding the role of some of the unconventional risk factors, signaling pathways and second messengers. This chapter addressed the role of vasoactive factors such as nitric oxide, endothelins and prostaglandins.

The literatutre relaed to role of nitric oxide in DN is complex and confusing in view of differences in the role of the three isoforms of NO synthases and the stage of the disease. The general consensus is that NO derived particularly from eNOS is activated early on in the course of DN, initiated by VEGF activation and uncontrolled hyperglycemia. The high renal NO generation may a role in hyperfiltration and development of microalbuminuria. As the renal disease progresses in diabetes a state of NO deficiency sets in, resulting from the NO inhibitory effects of TGF-β, reactive oxygen species and progressive accumulation of asymmetric dimethylarginine (ADMA). The NO quenching effects of advanced glycosylation end-products also contributes to decreased bioavailability of NO in the kidney in advanced DN. Manipulation of L-arginine-NO system has alluded many investigators as a therapeutic tool in DN for many years. While in general experimental studies in this direction have yielded positive results, human studies have not been promising partly since L-arginine is metabolized into multiple pathways in humans. Endothelins are incriminated in the pathogenesis of DN as multiple investigators reported increase in endothelins particularly ET-1 in human and experimental DN. The basis for such incrimination stems from not only the established hemodymanic effects of ETs in the diabetic microcirculation but also from the multiple and significant non-hemodynamic effects of ETs including inhibition of NO in vivo and in vitro. However more research is needed to establish the potential pathogenic role of ETs in DN and examine the therapeutic potential if any by manipulation of endothelins. Experimental and limited clinical evidence suggests that prostaglandins and thromboxanes may be involved in the pathogenesis of DN, since most such studies reported increased urinary excretion of prostaglandins. Therapeutic potential of manipulation of the eiscosanoids was also demonstrated by the interesting findings of structural and functional amelioration of DN by pharmacological inhibition of prostaglandins. Other vaso-reactive factors such as angiotensin and VEGF have been dealt in detail in other chapters. More extensive investigations are needed to establish the pathogenic potential of these vasoactive factors and for the myriad of these observations to transcend from scientific curiosity to clinical possibilities.

References

[1] Brosius, FC 3rd; Alpers, CE; Bottinger, EP; Breyer, MD; Coffman, TM; Gurley, SB; Harris, RC; Kakoki, M; Kretzler, M; Leiter, EH; Levi, M; McIndoe, RA; Sharma, K; Smithies, O; Susztak, K; Takahashi, N; Takahashi, T. Animal Models of Diabetic Complications Consortium. *J Am Soc Nephrol*, 2009 20(12),2503-12. Epub 2009 Sep 3. Mouse models of diabetic nephropathy.

[2] Cherney DZ; Scholey JW; Miller JA. Insights into the regulation of renal hemodynamic function in diabetic mellitus. *Curr Diabetes Rev,* 2008 4(4), 280-90.

[3] Schrijvers, BF; De Vriese, AS. Novel insights in the treatment of diabetic nephropathy. *Acta Clin Belg,* 2007 62(5), 278-90.

[4] Cherney, DZ; Scholey, JW; Miller, JA. Insights into the regulation of renal hemodynamic function in diabetic mellitus. *Curr Diabetes Rev*, 2008 4(4), 280-90.

[5] Bell, TD; DiBona, GF; Biemiller, R; Brands, MW. Continuously measured renal blood flow does not increase in diabetes if nitric oxide synthesis is blocked. *Am J Physiol Renal Physiol*, 2008 295(5), F1449-56. Epub 2008 Aug 27.

[6] Brosius, FC 3rd. New insights into the mechanisms of fibrosis and sclerosis in diabetic nephropathy. *Rev Endocr Metab Disord*, 2008 9(4), 245-54.

[7] Buschhausen, L; Seibold, S; Gross, O; Mathaeus, T; Weber, M; Schulze-Lohoff, E. Regulation of mesangial cell function by vasodilatory signaling molecules. *Cardiovasc Res*, 2001 51(3), 463-9.

[8] Gruden, G; Perin, PC; Camussi, G. Insight on the pathogenesis of diabetic nephropathy from the study of podocyte and mesangial cell biology. *Curr Diabetes Rev*, 2005 1(1), 27-40.

[9] Gruden, G; Perin, PC; Camussi, G. Insight on the pathogenesis of diabetic nephropathy from the study of podocyte and mesangial cell biology. *Curr Diabetes Rev*, 2005 1(1), 27-40.

[10] Hayden, MR; Whaley-Connell, A; Sowers JR. Renal redox stress and remodeling in metabolic syndrome, type 2 diabetes mellitus, and diabetic nephropathy: paying homage to the podocyte. *Am J Nephrol*, 2005 25(6), 553-69.

[11] Komers, R; Anderson, S. Glomerular endothelial NOS (eNOS) expression in type 2 diabetic patients with nephropathy. *Nephrol Dial Transplant*, 2008, 23(9), 3037; author reply 3037-8. Epub 2008 Jul 2. Comment on: Nephrol Dial Transplant, 2008 23(4), 1346-54.

[12] Hohenstein, B; Hugo, CP; Hausknecht, B; Boehmer, KP; Riess, RH; Schmieder, RE. Analysis of NO-synthase expression and clinical risk factors in human diabetic nephropathy. *Nephrol Dial Transplant*, 2008 23(4), 1346-54. Epub 2007 Dec 9.

[13] Levine, DZ; Iacovitti, M; Robertson, SJ. Modulation of single-nephron GFR in the db/db mouse model of type 2 diabetes mellitus II. Effects of renal mass reduction. *Am J Physiol Regul Integr Comp Physiol*, 2008 294(6), R1840-6. Epub 2008 Apr 16.

[14] Nakagawa, T. A new mouse model resembling human diabetic nephropathy: uncoupling of VEGF with eNOS as a novel pathogenic mechanism. *Clin Nephrol*, 2009 71(2),103-9.

[15] Kosugi, T; Heinig, M; Nakayama, T; Matsuo, S; Nakgawa, T. eNOS Knockout Mice with Advanced Diabetic Nephropathy Have Less Benefit from Renin-Angiotensin Blockade Than from Aldosterone Receptor Agonists. *Am J Pathol*, 2009. [Epub ahead of print]

[16] Mohan, S; Reddick, RL; Musi, N; Horn, DA; Yan, B; Prihoda, TJ; Natarajan, M; Abboud-Werner, SL. Diabetic eNOS knockout mice develop distinct macro- and microvascular complications. Lab Invest, 2008 88(5), 515-28. Epub 2008 Apr 7.

[17] Thaha, M; Pranawa; Yogiantoro, M; Sutjipto; Sunarjo; Tanimoto, M; Gohda, T; Tomino, Y. Association of endothelial nitric oxide synthase Glu298Asp polymorphism with end-stage renal disease. *Clin Nephrol*, 2008 70(2), 144-54.

[18] Ezzidi, I; Mtiraoui, N; Mohamed, MB; Mahjoub, T; Kacem, M; Almawi, WY. Association of endothelial nitric oxide synthase Glu298Asp, 4b/a, and -786T>C gene variants with diabetic nephropathy. *J Diabetes Complications*, 2008 22(5), 331-8. Epub 2008 Apr 16.

[19] Möllsten, A; Lajer, M; Jorsal, A; Tarnow, L. The endothelial nitric oxide synthase gene and risk of diabetic nephropathy and development of cardiovascular disease in type 1 diabetes. *Mol Genet Metab*, 2009 97(1), 80-4. Epub 2009 Feb 3

[20] Ritt, M; Ott, C; Delles, C; Schneider, MP; Schmieder, RE. Impact of the endothelial function in patients with type 2 diabetes. *Pharmacogenet Genomics*, 2008 18(8), 699-707.

[21] Chen, Y; Huang, H; Zhou, J; Doumatey, A; Lashley, K; Chen, G; Agyemin-Boateng, K; Eghan, BA; Acheampong, J; Fasanmade, O; Johnson, T; Akinsola, FB; Okafor, G; Oli, J; Ezepue, F; Amoah, A; Akafo, S; Adeyemo, A; Rotimi, CN. Polymorphism of the endothelial nitric oxide synthase gene is associated with diabetic retinopathy in a cohort of West Africans. *Mol Vis*, 2007 13, 2142-7.

[22] Zintzaras, E; Papathanasiou, AA; Stefanidis I. Endothelial nitric oxide synthase gene polymorphisms and diabetic nephropathy: a HuGE review and meta-analysis. *Genet Med*, 2009(10),695-706.

[23] Edgley, AJ; Tare, M; Evans, RG; Skordilis, C; Parkington, HC. In vivo regulation of endothelium-dependent vasodilation in the rat renal circulation and the effect of streptozotocin-induced diabetes. *Am J Physiol Regul Integr Comp Physiol*, 2008 295(3), R829-39. Epub 2008 Jul 16.

[24] McMahon, KW; Iznaola, O; Prabhakar, SS. Angiotensin-Nitric oxide interactions by in Angiotensin Research progress Ed: Hina Miura and Yuuto Saski Nova Science Publishers Inc 2008.

[25] Prabhakar, SS. tetrahydrobiopterin reverses high glucose mediated nitric oxide inhibition cultured murine mesangial cells. *Am J Physiol (Renal Physiology)*, 2001 281, F0179-F0188.

[26] Prabhakar, SS. Pathogenic role of nitric oxide alterations in diabetic nephropathy. *Curr Diab Rep*, 2005 5(6), 449-54.

[27] Allen, DA; Yaqoob, MM; Harwood, SM. Mechanisms of high glucose-induced apoptosis and its relationship to diabetic complications. *JNutr Biochem*, 2005 16(12), 705-13.

[28] Leon, CA; Raij, L. Interaction of haemodynamic and metabolic pathways in the genesis of diabetic nephropathy. *J Hypertens*, 2005 23(11), 1931-7.

[29] Nordquist, L; Palm, F. Diabetes-induced alterations in renal medullary microcirculation and metabolism. *Curr Diabetes Rev*, 2007 3(1), 53-65.

[30] Palm, F; Friederich, M; Carlsson, PO; Hansell, P; Teerlink, T; Liss, P. Reduced nitric oxide in diabetic kidneys due to increased hepatic arginine metabolism: implications for renomedullary oxygen availability. Am J Physiol Renal Physiol, 2008 294(1), F30-7. Epub 2007 Oct 17. Comment in: Am J Physiol Renal Physiol, 2008 294(1), F28-9.

[31] Pollock, JS; Carmines, PK. Diabetic nephropathy: nitric oxide and renal medullary hypoxia. *Am J Physiol Renal Physiol*, 2008 294(1), F28-9. Epub 2007 Nov 14. Comment on: Am J Physiol Renal Physiol, 2008 294(1), F30-7.

[32] Haidara, MA; Yassin, HZ; Rateb, M; Ammar, H; Zorkani, MA. Role of oxidative stress in development of cardiovascular complications in diabetes mellitus. *Curr Vasc Pharmacol*, 2006 43), 215-27.

[33] Goligorsky, MS; Chen, J; Brodsky, S. Workshop: endothelial cell dysfunction leading to diabetic nephropathy: focus on nitric oxide. Hypertension, 2001 37 (2Part 2), 744-8.

[34] Schrijvers, BF; De Vriese, AS; Flyvbjerg, A. From hyperglycemia to diabetic kidney disease: the role of metabolic, hemodynamic, intracellular factors and growth factors/cytokines. *Endocr Rev*, 2004 25(6), 971-1010.

[35] Raij, L. The pathophysiologic basis for blocking the rennin-angiotensin system in hypertensive patients with renal disease. *Am J Hypertens*, 2005 18(4 Pt 2), 95S-99S.

[36] Ksiazek, K; Witowski, J. [Dual rold of nitric oxide in the pathogens of diabetic nephropathy] [Article in Polish] *Przegl Lek*, 2002 59(3), 153-7.

[37] Prabhakar, SS. Pathogenic role of nitric oxide alterations in diabetic nephropathy. *Curr Diab Rep*, 2005 5(6), 449-54.

[38] Levine, DZ. Hyperfiltration, nitric oxide, and diabetic nephropathy. *Curr Hypertens Rep*, 2006 8(2), 153-7.

[39] Horoz, OO Yuksel, B; Bayazit, AK, Attila, G; Sertdemir, Y; Mungan, NO; Topaloglu, AK, Ozer, G.. Ambulatory blood pressure monitoring and serum nitric oxide concentration in type 1 diabetic children. *Endocr J*, 2009 56(3), 477-85.

[40] Komers, R; Anderson, S. Paradoxes of nitric oxide in the diabetic kidney. *Am J Physiol Renal Physiol*, 2003 284(6), F1121-37.

[41] Hanai, K; Babazono, T; Nyumura, I; Toya, K; Tanaka, N; Tanaka, M; Ishii, A; Iwamoto, Y. Asymmetric dimethylarginine is closely associated with the development and progression of nephropathy in patients with type 2 diabetes. *Nephrol Dial Transplant*, 2009 24(6), 1884-8. Epub 2009 Jan 7.

[42] Abhary, S; Kasmeridia, N; Burdon, DP; Kuot, A; Whiting, MJ; Yew, WP; Petrovsky, N; Craig, JE. Diabetic retinopahy is associated with elevated serum asymmetric and symmetric dimethylarginines. *Diabetes Care*, 2009 32(11), 2084-6. Epub 2009 Aug 12

[43] Yonem, A; Duran, C; Unal, M; Ipcioglu, OM; Ozcan, O. Plasma apelin asymmetric dimethylarginine levels in type 2 diabetic patients with diabetic retinopathy. *Diabetes Res Clin Pract*, 2009 84(3), 219-23.

[44] Sibal, L; Agarwal, SC; Schwedhelm, E; Lüneburg, N; Böger, RH; Home, PD. A study of endothelial function and circulating asymmetric dimethylarginine levels in people with Type 1 diabetes without macrovascular disease or microalbuminuria. *Cardiovasc Diabetol*, 2009 8, 27.

[45] Shibata, R; Ueda, S; Yamagishi, S; Kaida, Y; Matsumoto, Y; Fukami, K; Hayashida, A; Matsuoka, H; Kato, S; Kimoto, M; Okuda, S. Involvement of asymmetric dimethylarginine (ADMA) in tubulointerstitial ischaemia in the early phase of diabetic nephropathy. *Nephrol Dial Transplant*, 2009 24(4), 1162-9. Epub 2008 Nov 17.

[46] Santilli, F; Cipollone, F; Mezzetti, A; Chiarelli, F. The role of nitric oxide in the development of diabetic angiopathy. *Horm Metab Res*, 2004 36(5), 319-35.

[47] Huang, JS; Chuang, LY; Guh, JY; Huang, YJ. Effects of nitric oxide and antioxidants on advanced glycation end products-induced hypertrophic growth in human renal tubular cells. *Toxicol Sci*, 2009 111(1), 109-19.

[48] Cameron, NE; Gibson, TM; Nangle, MR; Cotter, MA. Inhibitors of advanced glycation end product formation and neurovascular dysfunction in experimental diabetes. *Ann N Y Acad Sci*, 2005 1043, 784-92.

[49] Thornalley, PJ. Use of aminoguanidine (Pimagedine) to prevent the formation of advanced glycation endproducts. *Arch Biochem Biophys*, 2003 419(1), 31-40.

[50] Gao, L; Mann GE. Vascular NAD(P)H oxidase activation in diabetes: a double-edged sword in redox signalling. *Cardiovasc Res*, 2009 82(1),9-20. Epub 2009 Jan 29.

[51] Satoh, M; Fujimoto, S; Arakawa, S; Yada, T; Namikoshi, T; Haruna, Y; Horike, H; Sasaki, T; Kashihara, N. Angiotensin II type 1 receptor blocker ameliorates uncouples endothelial nitric oxide synthase in rats with experimental diabetic nephropathy. *Nephrol Dial Tranplant*, 2008 23(12), 3806-13. Epub 2008 Jul 2.

[52] Araujo, M; Welch, WJ. Oxidate stress and nitric oxide in kidney function. *Curr Opin Npehrol Hypertens*, 2006 5(6), 449-54.

[53] Pacher, P; Szabó, C. Role of peroxynitrite in the pathogenesis of cardiovascular complications of diabetes. *Curr Opin Pharmacol*, 2006 6(2), 136-41. Epub 2006 Feb 17.

[54] Prabhakar, S; Starnes, J; Shi, S; Lonis, B; Tran, R. Diabetic nephropathy is associated with oxidative stress and decreased renal nitric oxide production. *J Am Soc Nephrol*, 2007 18(11), 2945-52. Epub 2007 Oct 10.

[55] Xiao, H; Li, Y; Qi, J; Wang, H; Liu, K. Peroxynitrite plays a key rold in glomerular lesions in diabetic rats. *J Nephrol*, 2009 22(6), 800-8.

[56] Wang, H; Li, Y; Liu, H; Liu, S; Liu, Q; Wang, X; Shi, Y; Duan H. Peroxynitrite mediates Glomerular Lesion of Diabetic Rat via JAK/STAT signaling pathway. *J Endocrinol Invest*, 2009 [Epub ahead of print]

[57] Pacher, P; Obrosova, IG; Mabley, JG, Szabó, C. Role of nitrosative stress and peroxynitrite in the pathogenesis of diabetic complications. Emerging new therapeutical strategies. *Curr Med Chem*, 2005 12(3), 267-75.

[58] Tooke, JE. Possible pathophysiological mechanisms for diabetic antiopathy in type 2 diabetes. *J Diabetes Complications*, 2000 14(4), 197-200.

[59] DeRubertis, FR; Craven, PA; Melhem, MF. Acceleration of diabetic renal injury in the superoxide dismutase knockout mouse: effect of tempol. *Metabolism*, 2007 56(9), 1256-64.

[60] Forbes, JM; Coughlan, MT; Cooper, ME. Oxidative stress as a major culprit in kidney disease in diabetes. *Diabetes*, 2008 57(6), 1446-54.

[61] Forbes, JM; Coughlan, MT; Cooper, ME. Oxidative stress as a major culprit in kidney disease in diabetes. *Diabetes*, 2008 57(6), 1446-54.

[62] Foster, JM; Carmines, PK; Pollock, JS. PP2B-dependent NO production in the medullary thick ascending limb during diabetes. *AM J Physiol Renal Physiol*, 2009 297(2), F471-80.

[63] Palm, F; Teerlink, T; Hansell, P. Nitric oxide and kidney oxygenation. *Curr Opin Nephrol Hypertens*, 2009 18(1), 68-73.

[64] Brosiums, FC 3rd. New Insights into the mechanisms of fibrosis and sclerosis in diabetic nephropathy. *Rev Endocr Metab Discord*, 2008 3(1), 53-65.

[65] Chiu, J; Khan, ZA; Farhangkhoee, H; Chakrabarti, S. Curcumin prevents diabetes-associated abnormalities in the kidneys by inhibiting p300 and nuclear factor-kappaB. *Nutrition*, 2009 25(9), 964-72.

[66] Bariş, N; Erdoğan, M; Sezer, E; Saygilli, F; Mert Ozgönül, A; Turgan, N; Ersöz, B. Alterations in L-arginine and inflammatory markers in type 2 diabetic patients with and without microalbuminuria. *Acta Diabetol*, 2009 46(4), 309-16. Epub 2009 Jan 28.

[67] Ritt, M; Ott, C; Raff, U; Schneider, MP; Schuster, I; Hilgers, KF; Schlaich, MP; Schmieder, RE. Renal vascular endothelial function in hypertensive patients with type 2 diabetes mellitus. *Am J Kidney Dis*, 2009 53(2), 281-9. Epub 2008 Dec 19.

[68] Nacci, C; Tarquinio, M; Montagnani, M. Molecular and clinical aspects of endothelial dysfunction in diabetes. *Intern Emerg Med*, 2009 4(2), 107-16.

[69] Schmieder, RE. Endothelial dysfunction: how can one intervene at the beginning of the cardiovascular continuum? *J Hypertens Suppl*, 2006 24(2), S31-5.

[70] Earle, KA; Harry, D; Madhavi, M; Zitouni, K; Barron, J. Nitric oxide bioavailability and its potential relevance to the variation in susceptibility to the renal and vascular complications in patients with type 2 diabetes. *Diabetes Care*, 2009 32(1), 138-40. Epub 2008 Oct 22.

[71] Anderson, S; Chapman, JG; Oyama, TT; Komers, R. Effect of Orchiectomy on Renal Function in Control and Diabetic Rats with Chronic Inhibition of Nitric Oxide. *Clin Exp Pharmacol Physiol,* 2009 [Epub ahead of print]

[72] Klahr, S; Morrissey, J. L-arginine as a therapeutic tool in kidney disease. *Semin Nephrol*, 2004 24(4), 389-94.

[73] Ohtake, K; Ishiyama, Y; Uchida, H; Muraki, E; Kobayashi, J. Dietary nitrite inhibits early glomerular injury in streptozotocin-induced diabetic nephropathy in rats. *Nitric Oxide,* 2007 17(2), 75-81. Epub 2007 Jul 4.

[74] Foster, RR. The importance of cellular VEGF bioactivity in the development of glomerular disease. *Nephron Exp Nephrol,* 2009;113(1),e8-e15. Epub 2009 Jul 9.

[75] Foster, RR. The importance of cellular VEGF bioactivity in the development of glomerular disease. *Nephron Exp Nephrol,* 2009;113(1),e8-e15. Epub 2009 Jul 9.

[76] Nakagawa, T; Segal, M; Croker, B; Johnson, RJ. A breakthrough in diabetic nephropathy: the role of endothelial dysfunction. *Nephrol Dial Transplant*, 2007 22(10), 2775-7. Epub 2007 Jun 25.

[77] Nakagawa, T. A new mouse model resembling human diabetic nephropathy: uncoupling of VEGF with eNOS as a novel pathogenic mechanism. *Clin Nephrol*, 2009 71(2), 103-9.

[78] Nakagawa, T. Uncoupling of VEGF with NO as a mechanism for diabetic nephropathy. *Diabetes Res Clin Pract*, 2008 82 Suppl 1, S67-9. Epub 2008 Oct 15.

[79] Sato, W; Kosugi, T; Zhang, L; Roncal, CA; Heinig, M; Campbell-Thompson, M; Yuzawa, Y; Atkinson, MA; Grant, MD; Coker, BP; Nakagawa, T. The pivotal role of VEGF on glomerular macrophage infiltration in advanced diabetic nephropathy. *Lab Invest*, 2008 88(9), 949-61. Epub 2008 Jul 7.

[80] Nakagawa, T. Uncoupling of the VEGF-endothelial nitric oxide axis in diabetic nephropathy: an explanation for the paradoxical effects of VEGF in renal disease. *J Physiol Renal Physiol,* 2007 292(6), F1665-72.

[81] Leehey, DJ; Singh, AK; Alavi, N; Singh, R. Role of angiotensin II in diabetic nephropathy. *Kidney Int Suppl*, 2000 77, S93-8.

[82] Ohtomo, S; Ito, M; Izuhara, Y; Van Ypersele De Strihou, C; Miyata, T. Reduction of albuminuria by angiotensin receptor blocker beyond blood pressure lowering: evaluation in megsin/receptor for advanced glycation end products/inducible nitric oxide synthase triple transgenic diabetic nephropathy mouse model. *Nephrology (Carlton),* 2008 13(6), 517-21. Epub 2008 Mar 17.

[83] Sarafidis, PA; Ruilope, LM. Insulin resistance, hyperinsulinemia, and renal injury: mechanisms and implications. *Am J Nephrol*, 2006 8(2), 153-7.

[84] Chakrabarti, S; Khan, ZA; Cukiernik, M; Fukuda, G; Chen, S; Mykherjee, S. Alteration of endothelins: a common pathogenetic mechanism in chronic diabetic complications. *Int J Exp Diabetes Res*, 2002 3(4), 217-31.
[85] Kalani, M. The importance of endothelin-1 for microvascular dysfunction in diabetes. *Vasc Health Risk Manag*, 2008 4(5),1061-8.
[86] Candido, R; Allen, TJ. Haemodynamics in microvascular complications in type 1 diabetes. *Diabetes Metab Res Rev*, 2002 18(4), 286-304.
[87] Kalani, M. The importance of endothelin-1 for microvascular dysfunction in diabetes. *Vasc Health Risk Manag*, 2008 4(5), 1061-8.
[88] Mikulić, I; Petrick, J; Galesić, K; Romić, Z; Cepelak, I; Zeljko-Tomić, M. Endothelin-1, big endothelin-1, and nitric oxide in patients with chronic renal disease and hypertension. *J Clin Lab Anal*, 2009 23(6), 347-56.
[89] Tomić, M; Galesić, K; Morović-Vergles, J; Romić, Z; Mikulić, I. The role of endothelin-1 and nitric oxide in the pathogenesis of hypertension in diabetic patients. *Coll Antropol*, 2008 32(1), 93-8.
[90] Kakoki,M; Smithies,O. The kallikrein-kinin system in health and in diseases of the kidney. *Kidney Int*, 2009 75(10),1019-30. Epub 2009 Feb 4.
[91] Kiritoshi, S; Nishikawa, T; Sonoda, K; Kukidome, D; Senokuchi, T; Matsuo, T; Matsumura, T; Tokunaga, H; Brownlee, M; Araki, E. Reactive oxygen species from mitochondria induce cyclooxygenase-2 gene expression in human mesangial cells: potential role in diabetic nephropathy. *Diabetes*, 2003 52(10), 2570-7.
[92] Owada, A; Suda, S; Hata, T. Effect of long-term administration of prostaglandin I(2) in incipient diabetic nephropathy. *Nephron*, 2002 92(4), 788-96.
[93] Xu, ZG; Li, SL; Lanting, L; Kim, YS; Shanmugam, N; Reddy, MA; Natarajan, R. Relationship between 12/15-lupoxygenase and COX-2 in mesangial cells: potential rold in diabetic nephropathy. *Kidney Int,* 2006 69(3), 512-9.
[94] Umeda, F; Kuroki, T; Nawata, H. Prostaglandins and diabetic nephropathy. *J Diabetes Complications*, 1995 9(4), 334-6.
[95] Mahadevan, P; Larkins, RG; Fraser, JR; Fosang, AJ; Dunlop, ME. Increased hyaluronan production in the glomeruli from diabetic rats: a link between glucose-induced prostaglandin production and reduced sulphated proteoglycan. *Diabetologia*, 1995 38(3), 298-305.
[96] Hayama, M; Akiba, S; Fukuzumi, M; Sato, T. High glucose-induced cytosolic phospholipase A2 activation responsible for eicosanoid production in rat mesangial cells. *J Biochem,* 1997 122(6), 1196-201.
[97] Okumura, M: Imanishi; M; Yamashita, T; Yamamura, Y; Kim, S; Kwao, H; Tanaka, S; Fujii, S. Renal production of thromboxane and prostaglandins in a rat model of type 2 diabetes. *Life Sci*, 2000 66(5), 371-7.
[98] Komers, R; Lindsley, JN; Oyama, TT; Schutzer, WE; Reed, JF; Mader, SL; Anderson, S. Immunohistochemical and functional correlation of reanl cyclooxygenase-2 in experimental diabetes. *J Clin Invest*, 2001 107(7), 889-98.
[99] Itoh, Y; Nakai, A; Kakizawa, H; Makino, M; Fujiwara, K; Kobayashi, T; Kato, T; Nagata, M; Oda, N; Katsumata, H; Nagasaka, A; Itoh, M. Alteration of endothelin-1 concentration in STZ-induced diabetic rat nephropathy. Effects of a PGI(2) derivative. *Horm Res*, 2001 56(5-6), 165-71.

[100] Zuo, Y; Gu, Y; Ma, J; Lin, S. [Effect of selective cyclooxygenase -2 inhibitor on the renal lesion of streptozotocin-induced diabetic rats and its possible mechanism] *Zhonghua Yi Xue Za Zhi,* 2002 82(4), 239-43.

[101] Yamashita, T; Shikata, K; Matsuda, M; Okada, S; Ogawa, D; Sugimoto, H; Wada, J; Makino, H. Beraprost sodium, prostacyclin analogue, attenuates glomerular hyperfiltration and glomerular macrophage infiltration by modulating ecNOS expression in diabetic rats. *Diabetes Res Clin Pract*, 2002 57(3), 149-61.

[102] Watanabe, M; Nakashima, H; Mochizuki, S; Abe, Y; Ishimura, A; Ito, K; Fukushima, T; Miyake, K; Ogahara, S; Saito, T. Amelioration of diabetic nephropathy in OLETF rats by prostaglandin I(2) analog, berapost sodium. *Am J Nephrol,* 2009 30(1), 1-11. Epub 2009 Jan 22.

[103] Nasrallah, R; Robertson, SJ; Hébert, RL. Chronic COX inhibition reduces diabetes-induced hyperfiltration, proteinuria, and renal pathological markers in 36-week B6-Ins2 (Akita) mice. *Am J Nephrol,* 2009 30(4), 346-53. Epub 2009 Jul 17.

[104] Makino, H; Tanaka, I; Mukoyama, M; Sugawara, A; Mori, K; Muro, S; Suganami, T; Yahata, K; Ishibashi, R; Ohuchida, S; Maruyama, T; Narumiya, S; Nakao, K. Prevention of diabetic nephropathy in rats by prostaglandin E receptor EP2-selective antagonist. *J Am Soc Nephrol,* 2002 13(7), 1757-65.

[105] Okumura, M; Imanishi, M; Okamura, M; Hosoi, M; Okada, N; Konishi, Y; Morikawa, T; Miura, K; Nakatani, T; Fujii, S. Role for thromboxane A2 from glomerular thrombi in nephropathy with type 2 diabetic rats. *Life Sci*, 2003 72(24), 2695-705.

[106] Cherney, DZ; Scholey, JW; Nasrallah, R; Dekker, MG; Slorach, C; Bradley, TJ; Hébert, RL; Sochett, EB; Miller, JA. Renal hemodynamic effect of cyclooxygenase 2 inhibition in young men and women with uncomplicated type 1 diabetes mellitus. *Am J Physiol Renal Physiol*, 2008 294(6), F1336-41. Epub 2008 Apr 9.

In: Advances in Pathogenesis of Diabetic Nephropathy
Editor: Sharma S. Prabhakar

ISBN: 978-1-61122-134-3
© 2012 Nova Science Publishers, Inc.

Chapter XI

Endothelial Dysfunction in Diabetic Nephropathy

Takamune Takahashi and Raymond C. Harris
Division of Nephrology and Hypertension, Vanderbilt University School of Medicine,
Nashville, TN 37232, US

Abstract

A hallmark of diabetic vascular complications is endothelial dysfunction which is characterized by impaired endothelium-dependent vasorelaxation, enhanced leukocyte-endothelial interactions, and thrombosis. There is compelling evidence that decreased nitric oxide (NO) bioavailability, which involves either inactivation of NO or a decrease in NO synthesis coupled with dysfunctional endothelial nitric oxide synthase (eNOS), play a major role in diabetic endothelial dysfunction and vascular injury. Furthermore, recent experimental studies using diabetic eNOS knockout mice have demonstrated an essential role of eNOS-derived NO in diabetic glomerular injury. In this chapter, we review the disorders in eNOS/NO system in DN, and discuss how dysfunctional eNOS/NO system contributes to DN, what molecules or pathways are involved in this disorder, and by what therapeutic approaches it could be restored.

Introduction

Diabetic nephropathy (DN) is one of the most serious end-organ complications in diabetes and the leading cause of end-stage renal disease in many countries. Endothelial dysfunction is a prevalent feature in diabetic vasculopathy and has also been shown to be an important pathophysiologic determinant for DN [1-3]. Endothelial cells play a key role in vascular homeostasis by generating paracrine factors that regulate vascular tone, inhibit platelet function, prevent adhesion of leukocytes, and limit proliferation of vascular smooth muscle cells as well as by constituting a selective barrier to the diffusion of macromolecules from the vessel lumen to the interstitial space. The dominant factor responsible for many of those functions is endothelial-derived nitric oxide (NO) generated by endothelial NO synthase (eNOS). Endothelial NO induces vasodilatation, suppresses platelet aggregation and adhesion, scavenges superoxide radicals, prevents oxidative modification of LDL cholesterol, limits vascular smooth muscle cell proliferation by specific actions on the cell cycle, and decreases the expression of proinflammatory genes in vascular cells [4-6]. Endothelial dysfunction and pathological changes seen in diabetic vasculature, including vasoconstriction, thrombosis, vascular inflammation, and proliferation of vascular smooth muscle cells, are believed to be caused largely by reduction of vascular NO bioavailability [5, 7]. Thus, the eNOS/NO system plays a central role in diabetic vascular disease including nephropathy and atherosclerosis. Here, we review disorders in the eNOS/NO system in diabetic kidney disease, and discuss how a dysfunctional eNOS/NO system contributes to this disease, what molecules or pathways are involved in this disorder, and by what therapeutic approaches it could be restored.

Mechanisms of Endothelial Dysfunction in Diabetes

Diabetes markedly increases the risk of all forms of cardiovascular disease. Endothelial dysfunction, which is characterized by defective endothelium-dependent relaxation, is a hall mark and an early sign of diabetic vascular complications. A large body of evidence in humans indicates that endothelial dysfunction is closely associated with microangiopathy and atherosclerosis in both type1 and type2 diabetes [8-10]. This association is particularly true in those patients with type 1 diabetes who have nephropathy. Decreases in endothelium-dependent relaxation are a common feature in both human and experimental diabetes. Furthermore, experimental studies have shown that endothelial dysfunction is found in both conduit and resistance arteries in diabetic animals[11]. These vascular beds showed normal relaxation to nitrovasodilatators, which relax vascular smooth muscle by activating guanylate cyclase but do not require an intact or normally functioning endothelium. These findings indicate that impaired vascular relaxation in diabetes cannot be explained by an intrinsic change in reactivity to NO or guanylate cyclase reactivity and that endothelial dysfunction is a primary event in diabetic vasculopathy. Thus, endothelial dysfunction is universal in diabetes and a critical determinant of DN.

Endothelial cells generate paracrine factors that induce vascular relaxation. These include NO, vasodilator prostanoids, and endothelium-derived hyperpolarizing factor (EDHF). Although the mechanisms underlying endothelial dysfunction in diabetes may be multifactorial[11-13], a large body of study has shown that endothelial dysfunction associated with diabetes is mainly due to a decrease in the bioavailability of NO, which involves either a decrease in NO synthesis or inactivation of NO. In vasculature, NO is synthesized by endothelial NO-synthase (eNOS, NOS3) in response to several stimuli, including receptor-dependent (bradykinin, acetylcholine, adenosine triphosphate/ATP) and mechanical stimuli (e.g. shear stress)[14, 15]. NO diffuses from the endothelium to the vascular smooth muscle cells, where it increases the concentration of cGMP by stimulating soluble guanylate cyclase and thereby induces vascular relaxation. A functional eNOS enzyme transfers electrons from nicotinamide adenine dinuleotide phosphate (NADPH) via flavin adenine dinucleotide (FAD) and flavin mononucleotide (FMN) in the carboxy-terminal reductase domain to the heme in the amino-terminal oxygenase domain where the substrate L-arginine is oxidized to L-citrulline and NO [16]. This normal flow of electrons requires "dimerization" of the enzyme, L-arginine (substrate), and tetrahydro-biopterin (BH_4, co-factor).

Diabetes stimulates production of reactive oxygen species (ROS) in endothelium. Hyperglycemia causes the production of superoxide ($O2^{\cdot-}$) through mitochondrial electron-transport chain, leading to formation of secondary ROS (17). Furthermore, superoxide is produced in vascular cells by multiple pathogenic stimuli and intracellular pathways in diabetes [17, 18]. These include advanced glycation end products (AGEs), angiotensin II (Ang-II), oxidized-LDL, inflammatory cytokines, free fatty acids, NADPH oxidase, xanthine oxygenase and cytochrome P450. Superoxide interacts avidly with NO to form peroxynitrite ($ONOO^-$). $ONOO^-$ reduces levels of BH_4, which is highly sensitive to oxidation, and causes eNOS "uncoupling"(6, 16, 19). In fact, supplementation with BH_4 or gene transfer of the GTP cyclohydrolase 1, the rate-limiting enzyme of BH4 synthesis, is able to correct the eNOS dysfunction in diabetes (20-24). Alternatively, oxidation of the zinc-thiolate complex of eNOS by $ONOO^-$ has been proposed as a mechanism of eNOS uncoupling. Uncoupled eNOS, in turn, generates superoxide instead of NO via the oxygenase domain, and further increases oxidative stress and decreases NO synthesis. Thus, uncoupling of eNOS changes eNOS from a protective enzyme to a contributor to oxidative stress. It is now thought that "uncoupled" eNOS and NADPH oxidase may serve as major source for superoxide overproduction in diabetic endothelium. Collectively, it is believed that endothelial dysfunction in diabetes is largely due to increased production of ROS, which will decrease the vascular bioavailability of NO.

In addition to this mechanism, it has been suggested that arginine deficiency and/or substrate utilization may cause vascular NO deficiency in diabetes [25]. Plasma arginine concentrations are decreased in diabetic rats and in some human patients[11], and the content of arginine is reduced in freshly isolated diabetic rat aorta [26]. There is increasing evidence both in vivo and in vitro that increasing concentration of arginine can improve endothelial dysfunction and NO production in diabetes, although it was ineffective in some studies[11]. L-arginine supplementation was shown to improve glomerular dysfunction and agonist-stimulated cGMP generation in diabetic rats [27, 28]. Moreover, recent studies have shown that arginase, an enzyme of the urea cycle hydrolyzing L-arginine to urea and L-ornithine, is expressed in vascular cells as well as in hepatic tissue and plays an important role in vascular NO homeostasis [29]. Some studies have shown that upregulation of arginase inhibits eNOS-mediated NO synthesis and may contribute to endothelial dysfunction in diabetes (30-32). Acute treatment of diabetic coronary arteries with arginase inhibitors was shown to reverse the impaired vasodilatation to acetylcholine [32]. Lastly, recent studies have shown that an endogenous competitive inhibitor of L-arginine, asymmetric dimethylarginine (ADMA), is increased in the patients with diabetes and may cause endothelial dysfunction [33-35]. ADMA was shown to be related to vascular complications in diabetic patients [36-38].

Endothelial Dysfunction and eNOS/NO Disorders in Diabetic Nephropathy

1) Human Diabetic Nephropathy

Microalbuminuria is a significant risk factor for cardiovascular mortality in type 1 and type 2 diabetes. Microalbuminuria predicts the development of overt DN in type 1 and type 2 diabetes [39], while the relationship in type 2 diabetes is less clear because of the greater heterogeneity of this condition and the presence of other risk factors for microalbuminuria in these, usually elderly patients. In type 1 diabetes, either microalbuminuria or macroalbuminuria is closely associated with systemic endothelial dysfunction [8, 10, 40]. In these patients, markers of endothelial dysfunction, including VCAM-1, ACE, ET-1, PAI-1, elevated urinary excretion of type IV collagen fragments, increased transcapillary escape rate of albumin and elevated serum vWF, are present before the onset of microalbuminuria and increase further in parallel with increasing endothelial dysfunction (10). While microalbuminuria may occur in the absence of endothelial dysfunction in some type 2 diabetes patients, in general, increased levels of thrombomodulin, PAI-1, serum type IV collagen and vWF predict its appearance [9]. Thus, endothelial dysfunction is correlated with, and precedes microalbuminuria, the best documented predictor for a high risk of development of DN in both type 1 and type 2 diabetes, indicating its critical involvement in the pathogenesis of human DN.

Altered serum or urine NO levels have been described in patients with DN [41-44]. Hiragushi et al. demonstrated that urine NO metabolites are increased in normo-and microalbuminuric diabetic patients with increased GFR and decline in macroalbuminuric patients [41]. Another study indicated that African-Asian type II diabetic patients with microalbuminuria, who are susceptible to end-stage renal failure, exhibit significantly decreased stable NO metabolites in the urine compared to a comparable group of Caucasian diabetic patients [45]. Furthermore, two studies have investigated serum NO levels and found increased levels of serum or plasma NO in micro- and macroalbuminuric nephropathy [43, 44]. Finally, immunohistochemical study of type 2 diabetic patients showed that eNOS expression is up-regulated in glomerular endothelium in nephropathy patients [41, 46] and declines in macroalbuminuric nephropathy [41]. These findings suggest that decreased endothelium-dependent vasodilation in early diabetic subjects is associated with the impaired action of NO secondary to its inactivation from increased oxidative stress, rather than decreased NO production from vascular endothelium and that NO production and eNOS expression decline as nephropathy advances.

2) eNOS Gene Polymorphisms Associated with Human Diabetic Nephropathy

Polymorphisms in the eNOS gene that lead to decreased eNOS expression have been found to be associated with advanced DN in both type 1 and type 2 diabetic patients. Genome wide scans have indicated that regions on 7q, 18q and 22q influence proteinuria and/or development of DN in type 2 diabetes [47]. Importantly, evidence for a region on 7q overlapped all studies (47). Notably the gene for eNOS is found on human chromosome 7q. Furthermore, recent studies have shown that eNOS gene polymorphisms affect eNOS activity and are associated with advanced DN in patients [47]. These polymorphisms include a Glu298Asp missense mutation, a 27-bp repeat in intron 4, and the T-786C single nucleotide polymorphism (SNP) in the promoter. Two eNOS polymorphisms, (−786) T > C and the 894G > T (Glu298Asp), have been shown to be associated with altered NOS activity in experimental studies. These polymorphisms have been reported to be associated with DN in type 1 and type 2 diabetic patients [48-51] and ESRD in some but not all studies (52-54). The progression of renal disease has also been reported to be influenced by (−786)T > C polymorphism (55). The variable number of tandem repeat (VNTR) polymorphism located in intron 4 of eNOS (eNOS4b/a polymorphism; 4b, five times repeats; 4a, four times repeats) was reported to be significantly associated with plasma NO concentration [56]. Carriers of the "a" allele in intron 4 were shown to exhibit lower plasma concentrations of NO metabolites. Variable results have been reported for the association of eNOS 4b/4a polymorphism with diabetic renal disease (57-60). Thus, the involvement of eNOS as a clinically relevant modifier for risk of human DN is supported by clinical studies showing that diabetes with an eNOS 894G > T (Glu298Asp) and (−786) T > C polymorphism exhibit not only decreased eNOS activity but also an accelerated risk of diabetic renal failure [49, 55, 61]. These studies suggest that genetic polymorphisms of eNOS also may play a role in the NO abnormalities that contribute to the development and progression of DN. However, these eNOS polymorphisms have not been associated with DN in all studies [62-66].

3) Experimental Diabetic Nephropathy

A number of studies have examined renal eNOS expression in diabetic animals [67]. The kidney expresses all three NOS isoforms; neuronal NOS (nNOS, NOS1), inducible NOS (iNOS, NOS2), and endothelial constitutive NOS (eNOS, NOS3)[68]. In rat and human kidney, eNOS is detected in the endothelium of preglomerular, glomerular, and postglomerular vessels, where iNOS and nNOS are hardly detected [69-71]; this finding indicates that eNOS is the major NOS isoform in renal endothelium. Most studies have demonstrated increased eNOS expression in early (1-6 weeks) diabetic kidney [72-78], although eNOS expression was unaltered in some studies [79-81]. Choi et al. reported markedly increased renal cortical expression of all NOS isoforms in streptozotocin (STZ) induced diabetic rats [72]. Sugimoto et al. showed enhanced eNOS expression and activity in endothelium of afferent arteriole and glomerulus, but not efferent arterioles, of STZ-induced diabetic rats by immunohistochemistry and NADPH diaphorase staining [73]. They also showed that enhanced NADPH diaphorase staining is associated with increases in afferent diameters, glomerular filtration rate (GFR) and glomerular hypertrophy. These changes were ameliorated either by insulin treatment or by treatment with L-NAME, a non-specific NOS inhibitor. Veelken et al. and de Vriese et al. also reported increased eNOS expression in the endothelium of preglomerular and glomerular vessels of hyperfiltering STZ-induced diabetic rats [75, 76]. Increased eNOS expression was also shown in purified renal vascular tress of diabetic rats [77]. Furthermore, Onozato et al. showed upregulation of eNOS in diabetic rat kidneys is corrected by an angiotensin-converting enzyme inhibitor (ACEI) or an angiotensin receptor blocker (ARB) treatment (78). In addition, Shin et al. reported that eNOS mRNA expression is increased in the outer medulla of STZ-induced diabetic rats treated with insulin (74). Thus, most of the available evidence suggests that eNOS expression is increased in the diabetic renal cortex early in the disease.

The mechanism of eNOS upregulation in diabetic kidney or glomeruli is still incompletely understood; however, several studies have implicated high-glucose and VEGF as mediators of the increased eNOS expression. In endothelial cell culture, Kasai et al. and Hoshiyama et al. have shown that high concentrations of D-glucose directly stimulate NO production concurrent with up-regulation of eNOS protein [82, 83]. Vascular endothelial growth factor (VEGF) is known to stimulate NO production in endothelial cells by up-regulating eNOS expression as well as by increasing eNOS activity through the PI3/Akt pathway [14, 15]. The expression of VEGF in visceral glomerular epithelial cells (podocytes) and of VEGF receptors in endothelial cells of glomerular capillaries and pre- and post-glomerular vessels is upregulated in diabetic rats as well as in human [76, 77, 84]. Vriese et al. have shown that anti-VEGF antibodies correct renal dysfunction (hyperfiltration, albuminuria, and hypertrophy) and prevent up-regulation of eNOS in early rat DN [76]. In addition to VEGF, Wang et al. showed that insulin-like growth factor-I (IGF-I), which is also increased in diabetic glomeruli, up-regulates glomerular eNOS expressions [85].

A characteristic hemodynamic alteration in early diabetic kidney is the development of glomerular hyperfiltration. Since NO may increase blood flow, it was suggested that increased vascular NO in early diabetes may serve as a mediator in diabetic glomerular hyperfiltration. Several lines of evidence suggested that renal NO generation and action may be increased early in diabetes, although decreased cortical NOS activity was demonstrated in some studies [79]. In streptozotocin-induced diabetic rats, renal cortical NOS activity measured by L-citrulline assay and plasma and urinary excretion levels of stable products NO oxidation (NOx) were shown to be significantly increased as compared with non-diabetic rats (27, 80). Moreover, experimental studies using non-selective NOS inhibitors provided further evidence regarding the NO status in diabetic kidney (these studies were nicely reviewed by Komers and Anderson [67]). Early studies have shown that $U_{NOx}V$ is increased in hyperfiltering diabetic rats, and NOS inhibition either with NLA or L-NAME decreases or normalizes GFR and RPF and induces greater vasoconstrictor responses in diabetic animals [27, 86], suggesting enhanced renal generation of NO in diabetes and its contribution to diabetic hyperfiltration. Furthermore, Komers et al. evaluated the effects of L-NAME in conscious control and hyperfiltering diabetic rats [87]. They showed that with a low dose of L-NAME, diabetic rats demonstrate a blunted mean arterial pressure response and significant reduction in GFR and RPF compared with controls. $U_{NOx}V$ was increased in diabetic rats and it was significantly reduced by low-dose L-NAME. In addition, diabetic rats demonstrated no response to the NO donor glyceryl trinitrate, while control rats showed significant renal vasodilatation. The authors interpreted the lack of a NO donor effect in the diabetic kidney as a further indication of enhanced NO production and/or signaling that can not be altered by additional NO. Similar results, i.e., significant reduction in hyperfiltration in response to L-NAME, have also been described in other studies [77, 88, 89]. These findings indicate increased NO production and action in diabetic kidney and its involvement in diabetic glomerular hyperfiltration, yet not all studies have found enhanced renal hemodynamic responses to NO inhibition (this may be due to techniques used for measurements of GFR and renal perfusion or the absence of insulin treatment as discussed by Komers and Andersons [67]).

There is also abundant literature indicating defective endothelium-dependent NO production and function in diabetes. Wang et al. evaluated responses to intravenous infusion of ACh and found that the renal vasodilator response to ACh was diminished in diabetic rats but not in normoglycemic diabetic rats [90]. Craven et al. demonstrated that generation of NO-dependent cyclic guanosine monophosphate is impaired in glomeruli isolated from diabetic rats (28). Furthermore, Sato et al. recently assessed glomerular NO synthesis in diabetic rats by direct NO measurements using the NO-sensitive fluorescent dye, dichlorofluorescein diacetate (DCFH-DA), and demonstrated decreased NO synthesis in diabetic glomeruli, whereas the mRNA and protein expression of eNOS was increased in the glomeruli [91]. They also suggested that superoxide production through NAD(P)H oxidase and uncoupled eNOS may serve as major sources of superoxide overproduction in diabetic glomeruli, and eNOS uncoupling is responsible for diminished NO bioavailability in the diabetic glomeruli. In addition, Chu and Bohlen showed that high glucose inhibits glomerular eNOS activity through a PKC mechanism, using a similar NO-sensitive fluorescent dye (4,5-diaminofluorescein diacetate) [92]. These findings suggest reduced NO bioavailability and/or defects in receptor-mediated eNOS activation in the renal vascular endothelium, apparently contrasting to observations of substantial NO dependency of renal hemodynamics in hyperfiltering rats, as revealed with nonspecific NOS inhibitors. Komers et al. hypothesized that increased nNOS activity could explain this paradox. This NOS form is expressed in macula densa cells and nNOS-derived NO was shown to decrease afferent arteriolar tone, contribute to control of intraglomerular pressure, and counteract afferent vasoconstriction induced by activation of tubular glomerular feedback [69, 93-95]. They examined the acute effects of systemic nNOS inhibition with the specific nNOS inhibitor S-methyl-L-thiocitrulline (SMTC) in diabetic rats, and found that SMTC induces stronger renal vasoconstriction responses in diabetic animals compared with control animals [96]. They also administered SMTC directly into the abdominal aorta above the left renal artery to diminish systemic effects of SMTC and demonstrated that SMTC nearly normalizes GFR in hyperfiltering diabetic rats without influencing MAP [97]. Renal hemodynamic effects of SMTC were attenuated in normoglycemic rats. Similar results were reported with a different nNOS inhibitors, 7-nitro indazole [98] or a different model, db/db mouse [99]. Conversely, the selective iNOS inhibitor, L-NIL, had no effects on renal hemodynamics in diabetic rats [75, 81]. Given the physiological roles of nNOS-derived NO and its higher production by macula densa cells in diabetes, these observations suggest that nNOS contributes to altered renal NO production and glomerular hyperfiltration in experimental diabetes. It is noteworthy that the nonspecific NOS inhibitor L-NAME did not influence GFR but further decreased RPF in diabetic rats pretreated with SMTC, suggesting a role of eNOS in the control of renal perfusion in diabetes. Therefore, it is likely that nNOS is the major NOS isoform responsible for diabetic glomerular hyperfiltration and that vascular NO bioavailability may be reduced in diabetic renal vasculature possibly due to increased vascular oxidative stress, despite an up-regulation of eNOS protein.

Lastly, several lines of evidence have suggested that progression of DN is associated with a state of progressive NO deficiency. By using thoracic aortic rings and vasoactive agents including acetylcholine, Pieper has demonstrated that the duration of diabetes may determine vascular NO production, from an increase at the early sages, followed by a period of normal production, and then to a progressive decrease [100]. Erdely et al. have suggested that advanced DN in Zucker rats, leading to severe proteinuria and declining renal function, is associated with decreases in renal cortical NO production [101]. They also showed that nNOS abundance declines as nephropathy progresses, whereas eNOS abundance is slightly increased. Khamaisi et al. also showed progressive reduction of renal cortical NOS activity in STZ-induced diabetic rats [102]. More recently, Yuzawa et al. showed that renal and glomerular eNOS expression is reduced in OVE26 transgenic diabetic mouse, which exhibits progressive nephropathy, whereas VEGF is upregulated in the kidney [103]. Furthermore, some studies have demonstrated that "chronic" inhibition of NO by a non-specific NOS inhibitor accelerates nephropathic changes in diabetic animals. Craven et al. showed that diabetic rats receiving nonpressor doses of L-NAME for four weeks exhibited significantly higher albuminuria and TGF-β expression(104), but another study showed no effects[105]. Kamijo et al. recently showed that long term L-NAME treatment (from 22 wks to 52 wks of age) drastically exacerbated diabetic nephropathy in Otsuka Long-Evans Tokushima fatty rats[106]. Taken together, these studies suggest that progressive NO deficiency may play a key role in the progression of DN.

Insights from Diabetic eNOS Knockout Mice

In early studies, the role of eNOS in DN was examined by using NOS inhibitors, comparing the effects of non-specific NOS inhibitors with those of isoform specific NOS inhibitors (nNOS or iNOS inhibitor). However, the conclusions reached were limited due to the lack of a specific eNOS inhibitor. During the past decades, targeted disruption of each of the NOS genes has been achieved, resulting in viable and fertile knockout mice for each NOS isoform [107]. These animals enabled us to investigate the specific functions of eNOS in DN. To date, four groups have investigated the renal effects of eNOS deficiency in diabetes by generating diabetic eNOS knockout mice. We and Mohan et al. have generated eNOS knockout mice with type II diabetes by backcross mating of eNOS knockout mouse to C57BLKS db/db strain [108, 109]. Two other studies have induced diabetes in C57BL6 strain eNOS knockout mice using STZ injection, either with high-dose [110] or multiple low dose STZ [111]. Compared with db/db eNOS +/+ (WT), the db/db eNOS -/- (knockout; KO) mice exhibited dramatic albuminuria, hypertension, reduced GFR (< 50% of db/db eNOS WT), and advanced renal histopathology including nodular mesangial expansion accompanied by fibronectin accumulation, mesangiolysis, focal segmental glomerulosclerosis, arteriolar hyalinosis, GBM thickening, glomerular macrophage infiltration, glomerular fibrin and hyaline deposition and mild tubulointerstitial fibrosis. It is noteworthy that the aorta was normal and atherogenic lesions were not observed in the db/db eNOSKO mice; this finding suggests that glomerular microvasculature is predominantly affected by eNOS deficiency. Interestingly, the db/db eNOSKO mice showed prominent hyperinsulinemia, large islets, and lower plasma glucose levels (109), yet the mechanism of this remains to be elucidated. The STZ-induced diabetic eNOS knockout mice also showed significant nephropathic changes as compared with STZ-induced diabetic eNOSWT and non-diabetic eNOSKO mice, although eNOS deficiency did not alter the severity of hyperglycemia. The renal abnormalities include significant albuminuria, hypertension, mesangial expansion, mesangiolysis, glomerular macrophage infiltration and fibrin deposition, arteriolar hyalinosis, and GBM thickening. It is noteworthy that high-dose STZ eNOSKO mice exhibited lower survival rate and a more severe renal phenotype than low-dose STZ eNOSKO mice, although low-dose STZ model showed higher blood glucose levels. These include overt albuminuria, lower GFR, nodular mesangial expansion, glomerular microaneurism, glomerulosclerosis, and tubulointerstitial injury. Glomerulosclerosis and tubulointerstitial injury were also observed in low-dose STZ eNOSKO mice; however, significant differences were not observed between diabetic and non-diabetic eNOSKO mice. These findings indicate that non-specific tissue toxicity of high-dose STZ may affect the renal phenotype in diabetic eNOSKO mice, while insulin treatment improves renal injury in high-dose STZ eNOSKO mice [110]. Indeed, Ins2^{Akita} eNOSKO diabetic mice that are F1 between C57BL/6 and 129SvEv develop nephropathy similar to what is seen in low-dose STZ eNOSKO mice (Takahashi N, University of North Carolina, personal communication). It is likely that both diabetes and eNOS deficiency are required for the renal toxicity of high-dose STZ.

The studies with diabetic eNOSKO mice clearly indicate a vital role of eNOS in the pathogenesis of DN; however, these diabetic eNOSKO studies have also raised several questions about the role of eNOS in DN.

1. Does hypertension account for advanced glomerular injury in diabetic eNOSKO mice? The diabetic eNOSKO mice exhibited elevated blood pressure as compared with diabetic eNOS WT mice, especially in high-dose STZ eNOSKO mice. Therefore, glomerular injury in the diabetic eNOSKO mice may be due in part by systemic hypertension and reduced renal blood flow. In fact, mesangiolysis is more frequently observed in the outer half of renal cortex in low-dose STZ eNOSKO mice (Takahashi T, unpublished observation). Kosugi et al. have recently examined the effects of blood pressure in the high-dose STZ eNOSKO model by treating the mice with hydralazine [112]. They have shown that hydralazine treatment remarkably suppresses albuminuria and glomerular injury, including mesangiolysis and microaneurysms, and improves renal function in high-dose STZ eNOSKO mice. In addition, our preliminary study showed that albuminuria and glomerular injury in db/db eNOSKO mice are markedly suppressed by ACE inhibition with captopril (Harris RC, unpublished observation). These findings demonstrate that systemic blood pressure and/or RAS system may have a profound effect on the glomerular injury in diabetic eNOSKO mice. In this context, it is noteworthy that eNOS-derived NO may negatively regulate Ang-II signaling [113]. It is known that most hypertensive animals do not produce mesangiolysis and nodular mesangial expansion. Furthermore, previous studies have suggested that endothelial dysfunction may alter autoregulation, and consequently predispose the animal to glomerular hypertension [114, 115] and that endothelial NO is an indispensable factor to regulate the intraglomerular pressure by modulating afferent and efferent arterioles [116, 117]. This could explain why a mild elevation of blood pressure (15-20 mmHg) in this model could have such a strong effect on glomerular injury. It would also be important to determine the effects of eNOS deficiency on renal perfusion in diabetic kidney. Reduction of cortical renal blood flow and subsequent renal ischemia may explain why mesangiolysis is observed mostly in outer cortex and why mesangiolysis is seen in only 7-10 % of glomeruli. In this context, it is noteworthy that glomerular hyperfiltration is not observed in diabetic eNOSKO mice [111].

2. What is the mechanism underlying glomerular injury in diabetic eNOSKO mice? Since NO regulates various biological responses including cell proliferation, apoptosis, and inflammation, multiple mechanisms could be involved in glomerular injury in diabetic eNOSKO mice. Endothelial NO was shown to prevent high glucose- mediated endothelial apoptosis by inhibiting NF-κB signaling [118, 119], decreasing cytokine-induced endothelial activation [120] as well as production of cytokines in endothelial cells [121], stimulating heme oxygenase-1 gene transcription [122], inhibiting high glucose-induced endothelial cellular senescence [123], and suppressing TGFβ production [124]. Disruption of these cell-protective activities of NO could accelerate glomerular injury in diabetic mice. Moreover, Nakagawa et al. has shown that NO negatively regulates VEGF receptor signaling in cultured endothelial cells exposed to high glucose [125]. They also observed up-regulated glomerular VEGF expression and endothelial cell proliferation in high-dose STZ eNOSKO mice [112]. Sato et al. has suggested that the loss of eNOS-derived NO in diabetes increases Flt-1 (VEGFR1) expression in macrophage, and stimulates glomerular macrophage infiltration concomitant with up-regulated glomerular VEGF and results in advanced diabetic glomerular injury [126]. In addition, we have shown that glomerular VE-cadherin is down-regulated in low-dose STZ eNOSKO mice [111]. These findings suggest that increased VEGF activity along with disruption of endothelial junctional integrity may result in abnormal endothelial growth and vascular leak and leads to advanced glomerular pathology (Figure). The precise mechanisms of VEGF up-regulation and VE-cadherin down-regulation in diabetic eNOSKO glomeruli are currently unknown. Since NO is known to suppress hypoxia inducible factor -1 (HIF1) expression [127], a potent inducer of VEGF, a potential mechanism may be that a deficit of eNOS-derived NO in diabetes may induce stable expression of HIF1 in glomeruli and lead to VEGF up-regulation. The increased VEGF signaling, in turn, may induce VE-cadherin redistribution and internalization by phosphorylating VE-cadherin [128], resulting in impaired endothelial cell-cell adhesion. This model is further supported by our preliminary observation of up-regulation of HIF1 in diabetic eNOSKO glomeruli (Takahashi T, unpublished observation). Further studies will be required to determine the mechanisms of advanced diabetic glomerular injury in diabetic eNOSKO mice.

3. *What is the mechanism of albuminuria in diabetic eNOSKO model?* The diabetic eNOSKO mice displayed preserved podocyte morphology and nephrin and VEGF expression. This is particularly true in low-dose STZ eNOSKO mice [111], suggesting that podocyte injury may not be the major cause of albuminuria in this model. The endothelial cell surface coat (known as the glycocalyx), which is composed of negatively charged proteoglycans and glycosaminoglycan, has recently been shown to serve as an important barrier to prevent passage of macromolecule at glomerular capillary wall by acting as a charge barrier [129, 130].

In addition, it was shown that chronic L-NAME treatment may cause albuminuria by impairing glomerular charge barrier as well as size selectivity [131]. We therefore evaluated anionic sites on the glomerular endothelial cell surface coat by cationic ferritin perfusion, and found a significant decrease in the density of anionic sites at the glomerular endothelial surface layer in diabetic eNOS KO mice [111]. Furthermore, our recent data demonstrate that the expression of heparanase, which cleaves heparan sulfate proteoglycans (HSPGs), a major component of anionic site in glomerular capillary wall, is up-regulated in the diabetic (low-dose STZ and db/db) eNOSKO glomeruli (Takahashi T, unpublished observation). These findings suggest a potential mechanism by which eNOS deficiency may up-regulate glomerular heparanase expression in the setting of diabetes and impair endothelial surface charge barrier, leading to albuminuria. It is noteworthy that similar heparanase induction is observed in the glomeruli of the diabetic patients with overt nephropathy [132, 133]. Adding to this mechanism, recent studies have suggested that NO may preserve the glomerular protein permeability by antagonizing superoxide and/or by activating soluble guanylyl cyclase (sGC) [134, 135]. Further studies will be required to determine the precise mechanism of albuminuria in diabetic eNOSKO mice.

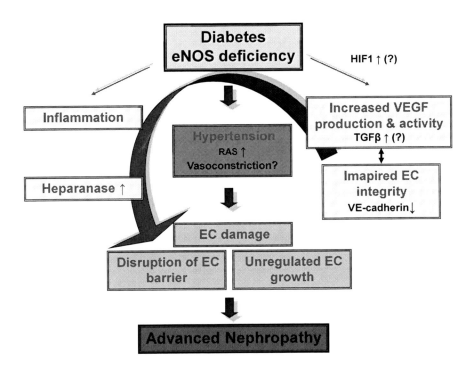

Figure. Schematic diagram illustrating the potential pathways involved in glomerular injury in diabetic eNOSKO mice. Hyperglycemia and eNOS deficiency elevate blood pressure, alter renal or glomerular perfusion, enhance inflammation, stimulate glomerular VEGF activity, down-regulate VE-cadherin, and induce heparanase expression in glomerulus. These changes may cause glomerular endothelial cell (EC) damage and unregulated endothelial cell growth, leading to advanced diabetic glomerular injury.

4. *Why do db/db eNOSKO mice show profound albuminuria and more severe renal lesions as compared with STZ-eNOS KO mice?* Although both db/db eNOSKO and STZ eNOSKO mice displayed a similar renal phenotype, clearly db/db eNOSKO mice showed a more severe renal phenotype involving profound albuminuria, reduced GFR, and glomerulosclerosis. The findings suggest that the genetic background (C57BLKS vs. C57BL6) and/or the type of diabetes (type II vs. type I) may significantly affect the renal phenotype of diabetic eNOSKO mice. It was shown that insulin receptor is expressed in vascular endothelium, and insulin transduces two distinct signals in endothelial cells [12, 136]. Insulin stimulates NO production in endothelial cells through PI3K/Akt activation and exhibits vasodilation and vascular protection. On the other hand, insulin was also shown to stimulate endothelial release of the vasoconstrictor endothelin-1 (ET-1), which counter-interacts with vascular NO [137], and upregulates VCAM-1 and E-selectin expression through MAP kinase activation, leading to vasoconstriction and inflammation. Thus, insulin has opposing hemodynamic actions, and the net effect on blood pressure negligible in physiological condition. It is conceivable that prominent hyperinsulinemia and eNOS deficiency in db/db eNOSKO mice may dominate and stimulate the vasoconstricting and

inflammatory insulin signaling pathway, leading to severe renal lesion. Further investigation would be required on this point.

5. *Do diabetic eNOSKO mice fully mimic human advanced DN?* Diabetic eNOSKO mice exhibited accelerated nephropathic changes and advanced glomerular pathology that overlap to human advanced DN, including reduced GFR. However, there seems to be some difference between diabetic eNOSKO model and human advanced DN. First, glomerular (podocytes) VEGF and nephrin expression are diminished in human advanced DN[138, 139], concurrent with podocyte detachment and reduced glomerular capillary endothelial fenestration (140). In contrast, glomerular VEGF is up-regulated in diabetic eNOSKO mouse [110, 126] and nephrin expression and podocyte morphology are well preserved in most of the glomeruli [111]. The finding suggests that high levels of VEGF may also have deleterious effects on diabetic glomeruli when eNOS-derived NO is absent. Second, mesangiolysis seen in diabetic eNOSKO mice is more severe than in human DN. Mesangiolysis is divided into three types in their mode of origin and morphological features [141]. The first type is severe mesangiolysis with glomerular microaneurysm, which is caused by severe mesangial cell injury (eg, anti-Thy1 model). The second type is mesangiolysis associated with extensive widening of the subendothelial space, which is thought to follow severe endothelial injury (eg, thrombotic microangiopathy). The third type is mesangiolysis with lamellated mesangial nodules, which is suggested to result from mild but persistent or recurrent mesangial and endothelial damage (eg, diabetic nephropathy). Morphological features of the mesangiolysis seen in diabetic eNOS KO mice are identical to the second type of mesangiolysis. The finding indicates that glomerular endothelial injury in diabetic eNOS KO mice is more severe than that in human DN. Finally, growing evidence demonstrates that uncoupled eNOS as well as NADPH oxidase serves as a major source of superoxide generation in diabetic endothelium (91). Hence, it is likely that eNOS deficiency may act to decrease diabetic endothelial oxidative stress. Indeed, decreased or unaltered oxidative stress in the diabetic eNOS KO glomeruli was suggested by immunohistochemistry for 8-hydroxydeoxy-guanosine and malondialdehyde, markers of cellular oxidative stress and DNA damage (Takahashi T., Takahashi N., unpublished observation). Thus, there seems to be some difference between diabetic eNOSKO model and human advanced DN. DN is a multifactorial disease, involving multiple genes, thereby a single gene deletion may not reconstitute all the spectrum of this disease. Accordingly, diabetic eNOSKO mice may be considered as a model of diabetic endothelial injury rather than a model of advanced DN.

6. *What study is required to determine further the role of eNOS in DN?* Diabetic eNOSKO studies have demonstrated a major role of eNOS in the pathogenesis of DN. However, the role of "endothelial" eNOS in this disease is still unclear, as eNOS has been shown to be expressed in various cell types including cardiomyocytes, hematopoietic cells, and renal tubular epithelial cells [14, 142]. In addition, eNOSKO mice have been shown to exhibit various congenital vascular anomalies with high frequency, including congenital septal defects and postnatal heart failure (143), abnormal aortic valve development [144], defective lung vascular development [145], and progressive focal renal scars (146). Therefore, a conditional knockout approach to target "endothelial" eNOS in adult diabetic mice will be required to determine the precise role of endothelial eNOS in DN. This effort will undoubtedly facilitate our understanding of the role of eNOS in DN.

Mediators Reducing eNOS Expression and Activity in Diabetic Endothelium

Human and animal studies have demonstrated that reduction of eNOS-derived NO is a key mechanism in the development and progression of DN. It would be therefore of great importance to determine the pathophysiologic pathways that contribute to the eNOS/NO disorders in diabetes. Besides gene expression, the activity of eNOS is known to be largely regulated by posttranslational modifications such as multisite phosphorylation, subcellular localization, calcium/calmodulin binding, S-Nitrosylation, and eNOS-protein interactions [15, 147, 148]. A variety of physiologic factors coupled with intracellular signaling pathways have been shown to promote NO release from endothelial cells. These include shear stress (via G proteins), ligands of G protein-coupled receptors (bradykinin, acetylcholine, histamine, adenosine, ATP/ADP, thrombin), VEGF, insulin, estrogen, sphingosine 1-phosphate, PI3-Akt, adenylate cyclase-PKA, and PLCγ (via calcium-calmodulin) pathways [14, 15]. Reductions of these physiologic stimuli and signaling could decrease vascular NO activity. Sphingosine 1-phosphate (S1P) has recently been identified as an important activator of eNOS. S1P regulates vascular homeostasis through its receptors including S1P1 and S1P2 (formally named EDG receptors). S1P stimulates NO production in endothelial cells through S1P1 coupled with elevation of intracellular calcium and Akt activation[149]. It is of note that S1P1 is down-regulated in diabetic rat glomeruli(150). Impaired endothelial insulin signaling (insulin resistance) as well as insulin deficiency was recently shown to blunt insulin-induced eNOS phosphorylation and cause endothelial dysfunction [151, 152].

Recent studies have identified various pathologic mediators that decrease the eNOS expression, activity and NO bioavailability in diabetic vasculature (summarized by Balakumar et al. [3]). These include hyperglycemia, activation of protein kinase C (PKC), advanced glycosylation end products (AGEs), tumor necrosis factor-alpha (TNFα), free fatty acids (FFA), asymmetric dimethylarginine (AMDA), angiotensin II (Ang-II), and endothelin-1 (ET-1) (3). Supr3physiological concentrations of D-glucose (30 mmol/L) were shown to be capable of scavenging NO [153]. Brodsky et al. have demonstrated that acute exposure of human endothelial cells to glucose, at levels found in plasma of diabetic patients, results in a significant blunting of NO responses to the eNOS agonists bradykinin and A23187[154]. In addition, Du et al. has demonstrated that hyperglycemia inhibits eNOS activity by posttranslational modification at the Akt site [155]. Activation of PKC (PKCβ1 and β2 isoforms in vascular cells), likely by de novo synthesis of diacylglycerol (DAG) from glucose or FFAs, decreases eNOS enzymatic activity by phosphorylating eNOS Thr495, a negative regulatory site, as well as by inhibiting insulin (or VEGF)-mediated Akt-dependent eNOS stimulation[156-159]. PKC also impairs insulin ability to release endothelial NO indirectly via oxidative stress and the subsequent activation of c-Jun N-terminal kinase [160]. The impact of PKC activation in the pathophysiology of DN has been well established(161). The link between PKC and eNOS activity supports the concept of NO insufficiency in the diabetic kidney. Accumulation of AGEs decreases NO bioavailability and eNOS expression by accelerating eNOS mRNA degradation as well as by producing ROS [162, 163]. AGEs were also shown to quench NO[164]. TNFα levels were shown to rise in diabetic kidney and urine prior to the onset of albuminuria. TNFα down-regulates eNOS mRNA, protein, and activity[165-168]. In addition, Goodwin et al. have recently shown that TNFα reduces argininosuccinate synthase expression, which provides the arginine pool for NO production, in endothelial cells [169]. FFAs are commonly elevated in diabetes and obesity and have been shown to impair NO production in endothelial cells by inhibiting insulin-stimulated eNOS activation [170, 171]. FFA also increases cellular levels of DAG and other lipid metabolites that in turn activate PKC, decreasing eNOS activity.

AMDA is an amino acid derived from the catabolism of proteins containing methylated arginine residues by the action of enzyme protein arginine methyltransferase (PRMT). ADMA acts as an eNOS inhibitor, by competitive inhibition of L-arginine oxidation, in a manner analogous to mono-methyl arginine [33, 172]. Alternatively, ADMA may cause eNOS uncoupling, leading not only to the loss of NO but also an increase in superoxide production in the vascular endothelium [173]. AMDA has been associated with endothelial dysfunction and is considered to be a risk factor for cardiovascular mortality and progression of chronic kidney disease [172]. Administration of L-arginine restores endothelial dysfunction associated with elevated plasma ADMA levels, consistent with the notion that ADMA is a competitive inhibitor [174, 175]. ADMA is elevated in patients with diabetes as well as in diabetic animals [33-35]. Two isoforms of dimethylarginine dimethylaminohydrolase (DDAH), DDAH1 and DDAH2, metabolize ADMA. In kidney, DDAH-1 is predominantly expressed in proximal tubules, whereas DDAH-2 is expressed in the vasculature and macula densa (176). *In vivo* gene silencing of DDAH-1 in the rat increased circulating ADMA, whereas gene silencing of DDAH-2 reduces vascular NO generation and endothelium-derived relaxation factor responses [177]. DDAH-1 +/- mice showed reduced endogenous capacity to generate and respond to endothelial NO, suggesting a potential contribution of DDAH-1 to endothelial dysfunction [178]. Onozato et al. has recently demonstrated that DDAH-1 is decreased in diabetic rat kidney, while DDAH-2 is increased[176]. These changes are normalized by administration of the angiotensin receptor blocker (telmisartan), which also reduces renal PRMT-1 expression. It was suggested that upregulation of DDAH-2 in the macula densa cells of the diabetic rat kidney may limit local ADMA accumulation, thereby enhancing nNOS-dependent afferent arteriolar vasodilatation and glomerular hyperfiltration, while a reduction in DDAH-1 in the proximal tubules may impair renal AMDA extraction, thereby increasing the circulating and renal parenchymal levels of ADMA that could contribute to the later development of hypertension [33]. Angiotensin type 1 receptor activation may mediate these DDAH alterations in diabetic kidney. Furthermore, a recent study has shown that the suppression of ADMA by DDAH overexpression could improve tubulointerstitial ischemia and subsequent renal damage in STZ-induced diabetic rat kidney [179]. High-glucose, TNFα, and AGEs were shown to reduce DDAH expression and activity in endothelial cells, promoting accumulation of ADMA and decreasing eNOS activity [180-182]. DDAH was also shown to be redox sensitive, and oxidative stress has been shown to increase the activity of PRMTs and decrease that of DDAH [183, 184]. Thus, increased production of ROS in diabetes could underlie increased ADMA levels. Collectively, these findings suggest a pivotal role of DDAH in diabetic kidney injury and vascular dysfunction [33].

Vasoconstrictor peptides such as Ang-II, ET-1, and urotensin-II, are upregulated in diabetes and promote ROS production and eNOS uncoupling, thereby reducing eNOS activity [3, 185, 186]. Ang-II mediated activation of Janus kinase (JAK) also inhibits the PI3 kinase-Akt pathway reducing eNOS activity and NO production[187]. Receptor antagonists of these vasoconstrictor peptides attenuates DN [188-190]. Angiotensin II type 1 receptor blocker

(Losartan) was recently shown to reduce ROS production in diabetic glomeruli and correct the eNOS uncoupling by increasing BH4 bioavailability [189]. It is of note that eNOS also inhibits Ang-II induced Rho kinase activation [113]. Given the fact that Rho kinase inhibition ameliorates diabetes-induced microvascular damage(191), the finding suggests an important role of Ang-II/eNOS cross-talk in diabetic vascular complication. Thus, various factors have been implicated in reduction in eNOS expression and activity in diabetes. These mediators have been extensively discussed and comprehensively reviewed elsewhere [3, 12, 14, 15, 33, 147, 148]. Additional and more detailed information may be found in these reviews.

Potential Mediators in the eNOS/NO Dysfunction in Diabetes

Adding to these well-studied mediators, recent studies have identified potential molecular pathways that may be importantly involved in decreases in endothelial NO production and NO bioavailability in diabetes, as described below. Although further studies are required to determine the role of these pathways in DN, these molecules could be new therapeutic targets for this disease.

1) AMPK

The AMP-activated protein kinase (AMPK) is a pivotal enzyme in the regulation of cellular energy balance [192, 193]. AMPK inhibits energy-consuming pathways upon decreased energy supply while it promotes energy producing pathways such as fatty acid oxidation and glycolysis. Furthermore, several AMPK-mediated signaling pathways were shown to govern glucose metabolism and improve glycemic control, implicating AMPK as a potential molecular target in the treatment of diabetes.

Recent studies have revealed that AMPK also plays an impotent role in vascular function(194). AMPK was shown to promote the production of endothelium-derived NO and preserve and protect vascular homeostasis and endothelial function. Moreover, recent studies have shown that AMPK enhances eNOS activity by direct phosphorylation at Ser1177[195] and Ser633(196) and by promoting its association with heat shock protein 90 [197]. Given the fact that NO itself can activate AMPK [198], AMPK-mediated eNOS activation might be essential for sustained NO release owing to a positive feedback loop. In fact, decreased eNOS-mediated NO production was recently shown in α2AMPK knockout mice [196]. AMPK-mediated eNOS activation is initiated by a variety of physiological stimuli including adiponectin, high-density lipoprotein, shear stress, hydrogen peroxide, thrombin, VEGF and estrogen [192]. The finding suggests that AMPK is constitutively active in the vasculature. It is noteworthy that AMPK is activated by hydrogen peroxide and peroxynitrite in endothelial cells and that AMPK reduces oxidative stress by stabilizing the mitochondrion and by inducing peroxisome proliferator coactivator 1α (PGC-1α)-dependent mitochondrial biogenesis [197]. The finding suggests that AMPK may function as an adaptive response to overcome the loss of NO bioavailability in this setting and that impaired AMPK activation causes excessive oxidative stress, leading to endothelial dysfunction. In this context, it is of interest that activation of AMPK reduces hyperglycemia-induced mitochondrial reactive oxygen species (ROS) production and promotes mitochondrial biogenesis in endothelial cells [199].

Although the alteration and the role of AMPK in diabetic vascular complications have not yet to be fully determined, these findings strongly suggest a critical role of AMPK in the pathogenesis of endothelial dysfunction in diabetes. In this context, it is of note that anti-diabetic drugs such as PPARγ agonists and metformin have AMPK activating properties and these drugs were shown to improve diabetic endothelial dysfunction [200-202]. It is conceivable that the observed vascular protective effects may result from AMPK-mediated eNOS activation. Therapy with AMPK-activating drugs may fulfill two important goals at the same time in diabetes, glycemic control and preservation of endothelial function. Further animal and human studies to determine the role of AMPK in DN and the development of specific AMPK activators that directly act on AMPK would be required to implicate this pathway as a novel molecular target in the treatment of DN.

2) SIRT1

Caloric restriction (CR) extends life span in organisms ranging from yeast to mammals. CR was also shown to decrease arterial blood pressure in healthy individuals and improves endothelium-dependent vasodilatation in obese and overweight individuals. Recent studies have shown that the SIRT1 protein deacetylase mediates the effects of CR on vascular function as well as on life span and metabolic pathway [203, 204]. SIRT1 is induced by CR *in vivo and in vitro* [205]. SIRT promotes endothelium-dependent vasodilatation by targeting eNOS for deacetylation. SIRT1 and eNOS colocalize and coprecipitate in endothelial cells, and SIRT1 deacetylates eNOS, stimulating eNOS activity and increasing endothelial NO production (206). In addition, recent studies have shown that NO regulates (increases) SIRT1 expression in endothelial cells [204, 207], suggesting that the SIRT1-eNOS axis may be a key pathway for maintaining vascular homeostasis (208, 209). Furthermore, a more recent study has shown a protective role of SIRT1 in diabetic vascular dysfunction [210]. Treatment of human endothelial cells with high glucose decreases SIRT1 expression and thus activates p53 (SIRT1 substrate) by increasing its acetylation. Introduction of SIRT1 or disruption of p53 inhibits high glucose-induced endothelial senescence and dysfunction in culture and in diabetic mice. Thus, SIRT1 have been implicated as a potential new molecular target for cardiovascular therapy and small molecule activators of SIRT1 (e.g. resveratol) may be used for the treatment of diabetic vascular complication.

3) TSP1, CD36, CD47

Thrombospondin-1 (TSP1) is a large secreted glycoprotein that has multiple biological activities including regulation of angiogenesis, cell proliferation, and apoptosis. TSP1 is upregulated in renal disease, whereas it is hardly detected in normal kidney [211]. TSP1 was shown to be upregulated in kidney biopsies as well as in blood mononuclear cells from patients with diabetic nephropathy [212, 213]. Recent studies have shown that TSP1 may suppress NO signaling in both endothelial and vascular smooth muscle cells through its receptor CD36 and CD47 [214-216]. Isenberg et al. have shown that TSP1 inhibits endothelial cell responses to NO in a cGMP-dependent manner [217]. Furthermore, their subsequent studies have shown that TSP1 acts primarily through its receptor CD47 to limit sGC activation [218]. At nanomolar concentrations, TSP1 also signals through CD36 to inhibit the same responses; however, CD47 is required for the CD36 signals to inhibit cGMP signaling [218, 219]. These findings indicate that engaging either CD47 or CD36 receptor inhibits vascular NO/cGMP signaling but CD47 is the necessary receptor of this TSP1 action. CD36 and CD47 could be new targets in diabetic vascular complication therapy [220].

4) Caveolin-1

eNOS is localized to specific subcellular domains. In resting endothelial cells, most eNOS proteins are localized to specialized invaginated domains of the cell membrane called caveolae [221]. Caveolae are characterized by the presence of a transmembrane scaffolding protein known as caveolin and caveolin-1 isoform is expressed in endothelial cells. eNOS is known to strongly and directly interacts with caveolin-1 and this protein interaction tonically inhibits eNOS activity by occupying the calmodulin binding site as well as by interfering with caveolin-associated receptors that stimulate eNOS activity [222, 223]. On the other hand, caveolin-1 was also shown to be required for regulation of eNOS activity by situating it in close physical proximity to other upstream signaling proteins present in caveolae. Thus, caveolin-1 is a major regulatory protein for eNOS activity. Either increased or decreased caveolin-1 expression could affect eNOS activity [224]. In diabetic animals, caveolin-1 expression was shown to be significantly increased in vasculature (225-227), indicating that high glucose levels cause an up-regulation of the endogenous eNOS inhibitory clamp by caveolin-1. This finding suggests that caveolin-1 may be a new therapeutic target in endothelial dysfunction associated with diabetes. However, there are few studies that have investigated caveolin-1 expression in diabetic kidney [228, 229], and further studies will be required on this subject.

Another important protein interaction in caveolae, which affects eNOS activity, is via heat shock protein 90 (HSP 90), an ATP-dependent chaperon. In contrast to caveolin-1, HSP90 was shown to function as an eNOS activator [230, 231]. Recently, it was suggested that translocation of HSP90 may reduce eNOS activity and contribute to diabetic endothelial dysfunction(232). However, its role in DN is currently unknown, since a recent study showed that total HSP90 expression is unaltered in diabetic rat glomeruli [233].

Conclusion and Perspective:

An abundance of evidence produced in recent years indicates that eNOS-derived NO plays a major role in the pathogenesis of DN. Endothelial dysfunction in diabetes is multifactorial, and various factors were shown to be involved in eNOS/NO dysfunction in diabetes. Increased production of reactive oxygen species (ROS) and subsequent eNOS uncoupling has been implicated in the central mechanism of decreased NO bioavailability in diabetic vasculature. Further studies will be required on the following points to better understand the role of this pathway in DN.

1. To determine the molecular and cellular mechanisms by which loss of eNOS-derived NO accelerate DN. It would also be important to determine the effects of eNOS deficiency on renal perfusion in diabetic kidney.
2. To determine the precise role of "endothelial" eNOS activity in DN by using conditional knockout mice.
3. To develop, test, and determine the therapeutic agents or strategies that effectively restore eNOS/NO dysfunction in DN. In this context, it would also be of great importance to explore new molecular target and pharmacological intervention that could increase eNOS activity to develop better treatment protocols for this disease. Diabetic eNOS knockout mouse would be effectively used for exploring the molecular pathways as well as pharmacological agents that restore diabetic renal vascular dysfunction caused by eNOS deficiency. Detailed information about current therapeutic approaches for diabetic endothelial dysfunction may be found in other reviews [5, 7, 234].
4. To develop and establish non-invasive methods and/or biomarkers to assess endothelial dysfunction and eNOS/NO activity in diabetic kidney. Imaging technique may be useful in this regard. Present methods and biomarkers are reviewed elsewhere [5, 197].

These efforts would greatly facilitate our understanding of the role of eNOS-derived NO in DN and may lead to better treatment protocols for this disease.

References

[1] Santilli F, Cipollone F, Mezzetti A, Chiarelli F. The role of nitric oxide in the development of diabetic angiopathy. *HormMetab. Res.*2004;36(5):319-35.

[2] Prabhakar SS. Role of nitric oxide in diabetic nephropathy. *SeminNephrol.*2004;24(4):333-44.

[3] Balakumar P, Chakkarwar VA, Krishan P, Singh M. Vascular endothelial dysfunction: a tug of war in diabetic nephropathy? *Biomed. Pharmacother.*2009 Mar;63(3):171-9.

[4] Albrecht EW, Stegeman CA, Heeringa P, Henning RH, van Goor H. Protective role of endothelial nitric oxide synthase. *J.Pathol.*2003;199(1):8-17.

[5] Calles-Escandon J, Cipolla M. Diabetes and endothelial dysfunction: a clinical perspective. *Endocr. Rev.*2001 Feb;22(1):36-52.

[6] Forstermann U. Endothelial NO synthase as a source of NO and superoxide. *Eur.J.Clin.Pharmacol.*2006;62 Suppl. 13:5-12.

[7] Hamilton SJ, Chew GT, Watts GF. Therapeutic regulation of endothelial dysfunction in type 2 diabetes mellitus. *Diab. Vasc. Dis. Res.*2007 Jun;4(2):89-102.

[8] Astrup AS, Tarnow L, Pietraszek L, Schalkwijk CG, Stehouwer CD, Parving HH, et al. Markers of endothelial dysfunction and inflammation in type 1 diabetic patients with or

without diabetic nephropathy followed for 10 years: association with mortality and decline of glomerular filtration rate. *Diabetes Care*2008 Jun;31(6):1170-6.

[9] Stehouwer CD, Gall MA, Twisk JW, Knudsen E, Emeis JJ, Parving HH. Increased urinary albumin excretion, endothelial dysfunction, and chronic low-grade inflammation in type 2 diabetes: progressive, interrelated, and independently associated with risk of death. *Diabetes*2002 Apr;51(4):1157-65.

[10] Schalkwijk CG, Poland DC, van Dijk W, Kok A, Emeis JJ, Drager AM, et al. Plasma concentration of C-reactive protein is increased in type I diabetic patients without clinical macroangiopathy and correlates with markers of endothelial dysfunction: evidence for chronic inflammation. *Diabetologia*1999 Mar;42(3):351-7.

[11] Pieper GM. Review of alterations in endothelial nitric oxide production in diabetes: protective role of arginine on endothelial dysfunction. *Hypertension*1998;31(5):1047-60.

[12] Nacci C, Tarquinio M, Montagnani M. Molecular and clinical aspects of endothelial dysfunction in diabetes. *Intern. Emerg. Med.* 2009 Apr;4(2):107-16.

[13] Rask-Madsen C, King GL. Mechanisms of Disease: endothelial dysfunction in insulin resistance and diabetes. *Nat. Clin. Pract. Endocrinol. Metab.*2007 Jan;3(1):46-56.

[14] Li H, Wallerath T, Forstermann U. Physiological mechanisms regulating the expression of endothelial-type NO synthase. *NitricOxide*2002;7(2):132-47.

[15] Dudzinski DM, Igarashi J, Greif D, Michel T. The regulation and pharmacology of endothelial nitric oxide synthase. *Annu.Rev.Pharmacol.Toxicol.*2006;46:235-76.

[16] Forstermann U, Munzel T. Endothelial nitric oxide synthase in vascular disease: from marvel to menace. *Circulation*2006 Apr 4;113(13):1708-14.

[17] Brownlee M. Biochemistry and molecular cell biology of diabetic complications. *Nature*2001;414(6865):813-20.

[18] Brownlee M. The pathobiology of diabetic complications: a unifying mechanism. *Diabetes*2005;54(6):1615-25.

[19] Zou MH, Cohen R, Ullrich V. Peroxynitrite and vascular endothelial dysfunction in diabetes mellitus. *Endothelium*2004;11(2):89-97.

[20] Moens AL, Kass DA. Tetrahydrobiopterin and cardiovascular disease. *Arterioscler. Thromb. Vasc. Biol.*2006 Nov;26(11):2439-44.

[21] Sasaki N, Yamashita T, Takaya T, Shinohara M, Shiraki R, Takeda M, et al. Augmentation of vascular remodeling by uncoupled endothelial nitric oxide synthase in a mouse model of diabetes mellitus. *Arterioscler. Thromb. Vasc. Biol.*2008 Jun;28(6):1068-76.

[22] Cai S, Khoo J, Channon KM. Augmented BH4 by gene transfer restores nitric oxide synthase function in hyperglycemic human endothelial cells. *Cardiovasc. Res.* 2005;65(4):823-31.

[23] Cai S, Khoo J, Mussa S, Alp NJ, Channon KM. Endothelial nitric oxide synthase dysfunction in diabetic mice: importance of tetrahydrobiopterin in eNOS dimerisation. *Diabetologia*2005;48(9):1933-40.

[24] Bauersachs J, Schafer A. Tetrahydrobiopterin and eNOS dimer/monomer ratio--a clue to eNOS uncoupling in diabetes? *Cardiovasc. Res.*2005;65(4):768-9.

[25] Goumas G, Tentolouris C, Tousoulis D, Stefanadis C, Toutouzas P. Therapeutic modification of the L-arginine-eNOS pathway in cardiovascular diseases. *Atherosclerosis* 2001 Feb 1;154(2):255-67.

[26] Pieper GM, Dondlinger LA. Plasma and vascular tissue arginine are decreased in diabetes: acute arginine supplementation restores endothelium-dependent relaxation by augmenting cGMP production. J Pharmacol Exp Ther1997 Nov;283(2):684-91.

[27] Bank N, Aynedjian HS. Role of EDRF (nitric oxide) in diabetic renal hyperfiltration. *Kidney Int*1993;43(6):1306-12.

[28] Craven PA, Studer RK, DeRubertis FR. Impaired nitric oxide-dependent cyclic guanosine monophosphate generation in glomeruli from diabetic rats. Evidence for protein kinase C-mediated suppression of the cholinergic response. *J. ClinInvest.* 1994;93(1):311-20.

[29] Durante W, Johnson FK, Johnson RA. Arginase: a critical regulator of nitric oxide synthesis and vascular function. Clin Exp Pharmacol Physiol2007 Sep;34(9):906-11.

[30] Bivalacqua TJ, Hellstrom WJ, Kadowitz PJ, Champion HC. Increased expression of arginase II in human diabetic corpus cavernosum: in diabetic-associated erectile dysfunction. *Biochem. Biophys. Res. Commun.*2001 May 18;283(4):923-7.

[31] Kampfer H, Pfeilschifter J, Frank S. Expression and activity of arginase isoenzymes during normal and diabetes-impaired skin repair. *J. Invest. Dermatol.*2003 Dec;121(6):1544-51.

[32] Romero MJ, Platt DH, Tawfik HE, Labazi M, El-Remessy AB, Bartoli M, et al. Diabetes-induced coronary vascular dysfunction involves increased arginase activity. *Circ. Res.*2008 Jan 4;102(1):95-102.

[33] Palm F, Onozato ML, Luo Z, Wilcox CS. Dimethylarginine dimethylaminohydrolase (DDAH): expression, regulation, and function in the cardiovascular and renal systems. *Am. J. Physiol. Heart. Circ. Physiol.*2007 Dec;293(6):H3227-45.

[34] Yamagishi S, Ueda S, Nakamura K, Matsui T, Okuda S. Role of asymmetric dimethylarginine (ADMA) in diabetic vascular complications. *Curr. Pharm. Des*2008;14(25):2613-8.

[35] Krzyzanowska K, Mittermayer F, Wolzt M, Schernthaner G. ADMA, cardiovascular disease and diabetes. *Diabetes Res. Clin. Pract.*2008 Dec 15;82 Suppl 2:S122-6.

[36] Tarnow L, Hovind P, Teerlink T, Stehouwer CD, Parving HH. Elevated plasma asymmetric dimethylarginine as a marker of cardiovascular morbidity in early diabetic nephropathy in type 1 diabetes. *Diabetes Care*2004 Mar;27(3):765-9.

[37] Krzyzanowska K, Mittermayer F, Krugluger W, Schnack C, Hofer M, Wolzt M, et al. Asymmetric dimethylarginine is associated with macrovascular disease and total homocysteine in patients with type 2 diabetes. *Atherosclerosis*2006 Nov;189(1):236-40.

[38] Krzyzanowska K, Mittermayer F, Shnawa N, Hofer M, Schnabler J, Etmuller Y, et al. Asymmetrical dimethylarginine is related to renal function, chronic inflammation and macroangiopathy in patients with Type 2 diabetes and albuminuria. *Diabet. Med.*2007 Jan;24(1):81-6.

[39] Satchell SC, Tooke JE. What is the mechanism of microalbuminuria in diabetes: a role for the glomerular endothelium? *Diabetologia*2008 May;51(5):714-25.

[40] Stehouwer CD, Fischer HR, van Kuijk AW, Polak BC, Donker AJ. Endothelial dysfunction precedes development of microalbuminuria in IDDM. *Diabetes*1995 May;44(5):561-4.

[41] Hiragushi K, Sugimoto H, Shikata K, Yamashita T, Miyatake N, Shikata Y, et al. Nitric oxide system is involved in glomerular hyperfiltration in Japanese normo- and micro-

albuminuric patients with type 2 diabetes. *Diabetes Res. Clin.* Pract2001 Sep;53(3):149-59.

[42] Delles C, Klingbeil AU, Schneider MP, Handrock R, Schaufele T, Schmieder RE. The role of nitric oxide in the regulation of glomerular haemodynamics in humans. *Nephrol Dial. Transplant.*2004 Jun;19(6):1392-7.

[43] Chiarelli F, Cipollone F, Romano F, Tumini S, Costantini F, di Ricco L, et al. Increased circulating nitric oxide in young patients with type 1 diabetes and persistent microalbuminuria: relation to glomerular hyperfiltration. *Diabetes*2000 Jul;49(7):1258-63.

[44] Maejima K, Nakano S, Himeno M, Tsuda S, Makiishi H, Ito T, et al. Increased basal levels of plasma nitric oxide in Type 2 diabetic subjects. Relationship to microvascular complications. *J. Diabetes Complications*2001 May-Jun;15(3):135-43.

[45] Earle KA, Mehrotra S, Dalton RN, Denver E, Swaminathan R. Defective nitric oxide production and functional renal reserve in patients with type 2 diabetes who have microalbuminuria of African and Asian compared with white origin. *J. Am. Soc. Nephrol.* 2001 Oct;12(10):2125-30.

[46] Hohenstein B, Hugo CP, Hausknecht B, Boehmer KP, Riess RH, Schmieder RE. Analysis of NO-synthase expression and clinical risk factors in human diabetic nephropathy. *Nephrol. Dial. Transplant.*2008 Apr;23(4):1346-54.

[47] Ng DP, Krolewski AS. Molecular genetic approaches for studying the etiology of diabetic nephropathy. *Curr. Mol. Med.*2005 Aug;5(5):509-25.

[48] Zanchi A, Moczulski DK, Hanna LS, Wantman M, Warram JH, Krolewski AS. Risk of advanced diabetic nephropathy in type 1 diabetes is associated with endothelial nitric oxide synthase gene polymorphism. *Kidney Int.*2000;57(2):405-13.

[49] Shin Shin Y, Baek SH, Chang KY, Park CW, Yang CW, Jin DC, et al. Relations between eNOS Glu298Asp polymorphism and progression of diabetic nephropathy. *Diabetes Res. Clin. Pract.*2004 Sep;65(3):257-65.

[50] Ahluwalia TS, Ahuja M, Rai TS, Kohli HS, Sud K, Bhansali A, et al. Endothelial nitric oxide synthase gene haplotypes and diabetic nephropathy among Asian Indians. *Mol. Cell Biochem.*2008 Jul;314(1-2):9-17.

[51] Liu Y, Burdon KP, Langefeld CD, Beck SR, Wagenknecht LE, Rich SS, et al. T-786C polymorphism of the endothelial nitric oxide synthase gene is associated with albuminuria in the diabetes heart study. *J.Am.Soc.Nephrol.*2005;16(4):1085-90.

[52] Noiri E, Satoh H, Taguchi J, Brodsky SV, Nakao A, Ogawa Y, et al. Association of eNOS Glu298Asp polymorphism with end-stage renal disease. *Hypertension*2002;40(4):535-40.

[53] Nagase S, Suzuki H, Wang Y, Kikuchi S, Hirayama A, Ueda A, et al. Association of ecNOS gene polymorphisms with end stage renal diseases. *Mol. Cell Biochem.*2003 Feb;244(1-2):113-8.

[54] Suzuki H, Nagase S, Kikuchi S, Wang Y, Koyama A. Association of a missense Glu298Asp mutation of the endothelial nitric oxide synthase gene with end stage renal disease. *Clin. Chem.*2000 Nov;46(11):1858-60.

[55] Asakimori Y, Yorioka N, Taniguchi Y, Ito T, Ogata S, Kyuden Y, et al. T(-786)-->C polymorphism of the endothelial nitric oxide synthase gene influences the progression of renal disease. *Nephron*2002 Aug;91(4):747-51.

[56] Wang XL, Mahaney MC, Sim AS, Wang J, Blangero J, Almasy L, et al. Genetic contribution of the endothelial constitutive nitric oxide synthase gene to plasma nitric oxide levels. *Arterioscler. Thromb. Vasc. Biol.*1997 Nov;17(11):3147-53.

[57] Asakimori Y, Yorioka N, Yamamoto I, Okumoto S, Doi S, Hirai T, et al. Endothelial nitric oxide synthase intron 4 polymorphism influences the progression of renal disease. *Nephron.*2001 Oct;89(2):219-23.

[58] Neugebauer S, Baba T, Watanabe T. Association of the nitric oxide synthase gene polymorphism with an increased risk for progression to diabetic nephropathy in type 2 diabetes. *Diabetes*2000;49(3):500-3.

[59] Ksiazek P, Wojewoda P, Muc K, Buraczynska M. Endothelial nitric oxide synthase gene intron 4 polymorphism in type 2 diabetes mellitus. MolDiagn2003;7(2):119-23.

[60] Fujita H, Narita T, Meguro H, Ishii T, Hanyu O, Suzuki K, et al. Lack of association between an ecNOS gene polymorphism and diabetic nephropathy in type 2 diabetic patients with proliferative diabetic retinopathy. *Horm. Metab. Res.*2000 Feb;32(2):80-3.

[61] Noiri E, Satoh H, Taguchi J, Brodsky SV, Nakao A, Ogawa Y, et al. Association of eNOS Glu298Asp polymorphism with end-stage renal disease. *Hypertension.*2002 Oct;40(4):535-40.

[62] Lin S, Qu H, Qiu M. Allele A in intron 4 of ecNOS gene will not increase the risk of diabetic nephropathy in type 2 diabetes of Chinese population. *Nephron*2002 Aug;91(4):768.

[63] Rippin JD, Patel A, Belyaev ND, Gill GV, Barnett AH, Bain SC. Nitric oxide synthase gene polymorphisms and diabetic nephropathy. *Diabetologia*2003 Mar;46(3):426-8.

[64] Degen B, Schmidt S, Ritz E. A polymorphism in the gene for the endothelial nitric oxide synthase and diabetic nephropathy. *Nephrol. Dial Transplant.*2001 Jan;16(1):185.

[65] Freedman BI, Yu H, Anderson PJ, Roh BH, Rich SS, Bowden DW. Genetic analysis of nitric oxide and endothelin in end-stage renal disease. *Nephrol. Dial. Transplant.*2000 Nov;15(11):1794-800.

[66] Shimizu T, Onuma T, Kawamori R, Makita Y, Tomino Y. Endothelial nitric oxide synthase gene and the development of diabetic nephropathy. *Diabetes Res. Clin. Pract.*2002 Dec;58(3):179-85.

[67] Komers R, Anderson S. Paradoxes of nitric oxide in the diabetic kidney. *Am.J.Physiol. Renal. Physiol.*2003;284(6):F1121-F37.

[68] Kone BC. Localization and regulation of nitric oxide synthase isoforms in the kidney. *Semin. Nephrol.*1999 May;19(3):230-41.

[69] Bachmann S, Bosse HM, Mundel P. Topography of nitric oxide synthesis by localizing constitutive NO synthases in mammalian kidney. *Am. .J Physiol.*1995 May;268(5 Pt 2):F885-98.

[70] Han KH, Lim JM, Kim WY, Kim H, Madsen KM, Kim J. Expression of endothelial nitric oxide synthase in developing rat kidney. *Am.J.Physiol. Renal Physiol.*2005;288(4):F694-F702.

[71] Furusu A, Miyazaki M, Abe K, Tsukasaki S, Shioshita K, Sasaki O, et al. Expression of endothelial and inducible nitric oxide synthase in human glomerulonephritis. *Kidney Int.*1998;53(6):1760-8.

[72] Choi KC, Kim NH, An MR, Kang DG, Kim SW, Lee J. Alterations of intrarenal renin-angiotensin and nitric oxide systems in streptozotocin-induced diabetic rats. *Kidney Int.* Suppl1997 Sep;60:S23-7.

[73] Sugimoto H, Shikata K, Matsuda M, Kushiro M, Hayashi Y, Hiragushi K, et al. Increased expression of endothelial cell nitric oxide synthase (ecNOS) in afferent and glomerular endothelial cells is involved in glomerular hyperfiltration of diabetic nephropathy. *Diabetologia*1998;41(12):1426-34.

[74] Shin SJ, Lai FJ, Wen JD, Hsiao PJ, Hsieh MC, Tzeng TF, et al. Neuronal and endothelial nitric oxide synthase expression in outer medulla of streptozotocin-induced diabetic rat kidney. *Diabetologia*2000;43(5):649-59.

[75] Veelken R, Hilgers KF, Hartner A, Haas A, Bohmer KP, Sterzel RB. Nitric oxide synthase isoforms and glomerular hyperfiltration in early diabetic nephropathy. *J. Am. Soc. Nephrol.*2000 Jan;11(1):71-9.

[76] Vriese AS, Tilton RG, Elger M, Stephan CC, Kriz W, Lameire NH. Antibodies against Vascular Endothelial Growth Factor Improve Early Renal Dysfunction in Experimental Diabetes. *J.Am.Soc.Nephrol.*2001May;12(5):993-1000.

[77] De Vriese AS, Stoenoiu MS, Elger M, Devuyst O, Vanholder R, Kriz W, et al. Diabetes-induced microvascular dysfunction in the hydronephrotic kidney: role of nitric oxide. *Kidney Int.*2001 Jul;60(1):202-10.

[78] Onozato ML, Tojo A, Goto A, Fujita T, Wilcox CS. Oxidative stress and nitric oxide synthase in rat diabetic nephropathy: effects of ACEI and ARB. *Kidney Int.*2002 Jan;61(1):186-94.

[79] Keynan S, Hirshberg B, Levin-Iaina N, Wexler ID, Dahan R, Reinhartz E, et al. Renal nitric oxide production during the early phase of experimental diabetes mellitus. *Kidney Int.* 2000;58(2):740-7.

[80] Ishii N, Patel KP, Lane PH, Taylor T, Bian K, Murad F, et al. Nitric oxide synthesis and oxidative stress in the renal cortex of rats with diabetes mellitus. *J. Am. Soc. Nephrol.* 2001 Aug;12(8):1630-9.

[81] Schwartz D, Schwartz IF, Blantz RC. An analysis of renal nitric oxide contribution to hyperfiltration in diabetic rats. *J. Lab. Clin. Med.*2001 Feb;137(2):107-14.

[82] Kasai N, Sugimoto K, Horiba N, Suda T. Effect of D-glucose on nitric oxide release from glomerular endothelial cells. *Diabetes Metab. Res. Rev.*2001 May-Jun;17(3):217-22.

[83] Hoshiyama M, Li B, Yao J, Harada T, Morioka T, Oite T. Effect of high glucose on nitric oxide production and endothelial nitric oxide synthase protein expression in human glomerular endothelial cells. *Nephron Exp.Nephrol.*2003;95(2):e62-e8.

[84] Cooper ME, Vranes D, Youssef S, Stacker SA, Cox AJ, Rizkalla B, et al. Increased renal expression of vascular endothelial growth factor (VEGF) and its receptor VEGFR-2 in experimental diabetes. *Diabetes*1999;48(11):2229-39.

[85] Wang Y, Nagase S, Koyama A. Stimulatory effect of IGF-I and VEGF on eNOS message, protein expression, eNOS phosphorylation and nitric oxide production in rat glomeruli, and the involvement of PI3-K signaling pathway. *Nitric.Oxide.*2004;10(1):25-35.

[86] Tolins JP, Shultz PJ, Raij L, Brown DM, Mauer SM. Abnormal renal hemodynamic response to reduced renal perfusion pressure in diabetic rats: role of NO. *Am. J. Physiol.*1993 Dec;265(6 Pt 2):F886-95.

[87] Komers R, Allen TJ, Cooper ME. Role of endothelium-derived nitric oxide in the pathogenesis of the renal hemodynamic changes of experimental diabetes. *Diabetes*1994 Oct;43(10):1190-7.

[88] Mattar AL, Fujihara CK, Ribeiro MO, de Nucci G, Zatz R. Renal effects of acute and chronic nitric oxide inhibition in experimental diabetes. *Nephron* 1996;74(1):136-43.

[89] Omer S, Shan J, Varma DR, Mulay S. Augmentation of diabetes-associated renal hyperfiltration and nitric oxide production by pregnancy in rats. *J. Endocrinol.* 1999 Apr;161(1):15-23.

[90] Wang YX, Brooks DP, Edwards RM. Attenuated glomerular cGMP production and renal vasodilation in streptozotocin-induced diabetic rats. *Am. J. Physiol.* 1993 May;264(5 Pt 2):R952-6.

[91] Satoh M, Fujimoto S, Haruna Y, Arakawa S, Horike H, Komai N, et al. NAD(P)H oxidase and uncoupled nitric oxide synthase are major sources of glomerular superoxide in rats with experimental diabetic nephropathy. *Am.J.Physiol. Renal. Physiol.* 2005;288(6):F1144-F52.

[92] Chu S, Bohlen HG. High concentration of glucose inhibits glomerular endothelial eNOS through a PKC mechanism. *Am.J.Physiol. Renal. Physiol.* 2004;287(3):F384-92.

[93] Wilcox CS, Welch WJ, Murad F, Gross SS, Taylor G, Levi R, et al. Nitric oxide synthase in macula densa regulates glomerular capillary pressure. *Proc. Natl. Acad. Sci. U S A* 1992 Dec 15;89(24):11993-7.

[94] Thorup C, Erik A, Persson G. Macula densa derived nitric oxide in regulation of glomerular capillary pressure. *Kidney Int.* 1996 Feb;49(2):430-6.

[95] Ichihara A, Inscho EW, Imig JD, Navar LG. Neuronal nitric oxide synthase modulates rat renal microvascular function. *Am. J. Physiol.* 1998 Mar;274(3 Pt 2):F516-24.

[96] Komers R, Oyama TT, Chapman JG, Allison KM, Anderson S. Effects of systemic inhibition of neuronal nitric oxide synthase in diabetic rats. *Hypertension* 2000 Feb;35(2):655-61.

[97] Komers R, Lindsley JN, Oyama TT, Allison KM, Anderson S. Role of neuronal nitric oxide synthase (NOS1) in the pathogenesis of renal hemodynamic changes in diabetes. *Am. J. Physiol. Renal. Physiol.* 2000 Sep;279(3):F573-83.

[98] Ito A, Uriu K, Inada Y, Qie YL, Takagi I, Ikeda M, et al. Inhibition of neuronal nitric oxide synthase ameliorates renal hyperfiltration in streptozotocin-induced diabetic rat. *J. Lab. Clin. Med.* 2001 Sep;138(3):177-85.

[99] Levine DZ, Iacovitti M, Robertson SJ, Mokhtar GA. Modulation of single-nephron GFR in the db/db mouse model of type 2 diabetes mellitus. *Am.J.Physiol. RegulIntegr.Comp. Physiol.* 2006;290(4):R975-R81.

[100] Pieper GM. Enhanced, unaltered and impaired nitric oxide-mediated endothelium-dependent relaxation in experimental diabetes mellitus: importance of disease duration. *Diabetologia* 1999;42(2):204-13.

[101] Erdely A, Freshour G, Maddox DA, Olson JL, Samsell L, Baylis C. Renal disease in rats with type 2 diabetes is associated with decreased renal nitric oxide production. *Diabetologia* 2004;47(10):1672-6.

[102] Khamaisi M, Keynan S, Bursztyn M, Dahan R, Reinhartz E, Ovadia H, et al. Role of Renal Nitric Oxide Synthase in Diabetic Kidney Disease during the Chronic Phase of Diabetes. *Nephron Physiol.* 2005;102(3-4):72-80.

[103] Yuzawa Y, Niki I, Kosugi T, Maruyama S, Yoshida F, Takeda M, et al. Overexpression of calmodulin in pancreatic beta cells induces diabetic nephropathy. *J. Am. Soc. Nephrol.* 2008 Sep;19(9):1701-11.

[104] Craven PA, DeRubertis FR, Melhem M. Nitric oxide in diabetic nephropathy. *Kidney Int.* Suppl1997 Sep;60:S46-53.

[105] Soulis T, Cooper ME, Sastra S, Thallas V, Panagiotopoulos S, Bjerrum OJ, et al. Relative contributions of advanced glycation and nitric oxide synthase inhibition to aminoguanidine-mediated renoprotection in diabetic rats. *Diabetologia*1997 Oct;40(10):1141-51.

[106] Kamijo H, Higuchi M, Hora K. Chronic inhibition of nitric oxide production aggravates diabetic nephropathy in Otsuka Long-Evans Tokushima Fatty rats. *Nephron. Physiol.*2006;104(1):p12-22.

[107] Huang PL. Mouse models of nitric oxide synthase deficiency. *J.Am.Soc.Nephrol.*2000;11 Suppl. 16:S120-3.

[108] Zhao HJ, Wang S, Cheng H, Zhang MZ, Takahashi T, Fogo AB, et al. Endothelial nitric oxide synthase deficiency produces accelerated nephropathy in diabetic mice. *J.Am.Soc.Nephrol.*2006;17(10):2664-9.

[109] Mohan S, Reddick RL, Musi N, Horn DA, Yan B, Prihoda TJ, et al. Diabetic eNOS knockout mice develop distinct macro- and microvascular complications. *Lab. Invest.*2008 May;88(5):515-28.

[110] Nakagawa T, Sato W, Glushakova O, Heinig M, Clarke T, Campbell-Thompson M, et al. Diabetic endothelial nitric oxide synthase knockout mice develop advanced diabetic nephropathy. *J.Am.Soc.Nephrol.*2007;18(2):539-50.

[111] Kanetsuna Y, Takahashi K, Nagata M, Gannon MA, Breyer MD, Harris RC, et al. Deficiency of endothelial nitric-oxide synthase confers susceptibility to diabetic nephropathy in nephropathy-resistant inbred mice. *Am.J.Pathol.2007*;170(5):1473-84.

[112] Kosugi T, Heinig M, Nakayama T, Connor T, Yuzawa Y, Li Q, et al. Lowering blood pressure blocks mesangiolysis and mesangial nodules, but not tubulointerstitial injury, in diabetic eNOS knockout mice. *Am. J. Pathol.*2009 Apr;174(4):1221-9.

[113] Suzuki H, Kimura K, Shirai H, Eguchi K, Higuchi S, Hinoki A, et al. Endothelial nitric oxide synthase inhibits G12/13 and rho-kinase activated by the angiotensin II type-1 receptor: implication in vascular migration. *Arterioscler. Thromb. Vasc. Biol.*2009 Feb;29(2):217-24.

[114] Johnson RJ, Herrera-Acosta J, Schreiner GF, Rodriguez-Iturbe B. Subtle acquired renal injury as a mechanism of salt-sensitive hypertension. *N. Engl. J. Med.*2002 Mar 21;346(12):913-23.

[115] Quiroz Y, Pons H, Gordon KL, Rincon J, Chavez M, Parra G, et al. Mycophenolate mofetil prevents salt-sensitive hypertension resulting from nitric oxide synthesis inhibition. *Am. J. Physiol. Renal. Physiol.*2001 Jul;281(1):F38-47.

[116] Edwards RM, Trizna W. Modulation of glomerular arteriolar tone by nitric oxide synthase inhibitors. *J. Am. Soc. Nephrol.*1993 Nov;4(5):1127-32.

[117] Patzak A, Kleinmann F, Lai EY, Kupsch E, Skelweit A, Mrowka R. Nitric oxide counteracts angiotensin II induced contraction in efferent arterioles in mice. *Acta Physiol. Scand.*2004 Aug;181(4):439-44.

[118] Ho FM, Lin WW, Chen BC, Chao CM, Yang CR, Lin LY, et al. High glucose-induced apoptosis in human vascular endothelial cells is mediated through NF-kappaB and c-Jun NH2-terminal kinase pathway and prevented by PI3K/Akt/eNOS pathway. *Cell Signal.*2006;18(3):391-9.

[119] Peng HB, Libby P, Liao JK. Induction and stabilization of I kappa B alpha by nitric oxide mediates inhibition of NF-kappa B. *J.Biol.Chem.*1995;270(23):14214-9.

[120] De Caterina R, Libby P, Peng HB, Thannickal VJ, Rajavashisth TB, Gimbrone MA, Jr., et al. Nitric oxide decreases cytokine-induced endothelial activation. Nitric oxide selectively reduces endothelial expression of adhesion molecules and proinflammatory cytokines. *J.ClinInvest.*1995;96(1):60-8.

[121] Peng HB, Rajavashisth TB, Libby P, Liao JK. Nitric oxide inhibits macrophage-colony stimulating factor gene transcription in vascular endothelial cells. *J.Biol.Chem.*1995;270(28):17050-5.

[122] Liu XM, Peyton KJ, Ensenat D, Wang H, Hannink M, Alam J, et al. Nitric oxide stimulates heme oxygenase-1 gene transcription via the Nrf2/ARE complex to promote vascular smooth muscle cell survival. *Cardiovasc. Res.*2007 Jul 15;75(2):381-9.

[123] Hayashi T, Matsui-Hirai H, Miyazaki-Akita A, Fukatsu A, Funami J, Ding QF, et al. Endothelial cellular senescence is inhibited by nitric oxide: implications in atherosclerosis associated with menopause and diabetes. *Proc. Natl. Acad. Sci. U S A.*2006 Nov 7;103(45):17018-23.

[124] Sanders PW. Vascular Consequences of Dietary Salt Intake. *Am. J. Physiol. Renal. Physiol.* 2009 Aug;297(2):F237-43.

[125] Nakagawa T, Sato W, Sautin YY, Glushakova O, Croker B, Atkinson MA, et al. Uncoupling of vascular endothelial growth factor with nitric oxide as a mechanism for diabetic vasculopathy. *J .Am. Soc. Nephrol.*2006 Mar;17(3):736-45.

[126] Sato W, Kosugi T, Zhang L, Roncal CA, Heinig M, Campbell-Thompson M, et al. The pivotal role of VEGF on glomerular macrophage infiltration in advanced diabetic nephropathy. *Lab. Invest.*2008 Sep;88(9):949-61.

[127] Haase VH. Hypoxia-inducible factors in the kidney. *Am. J. Physiol. Renal. Physiol.*2006 Aug;291(2):F271-81.

[128] London NR, Whitehead KJ, Li DY. Endogenous endothelial cell signaling systems maintain vascular stability. *Angiogenesis* 2009;12(2):149-58.

[129] Jeansson M, Haraldsson B. Glomerular size and charge selectivity in the mouse after exposure to glucosaminoglycan-degrading enzymes. *J. Am. Soc. Nephrol. 2003*; 14(7):1756-65.

[130] Jeansson M, Haraldsson B. Morphological and functional evidence for an important role of the endothelial cell glycocalyx in the glomerular barrier. *Am J Physiol Renal Physiol.* 2006;290(1):F111-6.

[131] Arcos MI, Fujihara CK, Sesso A, Almeida Prado EB, Almeida Prado MJ, De Nucci G, et al. Mechanisms of albuminuria in the chronic nitric oxide inhibition model. *Am. J.Physiol. Renal. Physiol.*2000;279(6):F1060-6.

[132] Maxhimer JB, Somenek M, Rao G, Pesce CE, Baldwin D, Jr., Gattuso P, et al. Heparanase-1 gene expression and regulation by high glucose in renal epithelial cells: a potential role in the pathogenesis of proteinuria in diabetic patients. *Diabetes*2005 Jul;54(7):2172-8.

[133] Lewis EJ, Xu X. Abnormal glomerular permeability characteristics in diabetic nephropathy: implications for the therapeutic use of low-molecular weight heparin. *Diabetes Care*2008 Feb;31 Suppl 2:S202-7.

[134] Sharma M, McCarthy ET, Savin VJ, Lianos EA. Nitric oxide preserves the glomerular protein permeability barrier by antagonizing superoxide. *Kidney Int.*2005 Dec;68(6):2735-44.

[135] Sharma M, Zou Z, Miura H, Papapetropoulos A, McCarthy ET, Sharma R, et al. ADMA Injures Glomerular Filtration Barrier: Role of Nitric Oxide and Superoxide. *Am J. Physiol. Renal. Physiol.* 2009 Jun;296(6):F1386-95.

[136] Fulton DJ. Mechanisms of vascular insulin resistance: a substitute Akt? *Circ. Res.*2009 May 8;104(9):1035-7.

[137] Quaschning T, Voss F, Relle K, Kalk P, Vignon-Zellweger N, Pfab T, et al. Lack of endothelial nitric oxide synthase promotes endothelin-induced hypertension: lessons from endothelin-1 transgenic/endothelial nitric oxide synthase knockout mice. *J. Am. Soc. Nephrol.*2007 Mar;18(3):730-40.

[138] Baelde HJ, Eikmans M, Lappin DW, Doran PP, Hohenadel D, Brinkkoetter PT, et al. Reduction of VEGF-A and CTGF expression in diabetic nephropathy is associated with podocyte loss. *Kidney Int.*2007 Apr;71(7):637-45.

[139] Doublier S, Salvidio G, Lupia E, Ruotsalainen V, Verzola D, Deferrari G, et al. Nephrin expression is reduced in human diabetic nephropathy: evidence for a distinct role for glycated albumin and angiotensin II. *Diabetes*2003 Apr;52(4):1023-30.

[140] Toyoda M, Najafian B, Kim Y, Caramori ML, Mauer M. Podocyte detachment and reduced glomerular capillary endothelial fenestration in human type 1 diabetic nephropathy. *Diabetes*2007 Aug;56(8):2155-60.

[141] Morita T, Yamamoto T, Churg J. Mesangiolysis: an update. *Am.J.Kidney Dis.*1998;31(4):559-73.

[142] Kleinbongard P, Schulz R, Rassaf T, Lauer T, Dejam A, Jax T, et al. Red blood cells express a functional endothelial nitric oxide synthase. *Blood*2006 Apr 1;107(7):2943-51.

[143] Feng Q, Song W, Lu X, Hamilton JA, Lei M, Peng T, et al. Development of heart failure and congenital septal defects in mice lacking endothelial nitric oxide synthase. *Circulation*2002;106(7):873-9.

[144] Lee TC, Zhao YD, Courtman DW, Stewart DJ. Abnormal aortic valve development in mice lacking endothelial nitric oxide synthase. *Circulation*2000;101(20):2345-8.

[145] Han RN, Babaei S, Robb M, Lee T, Ridsdale R, Ackerley C, et al. Defective lung vascular development and fatal respiratory distress in endothelial NO synthase-deficient mice: a model of alveolar capillary dysplasia? *Circ.Res.*2004;94(8):1115-23.

[146] Forbes MS, Thornhill BA, Park MH, Chevalier RL. Lack of endothelial nitric-oxide synthase leads to progressive focal renal injury. *Am .J. Pathol.*2007 Jan;170(1):87-99.

[147] Fleming I, Busse R. Molecular mechanisms involved in the regulation of the endothelial nitric oxide synthase. *Am J Physiol Regul Integr Comp Physiol*2003 Jan;284(1):R1-12.

[148] Govers R, Rabelink TJ. Cellular regulation of endothelial nitric oxide synthase. *Am. J. Physiol. Renal Physiol.*2001 Feb;280(2):F193-206.

[149] Igarashi J, Michel T. S1P and eNOS regulation. *Biochim. Biophys.* Acta2008 Sep;1781(9):489-95.

[150] Imasawa T, Kitamura H, Ohkawa R, Satoh Y, Miyashita A, Yatomi Y. Unbalanced expression of sphingosine 1-phosphate receptors in diabetic nephropathy. *Exp. Toxicol. Pathol.* 2010 Jan;62(1):53-60.

[151] Duncan ER, Crossey PA, Walker S, Anilkumar N, Poston L, Douglas G, et al. Effect of endothelium-specific insulin resistance on endothelial function in vivo. *Diabetes* 2008 Dec;57(12):3307-14.

[152] Kearney MT, Duncan ER, Kahn M, Wheatcroft SB. Insulin resistance and endothelial cell dysfunction: studies in mammalian models. *Exp. Physiol.* 2008 Jan;93(1):158-63.

[153] Giugliano D, Marfella R, Coppola L, Verrazzo G, Acampora R, Giunta R, et al. Vascular effects of acute hyperglycemia in humans are reversed by L-arginine. Evidence for reduced availability of nitric oxide during hyperglycemia. *Circulation* 1997 Apr 1;95(7):1783-90.

[154] Brodsky SV, Morrishow AM, Dharia N, Gross SS, Goligorsky MS. Glucose scavenging of nitric oxide. *Am.J.Physiol.Renal. Physiol.* 2001 Mar;280(3):F480-6;280(3):F480-6.

[155] Du XL, Edelstein D, Dimmeler S, Ju Q, Sui C, Brownlee M. Hyperglycemia inhibits endothelial nitric oxide synthase activity by posttranslational modification at the Akt site. *J.ClinInvest.* 2001;108(9):1341-8.

[156] Fleming I, Fisslthaler B, Dimmeler S, Kemp BE, Busse R. Phosphorylation of Thr(495) regulates Ca(2+)/calmodulin-dependent endothelial nitric oxide synthase activity. *Circ. Res.* 2001 Jun 8;88(11):E68-75.

[157] Michell BJ, Chen Z, Tiganis T, Stapleton D, Katsis F, Power DA, et al. Coordinated control of endothelial nitric-oxide synthase phosphorylation by protein kinase C and the cAMP-dependent protein kinase. *J. Biol. Chem.* 2001 May 25;276(21):17625-8.

[158] Matsubara M, Titani K, Taniguchi H. Interaction of calmodulin-binding domain peptides of nitric oxide synthase with membrane phospholipids: regulation by protein phosphorylation and Ca(2+)-calmodulin. *Biochemistry* 1996 Nov 19;35(46):14651-8.

[159] Naruse K, Rask-Madsen C, Takahara N, Ha SW, Suzuma K, Way KJ, et al. Activation of vascular protein kinase C-beta inhibits Akt-dependent endothelial nitric oxide synthase function in obesity-associated insulin resistance. *Diabetes* 2006 Mar;55(3):691-8.

[160] Ozcan U, Cao Q, Yilmaz E, Lee AH, Iwakoshi NN, Ozdelen E, et al. Endoplasmic reticulum stress links obesity, insulin action, and type 2 diabetes. *Science* 2004 Oct 15;306(5695):457-61.

[161] Koya D, King GL. Protein kinase C activation and the development of diabetic complications. *Diabetes* 1998 Jun;47(6):859-66.

[162] Xu B, Chibber R, Ruggiero D, Kohner E, Ritter J, Ferro A. Impairment of vascular endothelial nitric oxide synthase activity by advanced glycation end products. *FASEB J* 2003;17(10):1289-91.

[163] Rashid G, Benchetrit S, Fishman D, Bernheim J. Effect of advanced glycation end-products on gene expression and synthesis of TNF-alpha and endothelial nitric oxide synthase by endothelial cells. *Kidney Int.* 2004;66(3):1099-106.

[164] Bucala R, Tracey KJ, Cerami A. Advanced glycosylation products quench nitric oxide and mediate defective endothelium-dependent vasodilatation in experimental diabetes. *J.ClinInvest* 1991;87(2):432-8.

[165] Yoshizumi M, Perrella MA, Burnett JC, Jr., Lee ME. Tumor necrosis factor downregulates an endothelial nitric oxide synthase mRNA by shortening its half-life. *Circ. Res.* 1993 Jul;73(1):205-9.

[166] Li G, Barrett EJ, Barrett MO, Cao W, Liu Z. Tumor necrosis factor-alpha induces insulin resistance in endothelial cells via a p38 mitogen-activated protein kinase-dependent pathway. *Endocrinology* 2007 Jul;148(7):3356-63.

[167] Anderson HD, Rahmutula D, Gardner DG. Tumor necrosis factor-alpha inhibits endothelial nitric-oxide synthase gene promoter activity in bovine aortic endothelial cells. *J. Biol. Chem.* 2004 Jan 9;279(2):963-9.

[168] Makino N, Maeda T, Sugano M, Satoh S, Watanabe R, Abe N. High serum TNF-alpha level in Type 2 diabetic patients with microangiopathy is associated with eNOS down-regulation and apoptosis in endothelial cells. J Diabetes Complications 2005 Nov-Dec;19(6):347-55.

[169] Goodwin BL, Pendleton LC, Levy MM, Solomonson LP, Eichler DC. Tumor necrosis factor-alpha reduces argininosuccinate synthase expression and nitric oxide production in aortic endothelial cells. *Am. J. Physiol. Heart. Circ. Physiol.* 2007 Aug;293(2):H1115-21.

[170] Wang XL, Zhang L, Youker K, Zhang MX, Wang J, LeMaire SA, et al. Free fatty acids inhibit insulin signaling-stimulated endothelial nitric oxide synthase activation through upregulating PTEN or inhibiting Akt kinase. *Diabetes* 2006 Aug;55(8):2301-10.

[171] Kim F, Tysseling KA, Rice J, Pham M, Haji L, Gallis BM, et al. Free fatty acid impairment of nitric oxide production in endothelial cells is mediated by IKKbeta. *Arterioscler. Thromb. Vasc. Biol.* 2005 May;25(5):989-94.

[172] Cooke JP. Does ADMA cause endothelial dysfunction? *Arterioscler. Thromb. Vasc. Biol.* 2000 Sep;20(9):2032-7.

[173] Toutouzas K, Riga M, Stefanadi E, Stefanadis C. Asymmetric dimethylarginine (ADMA) and other endogenous nitric oxide synthase (NOS) inhibitors as an important cause of vascular insulin resistance. *Horm. Metab. Res.* 2008 Sep;40(9):655-9.

[174] Boger RH, Bode-Boger SM, Szuba A, Tsao PS, Chan JR, Tangphao O, et al. Asymmetric dimethylarginine (ADMA): a novel risk factor for endothelial dysfunction: its role in hypercholesterolemia. *Circulation* 1998 Nov 3;98(18):1842-7.

[175] Hand MF, Haynes WG, Webb DJ. Hemodialysis and L-arginine, but not D-arginine, correct renal failure-associated endothelial dysfunction. *Kidney Int.* 1998 Apr;53(4):1068-77.

[176] Onozato ML, Tojo A, Leiper J, Fujita T, Palm F, Wilcox CS. Expression of NG,NG-dimethylarginine dimethylaminohydrolase and protein arginine N-methyltransferase isoforms in diabetic rat kidney: effects of angiotensin II receptor blockers. *Diabetes* 2008 Jan;57(1):172-80.

[177] Wang D, Gill PS, Chabrashvili T, Onozato ML, Raggio J, Mendonca M, et al. Isoform-specific regulation by N(G),N(G)-dimethylarginine dimethylaminohydrolase of rat serum asymmetric dimethylarginine and vascular endothelium-derived relaxing factor/NO. *Circ. Res.* 2007 Sep 14;101(6):627-35.

[178] Leiper J, Nandi M, Torondel B, Murray-Rust J, Malaki M, O'Hara B, et al. Disruption of methylarginine metabolism impairs vascular homeostasis. *Nat. Med* 2007 Feb;13(2):198-203.

[179] Shibata R, Ueda S, Yamagishi S, Kaida Y, Matsumoto Y, Fukami K, et al. Involvement of asymmetric dimethylarginine (ADMA) in tubulointerstitial ischaemia in the early phase of diabetic nephropathy. *Nephrol. Dial. Transplant.* 2009 Apr;24(4):1162-9.

[180] Eid HM, Lyberg T, Arnesen H, Seljeflot I. Insulin and adiponectin inhibit the TNFalpha-induced ADMA accumulation in human endothelial cells: the role of DDAH. *Atherosclerosis*2007 Oct;194(2):e1-8.

[181] Sorrenti V, Mazza F, Campisi A, Vanella L, Li Volti G, Di Giacomo C. High glucose-mediated imbalance of nitric oxide synthase and dimethylarginine dimethylaminohydrolase expression in endothelial cells. *Curr. Neurovasc. Res.*2006 Feb;3(1):49-54.

[182] Lu CW, Xiong Y, He P. Dimethylarginine dimethylaminohydrolase-2 overexpression improves impaired nitric oxide synthesis of endothelial cells induced by glycated protein. Nitric Oxide2007 Feb;16(1):94-103.

[183] Sydow K, Munzel T. ADMA and oxidative stress. *Atheroscler. Suppl.*2003 Dec;4(4):41-51.

[184] Lin KY, Ito A, Asagami T, Tsao PS, Adimoolam S, Kimoto M, et al. Impaired nitric oxide synthase pathway in diabetes mellitus: role of asymmetric dimethylarginine and dimethylarginine dimethylaminohydrolase. *Circulation*2002 Aug 20;106(8):987-92.

[185] Loomis ED, Sullivan JC, Osmond DA, Pollock DM, Pollock JS. Endothelin mediates superoxide production and vasoconstriction through activation of NADPH oxidase and uncoupled nitric-oxide synthase in the rat aorta. *J. Pharmacol. Exp. Ther.*2005 Dec;315(3):1058-64.

[186] Pollock DM, Pollock JS. Endothelin and oxidative stress in the vascular system. *Curr. Vasc. Pharmacol.*2005 Oct;3(4):365-7.

[187] Marrero MB, Banes-Berceli AK, Stern DM, Eaton DC. Role of the JAK/STAT signaling pathway in diabetic nephropathy. *Am. J. Physiol. Renal. Physiol.*2006 Apr;290(4):F762-8.

[188] Hocher B, Schwarz A, Reinbacher D, Jacobi J, Lun A, Priem F, et al. Effects of endothelin receptor antagonists on the progression of diabetic nephropathy. *Nephron*2001 Feb;87(2):161-9.

[189] Satoh M, Fujimoto S, Arakawa S, Yada T, Namikoshi T, Haruna Y, et al. Angiotensin II type 1 receptor blocker ameliorates uncoupled endothelial nitric oxide synthase in rats with experimental diabetic nephropathy. *Nephrol. Dial. Transplant.*2008 Dec;23(12):3806-13.

[190] Sidharta PN, Wagner FD, Bohnemeier H, Jungnik A, Halabi A, Krahenbuhl S, et al. Pharmacodynamics and pharmacokinetics of the urotensin II receptor antagonist palosuran in macroalbuminuric, diabetic patients. *Clin. Pharmacol. Ther*2006 Sep;80(3):246-56.

[191] Arita R, Hata Y, Nakao S, Kita T, Miura M, Kawahara S, et al. Rho kinase inhibition by fasudil ameliorates diabetes-induced microvascular damage. *Diabetes*2009 Jan;58(1):215-26.

[192] Lage R, Dieguez C, Vidal-Puig A, Lopez M. AMPK: a metabolic gauge regulating whole-body energy homeostasis. *Trends Mol. Med.*2008 Dec;14(12):539-49.

[193] Zhang BB, Zhou G, Li C. AMPK: an emerging drug target for diabetes and the metabolic syndrome. *Cell Metab.*2009 May;9(5):407-16.

[194] Zou MH, Wu Y. AMP-activated protein kinase activation as a strategy for protecting vascular endothelial function. *Clin. Exp. Pharmacol. Physiol.*2008 May;35(5-6):535-45.

[195] Chen ZP, Mitchelhill KI, Michell BJ, Stapleton D, Rodriguez-Crespo I, Witters LA, et al. AMP-activated protein kinase phosphorylation of endothelial NO synthase. *FEBS Lett*1999 Jan 29;443(3):285-9.

[196] Chen Z, Peng IC, Sun W, Su MI, Hsu PH, Fu Y, et al. AMP-activated protein kinase functionally phosphorylates endothelial nitric oxide synthase Ser633. *Circ. Res.*2009 Feb 27;104(4):496-505.

[197] Schulz E, Dopheide J, Schuhmacher S, Thomas SR, Chen K, Daiber A, et al. Suppression of the JNK pathway by induction of a metabolic stress response prevents vascular injury and dysfunction. *Circulation*2008 Sep 23;118(13):1347-57.

[198] Zhang J, Xie Z, Dong Y, Wang S, Liu C, Zou MH. Identification of nitric oxide as an endogenous activator of the AMP-activated protein kinase in vascular endothelial cells. *J. Biol. Chem.*2008 Oct 10;283(41):27452-61.

[199] Kukidome D, Nishikawa T, Sonoda K, Imoto K, Fujisawa K, Yano M, et al. Activation of AMP-activated protein kinase reduces hyperglycemia-induced mitochondrial reactive oxygen species production and promotes mitochondrial biogenesis in human umbilical vein endothelial cells. *Diabetes*2006 Jan;55(1):120-7.

[200] Touyz RM, Schiffrin EL. Peroxisome proliferator-activated receptors in vascular biology-molecular mechanisms and clinical implications. *Vascul. Pharmacol.*2006 Jul;45(1):19-28.

[201] Okayasu T, Tomizawa A, Suzuki K, Manaka K, Hattori Y. PPARalpha activators upregulate eNOS activity and inhibit cytokine-induced NF-kappaB activation through AMP-activated protein kinase activation. *Life Sci.*2008 Apr 9;82(15-16):884-91.

[202] de Aguiar LG, Bahia LR, Villela N, Laflor C, Sicuro F, Wiernsperger N, et al. Metformin improves endothelial vascular reactivity in first-degree relatives of type 2 diabetic patients with metabolic syndrome and normal glucose tolerance. *Diabetes Care*2006 May;29(5):1083-9.

[203] Lavu S, Boss O, Elliott PJ, Lambert PD. Sirtuins--novel therapeutic targets to treat age-associated diseases. *Nat. Rev. Drug. Discov.*2008 Oct;7(10):841-53.

[204] Nisoli E, Tonello C, Cardile A, Cozzi V, Bracale R, Tedesco L, et al. Calorie restriction promotes mitochondrial biogenesis by inducing the expression of eNOS. *Science* 2005 Oct 14;310(5746):314-7.

[205] Ungvari Z, Parrado-Fernandez C, Csiszar A, de Cabo R. Mechanisms underlying caloric restriction and lifespan regulation: implications for vascular aging. *Circ. Res.*2008 Mar 14;102(5):519-28.

[206] Mattagajasingh I, Kim CS, Naqvi A, Yamamori T, Hoffman TA, Jung SB, et al. SIRT1 promotes endothelium-dependent vascular relaxation by activating endothelial nitric oxide synthase. *Proc. Natl .Acad. Sci .U S A.*2007 Sep 11;104(37):14855-60.

[207] Ota H, Eto M, Kano MR, Ogawa S, Iijima K, Akishita M, et al. Cilostazol inhibits oxidative stress-induced premature senescence via upregulation of Sirt1 in human endothelial cells. *Arterioscler. Thromb. Vasc. Biol.*2008 Sep;28(9):1634-9.

[208] Potente M, Dimmeler S. NO targets SIRT1: a novel signaling network in endothelial senescence. *Arterioscler. Thromb. Vasc. Biol.*2008 Sep;28(9):1577-9.

[209] Potente M, Dimmeler S. Emerging roles of SIRT1 in vascular endothelial homeostasis. *Cell Cycle* 2008 Jul 15;7(14):2117-22.

[210] Orimo M, Minamino T, Miyauchi H, Tateno K, Okada S, Moriya J, et al. Protective Role of SIRT1 in Diabetic Vascular Dysfunction. *Arterioscler. Thromb. Vasc .Biol.* 2009 Jun;29(6):889-94.

[211] Hugo C, Daniel C. Thrombospondin in renal disease. *Nephron. Exp. Nephrol.* 2009;111(3):e61-6.

[212] Hohenstein B, Daniel C, Hausknecht B, Boehmer K, Riess R, Amann KU, et al. Correlation of enhanced thrombospondin-1 expression, TGF-beta signalling and proteinuria in human type-2 diabetic nephropathy. *Nephrol. Dial. Transplant.* 2008 Dec;23(12):3880-7.

[213] Moczulski DK, Fojcik H, Wielgorecki A, Trautsolt W, Gawlik B, Kosiorz-Gorczynska S, et al. Expression pattern of genes in peripheral blood mononuclear cells in diabetic nephropathy. *Diabet Med.* 2007 Mar;24(3):266-71.

[214] Isenberg JS, Frazier WA, Roberts DD. Thrombospondin-1: a physiological regulator of nitric oxide signaling. *Cell Mol. Life Sci.* 2008 Mar;65(5):728-42.

[215] Isenberg JS, Roberts DD, Frazier WA. CD47: a new target in cardiovascular therapy. *Arterioscler Thromb. Vasc. Biol.* 2008 Apr;28(4):615-21.

[216] Isenberg JS, Martin-Manso G, Maxhimer JB, Roberts DD. Regulation of nitric oxide signalling by thrombospondin 1: implications for anti-angiogenic therapies. *Nat. Rev. Cancer* 2009 Mar;9(3):182-94.

[217] Isenberg JS, Ridnour LA, Perruccio EM, Espey MG, Wink DA, Roberts DD. Thrombospondin-1 inhibits endothelial cell responses to nitric oxide in a cGMP-dependent manner. *Proc. Natl. Acad. Sci. U S A.* 2005 Sep 13;102(37):13141-6.

[218] Isenberg JS, Ridnour LA, Dimitry J, Frazier WA, Wink DA, Roberts DD. CD47 is necessary for inhibition of nitric oxide-stimulated vascular cell responses by thrombospondin-1. *J. Biol. Chem.* 2006 Sep 8;281(36):26069-80.

[219] Isenberg JS, Jia Y, Fukuyama J, Switzer CH, Wink DA, Roberts DD. Thrombospondin-1 inhibits nitric oxide signaling via CD36 by inhibiting myristic acid uptake. *J. Biol. Chem.* 2007 May 25;282(21):15404-15.

[220] Isenberg JS, Frazier WA, Krishna MC, Wink DA, Roberts DD. Enhancing cardiovascular dynamics by inhibition of thrombospondin-1/CD47 signaling. *Curr. Drug. Targets* 2008 Oct;9(10):833-41.

[221] Goligorsky MS, Li H, Brodsky S, Chen J. Relationships between caveolae and eNOS: everything in proximity and the proximity of everything. *Am. J. Physiol. Renal. Physiol.* 2002 Jul;283(1):F1-10.

[222] Frank PG, Woodman SE, Park DS, Lisanti MP. Caveolin, caveolae, and endothelial cell function. Arterioscler *Thromb. Vasc. Biol.* 2003 Jul 1;23(7):1161-8.

[223] Li XA, Everson WV, Smart EJ. Caveolae, lipid rafts, and vascular disease. *Trends Cardiovasc. Med.* 2005 Apr;15(3):92-6.

[224] Xu Y, Buikema H, van Gilst WH, Henning RH. Caveolae and endothelial dysfunction: filling the caves in cardiovascular disease. *Eur. J. Pharmacol.* 2008 May 13;585(2-3):256-60.

[225] Pascariu M, Bendayan M, Ghitescu L. Correlated endothelial caveolin overexpression and increased transcytosis in experimental diabetes. *J. Histochem. Cytochem.* 2004 Jan;52(1):65-76.

[226] Bucci M, Roviezzo F, Brancaleone V, Lin MI, Di Lorenzo A, Cicala C, et al. Diabetic mouse angiopathy is linked to progressive sympathetic receptor deletion coupled to an

enhanced caveolin-1 expression. *Arterioscler. Thromb. Vasc. Biol.*2004 Apr;24(4):721-6.

[227] Lam TY, Seto SW, Lau YM, Au LS, Kwan YW, Ngai SM, et al. Impairment of the vascular relaxation and differential expression of caveolin-1 of the aorta of diabetic +db/+db mice. *Eur. J. Pharmacol.*2006 Sep 28;546(1-3):134-41.

[228] Komers R, Schutzer WE, Reed JF, Lindsley JN, Oyama TT, Buck DC, et al. Altered endothelial nitric oxide synthase targeting and conformation and caveolin-1 expression in the diabetic kidney. *Diabetes*2006 Jun;55(6):1651-9.

[229] Trujillo J, Ramirez V, Perez J, Torre-Villalvazo I, Torres N, Tovar AR, et al. Renal protection by a soy diet in obese Zucker rats is associated with restoration of nitric oxide generation. *Am. J. Physiol. Renal Physiol.*2005 Jan;288(1):F108-16.

[230] Garcia-Cardena G, Fan R, Shah V, Sorrentino R, Cirino G, Papapetropoulos A, et al. Dynamic activation of endothelial nitric oxide synthase by Hsp90. *Nature*1998 Apr 23;392(6678):821-4.

[231] Ou J, Fontana JT, Ou Z, Jones DW, Ackerman AW, Oldham KT, et al. Heat shock protein 90 and tyrosine kinase regulate eNOS NO* generation but not NO* bioactivity. *Am. J. Physiol. Heart Circ. Physiol.*2004 Feb;286(2):H561-9.

[232] Lei H, Venkatakrishnan A, Yu S, Kazlauskas A. Protein kinase A-dependent translocation of Hsp90 alpha impairs endothelial nitric-oxide synthase activity in high glucose and diabetes. *J. Biol. Chem.*2007 Mar 30;282(13):9364-71.

[233] Barutta F, Pinach S, Giunti S, Vittone F, Forbes JM, Chiarle R, et al. Heat shock protein expression in diabetic nephropathy. *Am. J. Physiol. Renal. Physiol.*2008 Dec;295(6):F1817-24.

[234] Potenza MA, Gagliardi S, Nacci C, Carratu MR, Montagnani M. Endothelial dysfunction in diabetes: from mechanisms to therapeutic targets. *Curr. Med. Chem.*2009;16(1):94-112.

Chapter XII

Recent Advances on Cell Biology of Podocytes and their Contribution to the Pathogenesis of Diabetic Glomerulosclerosis

Sandeep Magoon, Hitesh Shah, Saul Teichberg, and Pravin C. Singhal[*]

Department of Medicine and Pathology, North Shore LIJ Health System
Great Neck, NY 11021, US

Abstract

The podocyte strategically positioned along the outer aspect of the glomerular basement membrane, is a critical component of the glomerular filtration barrier (GFB), functioning in tandem with its associated slit diaphragm, to limit passage of albumin and plasma proteins into the urinary space. The absence of podocyte regeneration following cell injury or apoptosis, is a major limitation in the treatment to diabetic glomerular disease. In the past, because of its differentiated characteristics podocyte injury could not be studied in *in vitro* studies. However, availability of conditionally immortalized podocyte cell lines has advanced podocyte research to the next level. In the present study we have provided review of the literature pertaining to podocyte injury in general, and in diabetes in particular.

Normal Podocyte Structure and Biology

Podocytes are terminally differentiated and highly specialized epithelial cells of complex shape and are derived from the mesenchymal cells [1, 2]. The podocyte is characterized by a

---

[*] Address for correspondence: Pravin C. Singhal, M.D.Division of Kidney Diseases and Hypertension,100 Community Drive, Great Neck, NY 11021, Tel. 516-465-3010., Fax 516-465-3011, singhal@lij.edu.

central cell body which projects primary processes towards the glomerular capillaries. Primary processes further branch and differentiate into foot processes (Figure 1A), which interdigitate with the foot processes of other podocytes and are attached to GBM via integrins [3] and dystroglycans [4]. The junctional space between the adjacent foot processes are called filtration slits, and are bridged by a complex structure called slit diaphragm (Figs 1A and 1B). This functions as one of the important size selective barriers to protein translocaction from blood to urinary space. The complex architecture of the podocyte consists of Actin cytoskeleton, slit diaphragm, podocyte foot processes and transmembrane proteins.

Actin Cytoskeleton

Actin cytoskeleton forms the backbone of podocytes [5]. It is a dynamic structure which allows podocyte to modulate their shape and maintain normal function. The cytoskeleton is comprised of three ultra structural elements- microfilaments, intermediate filaments, and microtubules. Microfilaments contain a dense network of F-actin and myosin and are the predominant constituents of the foot process. Their functions include structural support, contraction and expansion, like a buffer to pressure and stretch within the glomerulus, as well as an anchorage for the other intracellular molecules are also involved in the cell signaling and communication.

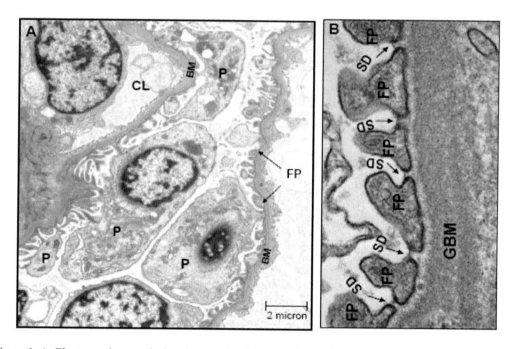

Figure 1. A. Electron micrograph showing relationship of podocyte foot processes with GBM. B. Higher magnification showing slit diaphragm. Glomerular basement membrane (CBM); podocyte (P); foot processes (FP); slit diaphragm (SD); capillary lumen (CL).

Slit Diaphragm

A number of characteristic proteins are essential for the normal functioning of the slit diaphragm, particularly nephrin, NEPH1, podocin, zona occludens-1 (ZO-1), CD2 adaptor protein (CD2AP), FAT, and P-cadherin (Figure 2) . Nephrin, a member of the Ig super family, was discovered by Tryggvason [6]. It is a transmembrane protein expressed by podocytes and localized within the slit diaphragm. Neprin interacts with and localizes to CD2AP and binds to podocin in the cytoplasm. It is required for the formation of the rod and the zipper-like structure of the slit diaphragm [7], and, it may play active role in podocyte signaling causing activation of a kinase cascade and thus inhibiting apoptosis [8,9]. Another Ig superfamily protein, NEPH-1[10, 11], has been identified, which interacts with nephrin, podocin and FAT1. Hence, the slit diaphragm and its components are important not only for regulating passage of protein, but also playing a crucial role in preventing apoptosis.

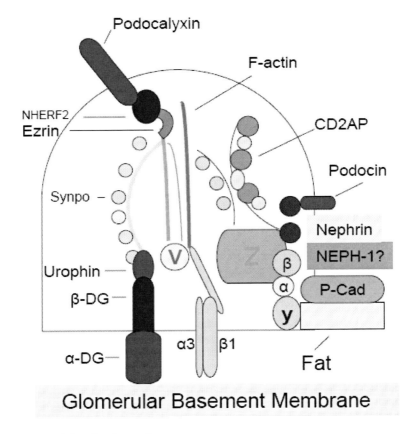

Figure 2. Podocyte and functional proteins.

Podocyte-Basement Membrane Interaction

The basal cell membrane of the foot process play very important role in propitiating attachment of podocytes to underlying glomerular basement membrane (GBM) through cell matrix contacts. The two most important consituents are α3β1 integrin and α and β dystroglycans [12]. The α chain contains a polyanionic binding site for the cationic laminin globular-binding domain common to many matrix proteins such as laminin, perlecan, proteoglycans and agrin. β chains link dystroglycan complex to the actin cytoskeleton non-covalently. Integrins, of which α3β1 is the predominant type, mediates cell matrix interaction and binds collagen, fibronectin, laminin and entactin/nidogen in the GBM [13]. Due to the interactive proximity of podocytes with the GBM, any mechanical force can be transmitted from the GBM to the cell body of the podocytes. Podocytes in the mature glomerulus, continue to synthesize and assemble basement membrane matrix molecules [14] and also secretes matrix-modifying enzymes like metalloproteinase 6, thus contributing to basement membrane matrix turnover.

Transmembrane Proteins

The plasma membrane of podocytes is composed of transmembrane proteins with negatively charged surface. Thus in addition to acting as size selective barrier to proteins, podocytes also prevent blood to urinary space protein leakage through negative charge barrier. The majority of the charge is provided by Podocalyxin [15], though Podoplanin [16] may also be important. Podocalyxin is a sialyated and sulfated membrane protein. Cytoplasmic domain of podocalyxin is attached to the actincytoskeleton through Na+/H+ exchanger regulatory factor 2(NHERF 2)/ezrin complexes [17].

Podocyte Dysfunction in Experimental Diabetes

A longitudinal record of the development of diabetic nephropathy has been obtained from animal experiments through repeated sampling. Gassler et al., [18] demonstrated that podocyte injury precedes the development of focal segmental glomerulosclerosis in obese fa/fa zucker rats, a model of type 2 diabetes. Coimbra et al., [19] also suggested that early progressive podocyte damage and macrophage infiltration is associated with type 2 diabetes and antedates both the development of glomerulosclerosis and tubulointerstitial damage. In the streptozotocin (STZ)-induced diabetic rat, a model of type 1 diabetes, Missud et al., [20] and Kelly et a., l[21] have reported effacement of foot processes along with decrease in podocyte number and reduction in Nephrin expression, which was attenuated with ACE inhibition.

Diabetes in Humans

Farquhar et al., [22] in 1957 were the first to report extensive foot process effacement in biopsies of patients with nephritic syndrome. In 1980Steffes et al., [23] described foot process widening in diabetic rats, which was confirmed by Ellis and colleagues [24] in patients with advanced type 1 diabetic nephropathy. Recent studies have described similar morphologic changes in type 1 diabetic subjects with microalbuminuria and a rate of urinary albumin excretion that was directly correlated with the width of foot processes [25]. Subsequent studies have also reported a decrease in the number and density of podocytes in addition to increased width of effaced foot processes in both type 1 and type 2 diabetes [26-29]. Podocytopenia can occur even in patients with diabetes of short duration [26]. As the podocyte number diminishes, there is a parallel increase in their width to cover the GBM [27, 30]. Meyer et al., [31] reported that the podocyte number predicts long term urinary albumin excretion in type 2 diabetes and suggested that among all morphological changes the strongest predictor of progressive renal disease is the decrease in the number of podocytes. At present, there is no standard protocol to estimate podocyte number in the biopsy specimens. However, approximations can be made using morphometric techniques. Dalla et al., [29] evaluated podocyte density and number in type 2 diabetic patients using electron microscopic morphometric analysis on biopsy specimens. They reported that changes in the structure and function occur in the early stages of diabetic nephropathy; moreover, it is the podocyte density and not the number, which is more predictive of albumiuria.An inverse correlation between proteinuria and podocyte number was also confirmed in another cross sectional study [32]. Nakamura et al., [33] studied the correlation between podocyte loss from the glomerulus and urinary excretion of podocytes in patients with type 2 diabetic nephropathy and concluded that urinary podocytes were present in 53% of patients with microalbuminuria and in 80% with macroalbuminuria; however, podocyturia was reduced with ACE inhibition. Normoalbuminuric patients and healthy control subjects had undetectable levels of urinary podocytes.

Pavenstadt and colleagues [34], in their review on the cell biology of podocytes, found a direct correlation between the development of proteinuria and podocytopenia. Once podocytes are decreased in number, the denuded GBM (without podocytes) develop synechial attachment with Bowman's capsule, an initial step in glomerulosclerosis. As foot processes are effaced, the length of slit diaphragm decreases, which might impede water filtration and decrease GFR. Olive Smithies [35] proposed an innovative theory, assuming the GBM was concentrated Gel, through which diffusion provides most of the protein and dilutent flow dependent. As GFR decreases, the concentration of protein in relation to water increases, which overwhelming the resorptive capacity of proximal tubular cells, resulting in proteinuria. The proposed theory reconciles with paradox of increasing proteinuria with declining renal function. However, theory remains unproven and controversial. Remuzzi et al., [36] in their landmark paper, explained the pathophysiology of progressive nephropathy with worsening proteinuria due to induction of tubular atrophy and interstitial fibrosis, together with glomerulosclerosis, leading to chronic renal failure.

In addition to structural changes, recent studies have looked at the functional abnormalities in podocytes. Nephrin excretion in the urine of type 2 diabetic subjects was seen in 17%, 28%, and 30% of patients with microalbuminuria, macroalbuminuria, and normoalbuminuria respectively [37]. In comparison, nondiabetic subjects did not leak any nephrin in the urine, suggesting that nephrin can be detected in the urine, as a marker of early podocyte injury, even before the onset of microalbuminuria. Diminution or Loss of mRNA for nephrin has also been reported in diabetic patients with proteinuria [38-40]. Proteinuria is inversely related to nephrin expression and a decrease in nephrin is correlated with increased foot processes effacement. However, in contrast, there was no reduction in the expression of CD2AP, suggesting a specific phenomenon, not related to podocyte injury or loss [39].

Podocyte Detachment and Apoptosis

Podocyes and podocyte specific protein products can be detected in the urine of patients with diabetic nephropathy. Two mechanisms i.e., detachment and/or apoptosis have been proposed; however the exact cause remains to be defined. Data on apoptosis, in both, experimental and human diabetic nephropathy is limited [41-44]. Podocytes adhere to the underlying GBM by integrins and dystroglycans and their attachment is critical for survival. Once they are detached, either they are shed live in the urine [45] or undergo apoptosis [46]. Podocyturia worsens with the progression of proteinuria [33]. Studies in rats and humans with diabetes, have shown that there is downregulation of alpha3B1 integrin receptor. Rat or human cultured podocytes decrease the expression of alpha3B1 integrin in the presence of hyperglycemia [47-49] and thus is thought to be mediated by TGF-β1[50,51]. Singhal et al. [52] reported Ang II induced apoptosis in cultured rat glomerular epithelial cells. Ang II has been demonstrated to play an important role in the progression of diabetic nephropathy [12, 13]. Moreover, Agents which inhibit the production of Ang II are being used extensively for slowing down the progression of diabetic nephropathy [12, 13]. In cell culture systems the proapoptotic effect of Ang II was abolished with anti TGF-β1 antibody, suggesting a role of TGF-B [52]. Non diabetic TGF-β overexpressing transgenic mice develop podocyte apoptosis in the glomerulus. TGF-β1 is characteristically increased in diabetes and may theoretically be causally associated with apoptosis [53]. TGF-β1 increases the expression of smad-7, which inhibits nuclear translocation and transcriptional activity of cell survival factor NF-kappaB [54,55].

Mechanisms of Podocyte Damage in Diabetes

Development of conditionally "Immortalized" podocyte cell lines have vastly improved our understanding of different molecular mechanisms causing injury to podocyte in diabetes [56, 57]. Podocytes normally do not divide and any attempt to induce the cells to re-enter the cell cycle leads to their dedifferentiation. The process of conditional immortalization involves the introduction of an oncogene whose gene product is temperature sensitive. At low temperature, the oncogene is active and will allow the cells to enter the cycle and divide. Once proliferation is complete, the oncogene is inactivated by moving the cells to higher temperature, allowing differentiation. Podocyte structural and functional changes are dependent on both the hemodynamic and metabolic consequences of diabetes. These conditionally immortalized podocytes express all markers of podocytes.

Hyperglycemia

Kim et a., [58] demonstrated that when podocytes in culture were exposed to high glucose concentration, there was up regulation of extracellular signal-regulated protein kinase ½ (ERK1/2) and Akt/protein kinase B (PKB), which are important for protein synthesis but not DNA synthesis. Susztak and colleagues [59] for the first time demonstrated podocyte apoptosis increased sharply with onset of hyperglycemia in Ins2 (Akita) (Akita) mice with type 1 diabetes and Lepr (db/db) (db/db) mice with obesity and type 2 diabetes. Increased extracellular glucose rapidly stimulated generation of intracellular reactive oxygen species (ROS) through NADPH oxidase and mitochondrial pathways and led to activation of proapoptotic p38 mitogen-activated protein kinase and caspase 3 and to apoptosis of conditionally immortalized podocytes in vitro. Podocyte apoptosis coincided with the onset of urinary albumin excretion (UAE) and preceded significant losses of podocytes in Akita (37% reduction) and db/db (27% reduction) mice. Kang et al. [60] emphasized the role of 12-lipooxygenase and the p38 MAPK signaling pathway in the synthesis of extracellular matrix in diabetes by podocytes. Diabetes in vivo and exposure of podocytes to high glucose in vitro stimulated 12-LO, p38 MAPK, and collagen alpha5 (IV) mRNA and (activated) protein. 12-LO inhibition by diminished the expression of podocyte phospho-p38 MAPK and collagen alpha5(IV) mRNA and protein. VEGF is up regulated early in diabetes, specifically in podocytes. In vivo, blockade of VEGF in diabetic rats abolished hyperfiltration and partially suppressed increased UAE, without affecting hyperglycemic control. RAGE, a receptor for advanced glycation end products (AGEs) displays enhanced expression in podocytes of genetically diabetic db/db mice [61]. RAGE-bearing podocytes express high levels of VEGF in parallel with enhanced recruitment of mononuclear phagocytes to the glomeruli. Activation of RAGE contributes to expression of VEGF and enhanced attraction/activation of inflammatory cells in the diabetic glomerulus, thereby setting the stage for mesangial activation and TGF-beta production; processes which converge to cause albuminuria and glomerulosclerosis.

ANG II

It has been reported, in animal models through pharmacological intervention, that increase in the Ang II activity is responsible for podocyte injury in diabetes. In STZ induced diabetic rats, AT1 receptor blockage and ACE inhibition decreased podocyte foot process widening. A study comparing aminoguanidine, blocker of advanced glycation end product formation with ACE inhibitor on nephrin expression showed attenuation of diabetes induced reduction in nephrin expression with ACE inhibition [62]. AngII is increased in glucose stimulated cultured podocytes and exogenous AngII increases mRNA and protein expression of p27, which inhibits cyclin dependent kinases [63]. In p27 knockout mice, there was attenuation of functional and morphological features of diabetic nephropathy.

Podocytes exposed to high concentration of AngII, in animal models of diabetes and in human diabetes, Ang II has been thought to be critically involved in the loss of nephrin from the slit diaphragm. Nephrin loss predisposes to increasing proteinuria and in reduction of electron dense slit diaphragm [64]. Effects of AngII are additive with glucose and it has been postulated that the final common pathway of injury may be through enhanced ROS production. AngII causes increased extracellular matrix production by stimulating alpha3 (IV) collagen through upregulating the expression of TGFb type II receptors and activating TGFb signaling system via Smad2 [65]. It also stimulates VGF secretion.

We have demonstrated that Ang II has potential to induce popdocyte apoptosis both in vitro as well as in vivo [52, 66]. In these studies, Ang II infusion not only decreased nephrin expression but also their site of expression.

TGF –β

It has been established by cell culture, experimental animal models and clinical trials, that hyperglycemia plays a central role in the pathogenesis of diabetic nephropathy. Among various cytokines that are stimulated, TFG- β appears to be most prominent fibrogenic cytokine [67]. In addition to overexpression of TGF- β in kidney, there is up regulation of TGF-β type II receptors and downstream smad signaling pathway, thus confirming the over activity of TGF- β system. Renal hypertrophy, mesangial matrix expansion and renal insufficiency were prevented in db/db diabetic mice by pan-selective neutralizing antibody (68, 69). However, if failed to show the similar effect on proteinuria.

Due to conflicting data, integral role of TGF- β in the pathogenesis of diabetic albuminuria can not be established. Kopp et al., [70] in transgenic mice with over expression of TGF- β, reported mesangial expansion, interstitial fibrosis, progressive renal insufficiency and proteinuria. Sharma and colleagues [71] observed increased albumin permeability in isolated rat glomeruli, when exposed to TGF- β ex-vivo. However, similar results could not be duplicated by Ziyadeh et al., [69], who failed to show significant reduction in albuminuria in db/db diabetic rats when treated with Anti TGF- β antibody. It was thought to be due to persistent increased expression of VGEF by other diabetic factors. Studies with Smad3 knock out mice have shown contradictory results as well. Sung et al., [72] failed to show amelioration of albuminuria in Smad 3 knock out mice rendered diabetic with STZ. However, Fujimoto [73] reported significant amelioration of albuminuria in Smad3 knockout mice with different background strain. Both studies reported prevention of mesangial expansion. Thus it appears that proteinuria is secondary to increased VGEF and TGF- β plays important role in the pathogenesis of glomerulosclerosis.

VEGF

VEGF is a specific mitogen for vascular endothelial cells and induces angiogenesis and increases permeability of blood vessels leading to proteinuria [74]. Diabetes has been shown to increase the podocyte expression of VEGF. The most convincing evidence that VEGF over expression in involved in the proteinuria comes from the studies in type I diabetic (STZ-induced) rats and in type 2 diabetic db/db mice. Neutralizing of VEGF with the anti-VEGF antibody resulte in amelioration of albuminuria as compared to untreated controls [75, 76]. Nitric oxide synthase also appears to be induced by VEGF, causing vasodilatation and hyperfiltration, hallmark of early diabetic nephropathy [75, 77].

VEGF appears to act through paracrine and autocrine loops. In the autocrine loop. Increase in the VEGF causes up regulation of type II TGFβ receptors, thus augmenting the effects of TGFβ1 which stimulates the production of various components of GBM, predominantly of alpha3(IV) collagen. VEGF signaling proceeds via autophophorylation of VEGF receptor-1 (VEGFR-1) and the activation of phosphatidylinositol 3-kinase(PI3K) pathway [78]. In the paracrine loop, VEGF increases the vascular permeability, likely by increasing the efferent tone, causing albuminuria. In human podocytes, VEGF interacts with nephrin to promote podocyte survival and inhibit apoptosis. This survival pathway involves VEGF induced phosphorylation of tyrosine residues at the intracellular domain of nephrin.

Mechanical Stretch

Studies have shown that mechanical stress modifies both morphology and protein expression in podocytes [79]. In diabetes, podocytes are exposed to elevated glucose concentrations as well as mechanical strain generated by high intracapillary pressures. Both these factors are responsible for podocyte injury, causing renal dysfunction. There is loss of α1β3 integrins which play a crucial role in anchoring podocyte to GBM. The loss of integrins is additive with stretch and high ambient glucose concentration. Decreased expression of GLUT2 and GLUT4 [80] on the surface of stretched cells suggests that the activity of other glucose transporters may be regulated by mechanical stress in podocytes. Mechanical stretch increases hypertrophy and decreases podocyte proliferation and these effects are mediated through activation of Erk1/2 and Akt and cell specific regulatory proteins [81, 82].

P66ShcA and Foxo Proteins

Recently, the p66ShcA protein has been demonstrated to play a critical role in the modulation of oxidative stress in a diabetic milieu [83-86]. Sv129p66ShcA$^{-/-}$ mice have been reported to express cardio-protective [86] and reno-protective phenotypes, in short-term studies following induction of streptozotocin (STZ)-induced diabetes mellitus. Most impressive was the protection exhibited at the cellular level for cardiac progenitor cells and cardiac muscle cells. In both cell populations, diabetic p66ShcA$^{-/-}$ mice show a striking reduction in apoptosis and entry to the senescent phenotype. Recently, a clearer understanding of p66ShcA gene has emerged, based on evidence the WTp66ShcA protein functionally interacts with the mammalian Forkhead homolog FOXO3a [87-90]. ROS induce phosphorylation at a critical CH2 Ser-36 residue, a modification that serves to promote the intracellular generation of ROS [87] and the recruitment of Akt/PKB, which directly phosphorylates and inactivates members of the highly conserved FOXO family of transcription factors [88]. FOXO family transcribes antioxidants such as MNSOD and catalase, DNA repair enzymes, cell cycle and apoptosis related proteins.

Summary

Proposed scheme for the role of podocyte injury and the development of diabetic glomerulosclerosis is shown in Figure 3. High glucose has potential to stimulate production of Ang II both by podocytes and mesangial cells. Ang II through its hemodynamic effect may lead to mechanical strech inducing podocyte ROS generation. Additionally, Ang II can directly stimulate ROS generation by podocytes. High glucose alone and in combination with Ang II invokes activation of p66ShcA pathway which induces phosphorylation of FOXO proteins and thus making them inactive for the transcription of antioxidants and DNA repair enzymes. Thus, high glucose milieu not only induces oxidative stress but also compromises cell survival phenotype by deactivating FOXP protein dependent stress response program. In addition, Ang II through TGF-β promotes podocyte apoptosis. Loss of podocyte will not only provide proximity of raw GBM to Bowman's capsule leading to adhesion but will also allow leakage of protein which has potential to promote tubulointerstitial lesions. Simultaneously, mesagial cell stimulation by high glucose will lead to the production of mesangial TGF-β leading to initial mesangial expansion and subsequent sclerosis. Thus, it appears though poodcyte play a predominant role in the development of diabetic glomerulosclerosis however its development is also contributed by adjacent kidney cells.

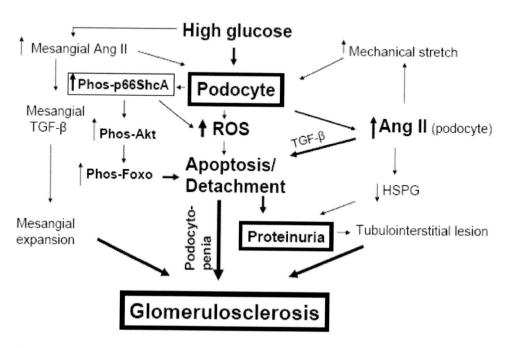

Figure 3. Proposed scheme forpodocyte injury leading to glomerulosclerosis.

References

[1] Shankland SJ, Al-Douahji M. Cell cycle regulatory proteins in glomerulardisease. *Exp. Nephrol.* 1999; 7: 207–211.

[2] Saxen L. Organogenesis of the Kidney. Cambridge University Press: Cambridge, 1997

[3] Adler S, Chen X. Anti-Fx1A antibody recognizes a beta-1-integrin on glomerular epithelial cells and inhibits adhesion and growth. *Am. J. Physiol* .1992; 262: F770–F776.

[4] Kojima K, Kerjaschki D. Is podocyte shape controlled by the dystroglycan complex? *Nephrol. Dial. Transplant* 2002; 17(Suppl 9): 23–24.

[5] Mundel P, Reiser J, Zuniga Mejia Borja A et al. Rearrangements of the cytoskeleton and cell contacts induce process formation during differentiation of conditionally immortalized mouse podocyte cell lines.*Exp. Cell Res.* 1997; 236: 248–258

[6] Ruotsalainen V, Ljungberg P, Wartiovaara J et al. Nephrin is specifically located at the slit diaphragm of glomerular podocytes. *Proc Natl Acad Sci USA* 1999; 96: 7962–7967.

[7] Ruotsalainen V, Patrakka J, Tissari P, Reponen P, Hess M, Kestila M, *et al*. Role of nephrin in cell junction formation in human nephrogenesis. *Am. J. Pathol.* 2000; 157: 1905-16

[8] Huber TB, Kottgen M, Schilling B, Walz G, Benzing T. Interaction with podocin facilitates nephrin signalling. *J. Biol. Chem.* 2001; 276:41543-6.

[9] Huber TB, Hartleben B, Kim J, Schmidts M, Schermer B, Keil A,*et al*. Nephrin and CD2AP associate with phosphoinositide 3-OH kinase and stimulate AKT-dependent signalling. *Mol. Cell Biol.*, 2003; 23: 4917-28

[10] Sellin L, Huber TB, Gerke P et al. NEPH1 defines a novel family of podocin interacting proteins. *FASEB J.* 2003; 17: 115–117.

[11] Benzing T. Signaling at the slit diaphragm. J Am Soc Nephrol 2004; 15:1382–1391

[12] Blanco S, Bonet J, Lopez D, Casa I, Romero R. ACE inhibitors improve nephrin expression in Zucker rats with glomerulosclerosis. *Kidney Int. Suppl* .2005; 93: S10-4.

[13] Mifsud SA, Allen TJ, Bertram JF, Hulthen UL, Kelly DJ, Cooper ME, *et al*. Podocyte foot process broadening in experimental diabetic nephropathy: amelioration with renin-angiotensin blockade. *Diabetologia* 2001; 44: 878-82.

[14] Miner JH. Renal basement membrane components. Kidney Int 1999; 56: 2016-24.

[15] Petermann AT, Pippin J, Krofft R, Blonski M, Griffin S, Durvasula R, *et al*. Viable podocytes detach in experimental diabetic nephropathy: potential mechanism underlying glomerulosclerosis.*Nephron. Exp. Nephrol.* 2004; 98: 14-23.

[16] Regoli M, Bendayan M. Alterations in the expression of the alpha 3 beta 1 integrin in certain membrane domains of the glomerular epithelial cells (podocytes) in diabetes mellitus. *Diabetologia* 1997; 40: 15-22

[17] Wang Z, Jiang T, Li J, Proctor G, McManaman JL, Licoa S, *et al*. Regulation of renal lipid metabolism, lipid accumulation, and glomerulosclerosis in FVBdb/db mice with type 2 diabetes. *Diabetes* 2005; 54: 2328-35.

[18] Gassler N, Elger M, Kranzlin B, Kriz W, Gretz N, Hahnel B, Hosser H, Hartmann I: Podocyte injury underlies the progression of focal segmental glomerulosclerosis in the fa/fa Zucker rat. *Kidney Int* 60:106 –116, 2001

[19] Coimbra TM, Janssen U, Grone HJ, Ostendorf T, Kunter U, Schmidt H, Brabant G, Floege J: Early events leading to renal injury in obese Zucker (fatty) rats with type II diabetes. *Kidney Int* 57:167–182, 2000

[20] Mifsud SA, Allen TJ, Bertram JF, Hulthen UL, Kelly DJ, Cooper ME, Wilkinson-Berka JL, Gilbert RE: Podocyte foot process broadening in experimental diabetic nephropathy: amelioration with renin-angiotensin blockade. *Diabetologia* 44:878–882, 2001

[21] Kelly DJ, Aaltonen P, Cox AJ, Rumble JR, Langham R, Panagiotopoulos S, Jerums G, Holthofer H, Gilbert RE: Expression of the slit-diaphragm protein, nephrin, in experimental diabetic nephropathy: differing effects of anti-proteinuric therapies. *Nephrol Dial Transplant* 17:1327–1332, 2002

[22] Farquhar MG, Vernier RL, Good RA. An electron microscope study of the glomerulus in nephrosis, glomerulonephritis, and lupus erythematosus. *J. Exp. Med.* 1957; 106: 649–660.

[23] Steffes MW, Leffert JD, Basgen JM, Brown DM, Mauer SM: Epithelia cell foot process width in intact and uninephrectomized diabetic and nondiabetic rats. *Lab. Invest.* 43:225–230, 1980

[24] Ellis EN, Steffes MW, Chavers B, Mauer SM: Observations of glomerular epithelial cell structure in patients wit type I diabetes mellitus. *Kidney Int.* 32:736–741, 1987

[25] Berg UB, Torbjornsdotter TB, Jaremko G, Thalme B: Kidney morphological changes in relation to long-term renal function and metabolic control in adolescents with IDDM. *Diabetologia* 41:1047–1056, 1998

[26] Steffes MW, Schmidt D, McCrery R, Basgen JM: Glomerular cell number in normal subjects and in type 1 diabetic patients. *Kidney Int.* 59:2104–2113, 2001

[27] Pagtalunan ME, Miller PL, Jumping-Eagle S, Nelson RG, Myers BD, Rennke HG, Coplon NS, Sun L, Meyer TW: Podocyte loss and progressive glomerular injury in type II diabetes. *J. Clin. Invest.* 99:342–348, 1997

[28] White KE, Bilous RW, Marshall SM, El Nahas M, Remuzzi G, Piras G, De Cosmo S, Viberti G: Podocyte number in normotensive type 1 diabetic patients with albuminuria. *Diabetes* 51:3083–3089, 2002

[29] Dalla Vestra M, Masiero A, Roiter AM, Saller A, Crepaldi G, Fioretto P: Is podocyte injury relevant in diabetic nephropathy? Studies in patients with type 2 diabetes. *Diabetes* 52:1031–1035, 2003

[30] .Nelson RG, Meyer TW, Myers BD, Bennett PH: Clinical and pathological course of renal disease in non-insulin-dependent diabetes mellitus: the Pima Indian experience. *Semin. Nephrol.* 17:124–131, 1997

[31] Meyer TW, Bennett GL, Nelson RG: Podocyte number predicts long-term urinary albumin excretion in Pima Indians with type II diabetes and microalbuminuria. *Diabetologia* 42:1341–1344, 1999

[32] White KE, Bilous RW: Structural alterations to the podocyte are related to proteinuria in type 2 diabetic patients. *Nephrol. Dial. Transplant* 19:1437–1440, 2004

[33] Nakamura T, Ushiyama C, Suzuki S, Hara M, Shimada N, Ebihara I, Koide H: Urinary excretion of podocytes in patients with diabetic nephropathy.*Nephrol. Dial. Transplant* 15:1379–1383, 2000

[34] Pavenstadt H, Kriz W, Kretzler M: Cell biology of the glomerular podocyte. *Physiol Rev.* 83:253–307, 2003

[35] Smithies O: Why the kidney glomerulus does not clog: a gel permeation/ diffusion hypothesis of renal function. *Proc .Natl. Acad. Sci .U S A* 100:410

[36] Remuzzi G, Bertani T: Pathophysiology of progressive nephropathies. *N. Engl. J. Med.* 339:1448–1456, 19988–4113, 2003

[37] Patari A, Forsblom C, Havana M, Taipale H, Groop PH, Holthofer H: Nephrinuria in diabetic nephropathy of type 1 diabetes. *Diabetes* 52: 2969–2974, 2003

[38] Koop K, Eikmans M, Baelde HJ, Kawachi H, De Heer E, Paul LC, Bruijn JA: Expression of podocyte-associated molecules in acquired humankidney diseases. *J. Am. Soc. Nephrol .*14:2063–2071, 2003

[39] Benigni A, Gagliardini E, Tomasoni S, Abbate M, Ruggenenti P, Kalluri R, Remuzzi G: Selective impairment of gene expression and assembly of nephrin in human diabetic nephropathy. *Kidney Int.* 65:2193–2200, 2004

[40] Langham RG, Kelly DJ, Cox AJ, Thomson NM, Holthofer H, Zaoui P, Pinel N, Cordonnier DJ, Gilbert RE: Proteinuria and the expression of the podocyte slit diaphragm protein, nephrin, in diabetic nephropathy: effectsof angiotensin converting enzyme inhibition. *Diabetologia* 45:1572–1576,2002

[41] Ortiz A, Ziyadeh FN, Neilson EG: Expression of apoptosis-regulatory genes in renal proximal tubular epithelial cells exposed to high ambient glucose and in diabetic kidneys. *J. Investig Med.* 45:50–56, 1997

[42] Murata I, Takemura G, Asano K, Sano H, Fujisawa K, Kagawa T, Baba K, Maruyama R, Minatoguchi S, Fujiwara T, Fujiwara H: Apoptotic cell loss following cell proliferation in renal glomeruli of Otsuka Long-Evans Tokushima Fatty rats, a model of human type 2 diabetes. *Am. J. Nephrol.* 22:587–595, 2002

[43] Kumar D, Zimpelmann J, Robertson S, Burns KD: Tubular and interstitial cell apoptosis in the streptozotocin-diabetic rat kidney. *Nephron. Exp. Nephrol.* 96:e77–e88, 2004

[44] Kumar D, Robertson S, Burns KD: Evidence of apoptosis in human diabetic kidney. *Mol. Cell Biochem* .259:67–70, 2004

[45] Vogelmann SU, Nelson WJ, Myers BD, Lemley KV: Urinary excretion of viable podocytes in health and renal disease. *Am. J. Physiol Renal. Physiol.* 285:F40–F48, 2003

[46] Kretzler M: Regulation of adhesive interaction between podocytes and glomerular basement membrane. *Microsc. Res. Tech.* 57:247–253, 2002

[47] Chen HC, Chen CA, Guh JY, Chang JM, Shin SJ, Lai YH: Altering expression of alpha3beta1 integrin on podocytes of human and rats with diabetes. *Life Sci* 67:2345–2353, 2000

[48] Regoli M, Bendayan M: Alterations in the expression of the alpha 3 beta 1 integrin in certain membrane domains of the glomerular epithelial cells (podocytes) in diabetes mellitus. *Diabetologia* 40:15–22, 1997

[49] Kitsiou PV, Tzinia AK, Stetler-Stevenson WG, Michael AF, Fan WW, Zhou B, Tsilibary EC: Glucose-induced changes in integrins and matrix-related functions in cultured human glomerular epithelial cells. *Am. J. Physiol. Renal. Physiol.* 284:F671–F679, 2003

[50] Kagami S, Border WA, Ruoslahti E, Noble NA: Coordinated expression of beta 1 integrins and transforming growth factor-beta-induced matrix proteins in glomerulonephritis. *La.b Invest.* 69:68–76, 1993

[51] Kumar NM, Sigurdson SL, Sheppard D, Lwebuga-Mukasa JS: Differential modulation of integrin receptors and extracellular matrix laminin by transforming growth factor-beta 1 in rat alveolar epithelial cells. *Exp. Cell Res.* 221:385–394, 1995

[52] Ding G, Reddy K, Kapasi AA, Franki N, Gibbons N, Kasinath BS, Singhal PC: Angiotensin II induces apoptosis in rat glomerular epithelial cells. *Am. J. Physiol. Renal. Physiol.* 283:F173–F180, 2002

[53] Yoo J, Ghiassi M, Jirmanova L, Balliet AG, Hoffman B, Fornace AJ Jr, Liebermann DA, Bottinger EP, Roberts AB: Transforming growth factorbeta-induced apoptosis is mediated by Smad-dependent expression of GADD45b through p38 activation. *J. Biol. Chem.* 278:43001–43007, 2003

[54] Schiffer M, Bitzer M, Roberts IS, Kopp JB, ten Dijke P, Mundel P, Bottinger EP: Apoptosis in podocytes induced by TGF-beta and Smad7.*J. Clin. Invest.* 108:807–816, 2001

[55] Schiffer M, Mundel P, Shaw AS, Bottinger EP: A novel role for the adaptor molecule CD2-associated protein in transforming growth factor-betainduced apoptosis. *J Biol Chem.* 279:37004–37012, 2004

[56] Mundel P, Reiser J, Zunuga-Mejia-Borja A, Pavenstadt H, Davidson G, Kritz W, et al. Rearrangements of the cytoskeleton and cell contacts induce process formation during differentiation of conditionally immortalized mouse podocyte cell lines. *Exp. Cell Res.* 1997; 236: 248-58.

[57] Jat PS, Sharp PA. Cell lines established by a temperature-sensitive simian virus 40 large-T-antigen gene are growth restricted at the nonpermissive temperature. *Mol. Cell. Biol.* 1989; 9: 1672-81.

[58] Kim NH, Rincon-Choles H, Bhandari B, Ghosh Choudhury G, Abboud HE, Gorin Y. Redox dependence of glomerular epithelial cell hypertrophy in response to glucose. Am *J. Physiol. Renal. Physiol.* 2006; 290: F741-51

[59] Susztak K, Raff AC, Schiffer M, Bottinger EP. Glucose-induced reactive oxygen species cause apoptosis of pdoocytes and podocyte depletion at the onset of diabetic nephropathy. *Diabetes* 2006; 55:225-33.

[60] Kang SW, Natarajan R, Shahed A, Nast CC, LaPage J, Mundel P, et al. Role of 12-lipoxygenase in the stimulation of p38 mitogenactivated protein kinase and collagen alpha5(IV) in experimental diabetic nephropathy and in glucose-stimulated podocytes. *J. Am. Soc. Nephrol.* 2003; 14: 3178-87.

[61] Wendt TM, Tanji N, Guo J, Kislinger TR, Qu W, Lu Y, et al.RAGE drives the development of glomerulosclerosis and indicates podocyte activation in the pathogenesis of diabetic nephropathy.*Am. J. Pathol.* 2003; 162: 1123-37

[62] Mifsud SA, Allen TJ, Bertram JF, Hulthen UL, Kelly DJ, Cooper ME, Wilkinson-Berka JL, Gilbert RE: Podocyte foot process broadening in experimental diabetic nephropathy: amelioration with renin-angiotensin blockade. *Diabetologia* 44:878–882, 2001

[63] Xu ZG, Yoo TH, Ryu DR, Cheon Park H, Ha SK, Han DS, et al. Angiotensin II receptor blocker inhibits p27Kip1 expression in glucose-stimulated podocytes and in diabetic glomeruli. Kidney Int 2005; 67: 944-52.

[64] Benigni A, Gagliardini E, Tomasoni S, Abbate M, Ruggenenti P, Kalluri R, et al. Selective impairment of gene expression and assembly of nephrin in human diabetic nephropathy. Kidney Int 2004; 65: 2193-200.

[65] Chen S, Lee JS, Iglesias-de la, Cruz MC, Wang A, Izquierdo-Lahuerta, et al. Angiotensin II stimulates alpha3(IV) collagen production in mouse podocytes via TGF-beta and VEGF signalling: implications for diabetic nephropathy. *Nephrol. Dial. Transplant.* 2005; 20: 1320-8.

[66] Jia J, Ding G, Zhu J, Chen C, Liang W, Franki N, Singhal PC. Angiotensin II Infusion Induces Nephrin Expression Changes and Podocyte Apoptosis. *Am. J. Nephrol.* 28:500-507, 2008

[67] Ziyadeh FN: Mediators of diabetic renal disease: the case for TGF-_ as the major mediator. *J Am Soc Nephrol* 15 (Suppl. 1):S55–S57, 2004

[68] Hong SW, Isono M, Chen S, Iglesias-de la Cruz MC, Han DC, Ziyadeh FN: Increased glomerular and tubular expression of TGF-beta1, its type II receptor, and activation of the Smad signaling pathway in the db/dbmouse. *Am. J. Pathol.* 158:1653–1663, 2001

[69] 69. Ziyadeh FN, Hoffman BB, Han DC, Iglesias-de la Cruz MC, Hong SW, Isono M, Chen S, McGowan TA, Sharma K: Long-term prevention of renal insufficiency, excess matrix gene expression, and glomerular mesangial matrix expansion by treatment with

monoclonal antitransforming growth factor-_ antibody in db/db diabetic mice. *Proc Natl. Acad. Sci. U S A* 97:8015– 8020, 2000

[70] Kopp JB, Factor VM, Mozes M, Nagy P, Sanderson N, Bottinger EP, Klotman PE, Thorgeirsson SS: Transgenic mice with increased plasma levels of TGF-beta 1 develop progressive renal disease. *Lab Invest.* 74:991–1003, 1996

[71] Sharma R, Khanna A, Sharma M, Savin VJ: Transforming growth factorbeta1 increases albumin permeability of isolated rat glomeruli via hydroxyl radicals. *Kidney Int.* 58:131–136, 2000

[72] Sung SH, Chen S, Laping NJ, Ziyadeh FN: Albuminuria is ameliorated by an inhibitor of VEGF receptors, SU5416, in diabetic db/db mice but is unaffected in Smad3-knockout mice rendered diabetic with streptozotocin(Abstract). *J. Am. Soc. Nephrol.* 15:720A–721A, 2004

[73] Fujimoto M, Maezawa Y, Yokote K, Joh K, Kobayashi K, Kawamura H, Nishimura M, Roberts AB, Saito Y, Mori S: Mice lacking Smad3 are protected against streptozotocin-induced diabetic glomerulopathy. *Biochem Biophys. Res Commun* 305:1002–1007, 2003

[74] Neufeld G, Cohen T, Gengrinovitch S, Potorak Z: Vascular endothelial growth factor and its receptors. *FASEB J* 13:9 –22, 1999

[75] De Vriese AS, Tilton RG, Elger M, Stephan CC, Kriz W, Lameire NH: Antibodies against vascular endothelial growth factor improve early renal dysfunction in experimental diabetes. *J. Am. Soc. Nephrol .*12:993–1000, 2001

[76] Flyvbjerg A, Dagnaes-Hansen F, De Vriese AS, Schrijvers BF, Tilton RG, Rasch R: Amelioration of long-term renal changes in obese type 2 diabetic mice by a neutralizing vascular endothelial growth factor antibody.*Diabetes* 51:3090 –3094, 2002

[77] Schrijvers BF, Flyvbjerg A, De Vriese AS: The role of vascular endothelial growth factor (VEGF) in renal pathophysiology. *Kidney Int* 65:2003–2017, 2004

[78] Chen S, Kasama Y, Lee JS, Jim B, Marin M, Ziyadeh FN. Podocyte-derived vascular endothelial growth factor mediates the stimulation of alpha3 (IV) collage production by transforming growth factor-beta1 in mouse podocytes. *Diabetes* 2004; 53: 2939-49.

[79] Dessapt C, Hargreaves R, Dei Cas A, Marshall J, Hayward A, Viberti G, *et al.* Modulation of alpha3-beta1 integrin expression and cell adhesion in glomeurlar podocytes by glucose and mechanical stretch. *Diabetic Med.* 2004; 21(suppl 2): 10-11.

[80] Lewko B, Bryl E, Witkowski JM, Latawiec E, Angielski S, Stepinski J. Mechanical stress and glucose concentration modulate glucose transport in cultured rat podocytes. *Nephrol. Dial. Transplant.* 2005; 20: 306-11.

[81] Petermann AT, Hiromura K, Bionski M, Pippin J, Monkawa T, Durvasula R, *et al.* Mechanical stress reduces podocyte proliferation *in vitro*. Kidney Int 2002; 61: 40-50.

[82] Petermann AT, Pippin J, Durvasula R, Pichler R, Hiromura K, Monkawa T, *et al.* Mechanical stretch induces podocyte hypertrophy *in vitro*. *Kidney Int.* 2005; 67: 157-66.

[83] Menini S, Amadio L, Oddi G, Ricci C, Pesce C, Pugliese F, Giorgio M, Migliaccio E, Pelicci P, Iacobini C, Pugliese G. Deletion of p66Shc longevity gene protects against experimental diabetic glomerulopathy by preventing diabetes-induced oxidative stress. *Diabetes* 55:1642-1650, 2006.

[84] Camici GG, Schiavoni M, Francia P, Bachschmid M, Martin-Padura I, Hersberger M, Tanner FC, Pelicci P, Volpe M, Anversa P, Luscher TF, Cosentino F. Genetic deletion

of p66(Shc) adaptor protein prevents hyperglycemia-induced endothelial dysfunction and oxidative stress. *Proc. Natl. Acad. Sci. USA* 104:5217-5222, 2007.

[85] Napoli C, Martin-Padura I, de Nigris F, Giorgio M, Mansueto G, Somma P, Condorelli M, Sica G, De Rosa G, Pelicci P. Deletion of the p66Shc longevity gene reduces systemic and tissue oxidative stress, vascular cell apoptosis, and early atherogenesis in mice fed a high-fat diet. *Proc Natl Acad Sci USA* 100: 2112–2116, 2003

[86] Francia P, delli Gatti C, Bachschmid M, Martin-Padura I, Savoia C, Migliaccio E, Pelicci PG, Schiavoni M, Lüscher TF, Volpe M, Cosentino F. Deletion of p66shc gene protects against age-related endothelial dysfunction Circulation. 110:2889-95, 2004

[87] 87.Nemoto S, Finkel T. Redox regulation of forkhead proteins through a p66shc-dependent signaling pathway. *Science* 295:2450-452, 2002.

[88] Hu Y, Wang X, Zeng L, Cai DY, Sabapathy K, Goff SP, Firpo EJ, Li B. ERK phosphorylates p66shcA on Ser36 and subsequently regulates p27kip1 expression via the Akt-FOXO3a pathway: implication of p27kip1 in cell response to oxidative stress. *Mol. Biol. Cell* 16:3705-3718, 2005.

[89] Salih DA, Brunet A. 2008. FoxO transcription factors in the maintenance of cellular homeostasis during aging. *Curr. Opin. Cell Biol.* 20:126-36, 2008.

[90] Burgering BMT and Kops GJP. Cell cycle and death control: long live Forkheads. *Trends Biochem. Sci.* 27:352-360, 2002

Chapter XIII

Role of Translational Dysregulation in Diabetic Nephropathy

Denis Feliers and B.S. Kasinath
Department of Medicine, University of Texas Health Science Center, South Texas Veterans Health Care System, San Antonio, Texas 78229, US

Introduction

Gene expression includes transcription of genes into a pre-mRNAs, maturation of pre-mRNAs into mature mRNAs, and translation of mRNAs into proteins. All these steps are complex processes, that are highly orchestrated and regulated.

Contrary to transcriptional regulation, translational control of pre-existing mRNAs allows for rapid up-regulation of the encoded proteins in response to transitory signals. Once believed to be coupled to transcriptional regulation, translation control of gene expression is being increasingly recognized as an independent and important phenomenon.

Mechanisms of mRNA Translation

Overview

The process of mRNA translation can be divided into 3 phases: initiation, elongation, and termination. The initiation stage consists of binding of the small (40S) ribosomal subunit loaded with Met-tRNAi in a preinitiation complex (PIC) to the 5' untranslated region (UTR). This complex scans the 5' UTR until it reaches the AUG start codon. When the start codon (AUG) is identified by the PIC and bound by the methionyl tRNA (Met-tRNAi), the process of elongation starts. This process can be divided into three distinct and consecutive steps: codon-directed binding of aminoacyl tRNA, translocation and peptide bond formation. At the P site, a peptide bond is created between the previous amino acid and the one that has arrived newly and releases tRNA from the previous amino acid. The released tRNA can then be reused to deliver the specific amino acid as dictated by the codon sequence on the mRNA.

The termination phase begins with the arrival of the 80S ribosome at the termination codon of the mRNA. The release of the nascent chain is mediated by the ribosomal release factor, which has structural similarities with the tRNA. After this, the 80S ribosome is split into the 60S and the 40S subunits with the assistance of initiation factors eIF6, and is recycled for another round of peptide synthesis.

Initiation of mRNA Translation

The most regulated stage of mRNA translation is the initiation stage. It requires numerous factors (initiation factors) arranged in macromolecular complexes that interact physically and functionally with exquisite precision.

Formation of the Pre-Initiation Complex and Binding to mRNA

The PIC is formed in the absence of mRNA, by association of Met-tRNAi and eIF2 in its GTP-bound form (eIF2-GTP). The binding of this complex to the 40S ribosomal subunit requires eIF3, a factor which binds to the 18S RNA [1] and several ribosomal proteins [2,3], close to the attachment site for eIF2, the mRNA and the 60S subunit [4]. eIF3 plays an important role either in the formation or the stability of the 43S PIC. In addition to eIF3, eIF1 plays a role in the 43S PIC formation [5,6], apparently by stabilizing the 40S pre-initiation complex intermediates [7]. The 43S PIC is an extremely large and complex structure; it is estimated that about 700 kDa of non-ribosomal proteins are complexed to the 40S subunit [7].

The mRNA can now bind the PIC, and this is the step that is the most regulated event in the intiation of mRNA translation. It is important to understand that the mRNA is already associated with other initiation factors, including eIF4F, when it binds the PIC. There are 3 highly regulated mechanisms of binding of these initiation factors to the mRNA - cap-dependent initiation, internal ribosome entry system (IRES)-driven initiation, and upstream Open Reading Frame (uORFs)-driven initiation that will be discussed below. eIF4F is a multimeric protein complex composed of eIF4E, a protein the binds the cap structure at the 5' terminus of the mRNA, eIF4A, a DEAD box containing protein and eIF4G, a large scaffolding protein. In addition to binding to eIF4E and 4A, eIF4G also contains binding sites for eIF3, and their association could bridge the mRNA and the PIC and stabilize the complex [8]. In addition, eIF4G can bind the poly(A)-binding protein 1 (PA-BP1), which binds the poly(A) tail at the extreme end of the 3' UTR [9]. This association allows circularization of the mRNA in a closed loop configuration, which is believed to increase the efficiency of mRNA translation [10].

Scanning and Selection of Start Codon

Most mRNAs have a highly complex 5' UTR with many secondary structures that hinder scanning of the 43S PIC to the AUG start codon. These structures are resolved by eIF4A, which is part of the eIF4F complex and possesses an ATP-dependent helicase activity [11]. eIF4B, which also binds to eIF3 [12] and PA-BP1 [13], is a cofactor of eIF4A in the unwinding of the 5' UTR [14]. The 43S PIC scans the 5' UTR of the mRNA until reaches the AUG start codon. Formation of a 43S complex positioned at the AUG start codon is dependent on eIF1, eIF1A, eIF4A and eIF4B, in addition to eIF2, eIF3 and eIF4F [15]. At that point, the scanning stops and the 60S ribosomal subunit joins the 43S PIC. This step is facilitated by eIF5 which, through binding to eIF2β [16] and eIF3 [17], associates with the 43S PIC positioned at the start codon and stimulates GTP hydrolysis by eIF2, acting as a GTPase-activating protein (GAP), prior to ejection of all eIFs and joining of the 60S subunit [18,19]. A tight coupling between the GAP activity of eIF5 and base pairing between Met-tRNAi and the start codon is essential for the accuracy of translation initiation [20].

Peptide Chain Elongation

The Met-tRNAi is bound to a ribosomal site called the P site (donor site), and the next codon to be translated, the first internal codon, is in an open ribosomal position adjacent to the P site, referred to as the A site (acceptor site). The tRNA corresponding to this codon binds to that site, a reaction that requires eEF1A-GTP [7]. When the two ribosomal sites are filled, a peptide bond is formed between the methionine residue and the incoming amino-acid. Peptide bond formation results in the synthesis of a dipeptide attached to the tRNA at the A site, and the P site is left with a deacylated tRNA. This reaction is mediated mostly by the 60S subunit of the ribosome and does not require any additional factor. It seems that appropriate binding and alignment of the peptidyl-tRNA at the P site and of the aminoacyl-tRNA at the A site is sufficient to allow the reaction components to bind in the appropriate stereochemical configuration to allow for the spontaneous synthesis of the peptide bond [7].

In order to be translated, the next codon must move to the A site. This movement, referred to as translocation, requires eEF2 which catalyzes the movement of the ribosome and the mRNA in opposite direction, by the equivalent of three bases (one codon) [21] During translocation, the aminoacyl-tRNA moves from the A to the P site, the next codon is positioned at the A site, and the deacylated tRNA is released. In this manner, aminoacids from the aminoacyl-tRNA pool are added one at a time to the nascent peptidyl chain, and synthesis occurs from the aminoterminal residue to the carboxyterminal residue.

Termination and Ribosome Subunit Dissociation

When all the codons of the open reading frame have been translated, the translation of the last peptide results in a polypeptide chain attached to a tRNA at the A site through its C-terminal aminoacid residue. Translocation then shifts the polypeptidyl-tRNA to the P site and brings to the A site the termination codon (UAA, UAG, UGA), for which there are no tRNAs with complementary anticodons. A release factor (RF4) then binds the A site, and catalyzes the termination reaction, along with the termination factor RF3 [22]. This reaction involves hydrolysis of the peptidyl-tRNA ester bond, and release of the completed polypeptide chain, the deacylated tRNA and the ribosome from the mRNA. After this, the 40S and 60S ribosomal subunits are dissociated, a process facilitated by eIF6 [23]. The precise mechanism of this process is still poorly understood.

Regulation of mRNA Translation: Initiation Stage

Cap-Dependent Translation Initiation

The principal mechanism to control the rate of translation initiation involves the mRNA 5'-cap recognition process by the eIF4F complex, composed of eIF4E, eIF4G and eIF4A. Binding of eIF4F to the cap structure is mediated by eIF4E. In order to prevent premature translation of mRNAs, cells have developed strategies to prevent untimely binding of eIF4E to the cap structure.

a) eIF4E-binding proteins (4E-BPs): The 4E-BPs compete with eIF4G for a shared binding site on eIF4E [24]. Binding of 4E-BPs to eIF4E is controlled by phosphorylation: hypophosphorylated 4E-BPs bind strongly to eIF4E, whereas phosphorylation of 4E-BPs on various serine and threonine residues weakens their interaction with eIF4E [25]. Several kinases target 4E-BPs [25], but the most critical seems to be mammalian target of rapamycin (mTOR), which is activated by the PI3K/Akt signaling pathway, but also senses and integrates signals from extracellular stimuli, amino acid availability, and oxygen and energy status of the cells. mTOR is also directly or indirectly responsible for the phosphorylation of several substrates, which are relevant to translation, including eIF4G, p70S6K [26], and eukaryotic elongation factor-2 kinase (eEF2K). S6Ks also phosphorylate Pdcd4, which is a tumor suppressor that binds and suppresses eIF4A activity [27]. Phosphorylation of Pdcd4 leads to its ubiquitination and degradation by the proteasome [28]. Another major cellular signaling pathway that strongly impacts translation is the Ras-MAPK pathway. It is responsible for the phosphorylation of eIF4E and eIF4B. eIF4B phosphorylation occurs at Ser422, the site which is phosphorylated by p70S6K [26].

IRES-Driven mRNA Translation

Contrary to cellular mRNAs, viral mRNAs bypass the conventional scanning mechanism and at least a subset of initiation factors by using internal ribosome entry sites (IRESs) to recruit the 40S subunit more directly to the initiation region. IRESs are ~450 nucleotide-long, highly structured elements, originally found in the 5'UTR of poliovirus mRNAs [29,30], that are stimulated by noncanonical IRES trans-activating factors (ITAFs), including the polypyrimidine tract binding protein (PTB), ITAF45, or the La autoantigen, most likely to stabilize their active conformations [31]. The poliovirus IRES recruits directly several initiation factors and the 40S ribosomal subunit to an internal viral translation initiation codon. Therefore, the translation of poliovirus mRNA does not require eIF4E [32], but requires the carboxy-terminal fragment of eIF4G that is generated by the proteolytic cleavage of eIF4G by a virus-encoded protease. Because cap-dependent translation requires full-length eIF4G, cleavage of eIF4G inhibits translation of cellular mRNAs, to the benefit of viral mRNA translation [33]. It is now known that different viruses possess different classes of IRESs. For example, binding of 40S ribosomal subunit to the HCV IRES does not require initiation factors, although they do participate in the process of translation initiation [33]. The IRES found in cricket paralysis virus (CrPV) recruits both the 40S and 60S ribosomal subunits and also acts as a mimic of Met-tRNAi to permit initiation of the translation of viral capsid proteins in the absence of Met-tRNAi. The IRESs of hepatitis C virus (HCV) bind directly to the 40S subunit, in the absence of eIF4F, but require eIF3 and either eIF2/eIF5 or eIF5B to form a 43S PIC competent for subunit joining [34,35]. The ability to use eIF5B instead of eIF2 for tRNAi recruitment may allow initiation to proceed in virus-infected cells when eIF2 is inactivated by phosphorylation.

It is now clear that a subset of cellular mRNAs also contain IRESs. Cellular IRESs seem to be present in mRNAs whose expression is activated by stress, when cap-dependent translation may be inefficient [36]. Many IRES-containing host mRNAs encode proteins that protect cells from stress, such as c-myc, X chromosome-linked inhibitor of apoptosis protein (XIAP), inhibitor of apoptosis protein 2 (HIAP2/c-IAP1), Hsp70, Bcl-2, Survivin and VEGF, whereas the proteins encoded by other IRES-containing cellular mRNAs seem to be important during apoptosis, such as death-associated protein 5 (DAP5), Reaper, protein kinase Cδ, and the apoptotic protease activating factor 1 (Apaf-1) [37].

Other mechanisms (uORFs)

Several mRNAs contain upstream Open Reading Frame (uORFs) that repress their translation. The mechanisms of translation repression vary with different uORFs. One mechanism involves a "roadblock" to scanning PICs produced by an 80S ribosome that stalls while translating the uORF in a manner dictated by the amino acid sequence of the attenuator peptide encoded by the uORF [31]. In another case, the uORF-encoded peptidyl-tRNA interacts with release factor eRF1 to block polypeptide hydrolysis and stall the ribosome at the stop codon [38]. These uORF-containing mRNAs are not translated under normal conditions, but become translated under stress conditions. Their translation requires the phosphorylation of eIF2α on Ser51, which converts eIF2-GDP into a competitive inhibitor of eIF2B, the eIF2-GEF (guanine nucleotide exchange factor), eIF2B, and inhibits the ternary complex assembly. Phosphorylation of eIF2 reduces global translation, allowing cells to conserve resources and to initiate a reconfiguration of gene expression to effectively manage stress conditions. Phosphorylated eIF2α induces translation of specific mRNAs, such as that encoding the bZIP (basic leucine zipper) transcriptional regulator ATF4 (activating transcription factor 4), and GCN4, all of which contain uORFs. Phosphorylated eIF2α can overcome the inhibitory effects of the uORFs by a complex mechanism. In the case of GCN4 mRNA which contains 4 uORFs, after translation of the 5'-most uORF (uORF1), post-termination 40S subunits can resume scanning and reinitiate downstream at uORFs 2, 3, or 4 after rebinding the ternary complex. But the scanning is blocked after termination at these uORFs. Reduction of ternary complex formation following eIF2α phosphorylation leads a fraction of post-termination 40S subunits to rebind the ternary complex only after bypassing uORFs 2–4 and reinitiate at the GCN4 start codon, leading to GCN4 mRNA translation [39]. In turn, transcription factors like ATF4 also enhances the expression of additional transcription factors, ATF3 and CHOP (CCAAT/enhancer-binding protein homologous protein)/GADD153 (growth arrest and DNA-damage-inducible protein), that assist in the regulation of genes involved in metabolism, the redox status of the cells and apoptosis [40].

Elongation Stage

The recruitment of aminoacyl tRNA to the A (aminoacyl) site on the 80S ribosomal complex is facilitated by eEF1A.GTP [41]. Whether the GTP loading of eEF1A is regulated is not known, but it seems that eEF1A is constitutively active; therefore its regulation occurs through modulation of its protein expression. The next step, translocation of the peptidyl-tRNA from the A to the P site, is helped by eEF2 [21]. Under unstimulated conditions, the activity of eEF2 is inhibited by phosphorylation on Thr56 by eEF2K [42], a calcium/calmodulin-dependent kinase, and actively dephosphorylated by PP2A [43]. Activation of PP2A is extremely complex; PP2A is a heterotrimeric serine/threonine phosphatase, consisting of a dimeric core enzyme containing the structural A and catalytic C subunits, and a regulatory B subunit. When the catalytic C subunit associates with the A and B subunits, several species of holoenzymes are produced with distinct functions and characteristics. The A subunit is the scaffold required for the formation of the heterotrimeric complex. When the A subunit binds it alters the enzymatic activity of the catalytic C subunit, even if the B subunit is absent (see [44] for a review). The regulation of eEF2 inactivation by eEF2K is better understood: eEF2K is itself inactivated by phosphorylation by p70S6K [45] and other kinases [46,47]. Because p70S6K is a directly activated by phosphorylation by mTOR, activation of the latter can stimulate both the intiation and the elongation phases of mRNA translation through inactivation of 4E-BP1 and activation of eEF2, respectively.

Regulation by miRNAs

Biogenesis of miRNAs

Transcription of miRNAs is typically performed by RNA polymerase II, and transcripts are capped and polyadenylated [48]. Most miRNAs are produced from transcription units that contain more than one miRNA [49]. The primary transcript (pri-miRNA) consists of an imperfectly paired stem of ~33 bp, with a terminal loop and flanking segments [49]. The pri-miRNA is then processed to yield the mature miRNA. The first processing step, which occurs in the nucleus and excises the loop from the remainder of the transcript to create a pre-miRNA is carried out by Drosha [48]. Drosha catalyzes pri-miRNA processing [50] with a protein called DGCR8 which stably associates with the ribonuclease to form the Microprocessor complex. The pre-miRNA is exported from the nucleus to the cytoplasm, where it forms a miRNA/miRNA duplex. The second processing step, which excises the terminal loop from the pre-miRNA stem to create a mature miRNA duplex of approximately 22 bp in length [49], is carried out by Dicer [48], in complex with Ago2 and TRBP [51]. The mammalian Dicer/Ago/miRNA complex is associated with other proteins, such as Gemin3, Gemin4, Mov10, and Imp8 [49,52,53], as well as GW182 [52,54,55]. GW182 is both necessary and sufficient for miRNA-bound Ago to silence gene expression [54,56,57]. Thus, miRNA-bound Ago in association with GW182 can be thought of as the "miRISC complex".

Regulation of miRNA biogenesis has become the subject of extensive studies. The synthesis of many miRNAs is under the control of the targets that they regulate. For example, in Drosophila, miR-7 represses the translation of a transcription factor called Yan, which itself represses the transcription of the miR-7 gene [58], in a mutual negative feedback mechanism. A rationale for these mutual negative feedbacks lays in the fact that tight regulation of miRNA biogenesis is crucial. Misexpression of miRNAs frequently mimics loss-of-function phenotypes for their targets. This would be prevented if biogenesis of a miRNA is strictly controlled by its targets. The restriction would also explain how off-targeting effects by wayward miRNAs are carefully limited.

miRNAs Repress mRNA Translation

With few exceptions, miRNA-binding sites in animal mRNAs lie in the 3' UTR and are usually present in multiple copies. Most animal miRNAs bind with mismatches and bulges, with the exception of the "seed region" at nucleotide 28, which involves Watson-Crick base pairing of miRNA and mRNA. The degree of miRNA-mRNA complementarity seems to be a key determinant of the regulatory mechanism: perfect complementarity allows Ago-catalyzed cleavage of the mRNA strand, whereas central mismatches exclude cleavage and promote repression of mRNA translation. Some studies have found evidence that miRISC represses the initiation phase of mRNA translation [59-63]. Other studies have found evidence for repression of post-initiation processes [64-67].

Regardless of the stage at which repression occurs, there are several possible mechanisms of miRISC-mediated repression. 1) miRISC could promote premature ribosome dissociation from mRNAs [67]. 2) miRISC could stimulate deadenylation of the mRNA tail and cause PA-BP1 to dissociate from the tail and prevent mRNA circularization; in this model, deadenylation is promoted by GW182, which triggers deadenylation and translation repression in Drosophila cells [68]. 3) miRISC could block association of the 60S ribosomal subunit with the 40S preinitiation complex, through physical associates between Ago2 and eIF6 [69]. It is important to remember that in most cases, translational repression is not accompanied by mRNA destabilization, so that repression of translation by miRNA is only transitory and that mRNA translation can resume when miRNAs, whose half-life is very short, are degraded.

mRNA Translation in Diabetic Kidney Disease

Cardinal aspects of diabetic nephropathy include hypertrophy evident in early stages and matrix accumulation and renal fibrosis that occur with longer duration of disease. Both these events require upregulation of structural proteins and extracellular matrix proteins, which is achieved by a combination of increased synthesis and decreased degradation. Kidney injury in diabetes is mediated by several growth factors which are themselves upregulated, e.g., angiotensin II (Ang II), TGFβ, VEGF, connective tissue growth factor. Until recently, increased protein synthesis was thought to be due only to increased transcription of their genes. Recent investigations from many laboratories including ours have revealed an important role for mRNA translation as an independent or coordinated site of regulation of protein synthesis. There is an additional reason for translation to be a target of regulation in diabetes.

Hypertrophy in Diabetic Nephropathy

Cellular hypertrophy is defined by cellular enlargement, accompanied with increased protein and RNA content without change in DNA content. Kidney growth in diabetes is mostly due to hypertrophy, after a brief period of hyperplasia, mostly involving mesangial cells [70-72]. Renal hypertrophy is observed in other conditions, such as unilateral nephrectomy, and following high protein diet consumption or steroid administration; however, progressive renal disease is not seen with these conditions. Association of renal hypertrophy with progressive renal injury in diabetes could be due to increased oxidative stress [73]. Renal hypertrophy is the earliest structural abnormality in diabetes and coincides with increased glomerular filtration rate. In addition to Ang II and TGFβ, insulin like growth factor (IGF-I), hepatocyte growth factor and epidermal growth factor, could also play a role in diabetes-induced renal hypertrophy [73]. Upregulation of IGF-I in renal cortex coincides with renal hypertrophy in rodents with type 1 or type 2 diabetes, suggesting that IGF-I could play a role in the stimulation of protein synthesis. In renal proximal tubular epithelial cells in culture, IGF-I stimulation of protein synthesis was mediated by the PI3K-Akt-mammalian target of rapamycin (mTOR) signaling pathway that culminated in 4E-BP1 hyperphosphorylation and inactivation [74].

Cell Cycle in Diabetic Renal Hypertrophy

Cell cycle is a very complex process that requires passage through "gap" or G phases before initiation of DNA synthesis (S phase) and separation of the two sister cells (M phase). The G1 phase precedes the S phase, and during this phase, the cell increases the synthesis of its structural protein and increases in size until it reaches a size that allows formation of the two daughter cells [75]. Passage through G1 phase is coordinated by cyclin-dependent kinases (Cdks) that are themselves regulated by cyclin-dependent kinase inhibitors (CKIs) (for a review, see [76]). Feliers et al. have shown that overexpression of the retinoblastoma protein in mesangial cells, which blocks the cells in late G1 phase, induces a cellular hypertrophy similar to that induced by high glucose, and that high glucose-induced hypertrophy was due to activation of Cdk4, but not of Cdk2, which is required for passage into S phase [77]. Other studies have shown that p27Kip1, a CKI that prevents passage of cells into S phase, is upregulated in hypertrophic, diabetic kidneys and that in mice deficient in p27kip1 renal hypertrophy is inhibited following 6–12 weeks of diabetes induced by streptozotocin [78,79], confirming that blockade of renal cells in late G1 phase is required for renal hypertrophy.

AMP Activated Protein Kinase in Diabetic Renal Hypertrophy

Since mRNA translation is a rate-limiting step in protein synthesis and increased protein synthesis is essential for cellular hypertrophy, we have studied the regulation of mRNA translation in models relevant to diabetic nephropathy. High glucose-induced hypertrophy of glomerular epithelial cells in vitro was accompanied by inactivating phosphorylation of 4E-BP1 on Thr37/46 and activating dephosphorylation of eEF2 on Thr56, indicating that both the initiation phase and elongation phases of mRNA translation were stimulated during cell hypertrophy [80]. Because mRNA translation consumes large amounts of energy, in the form of ATP, we studied the role of AMP-activated protein kinase (AMPK) in high glucose induced glomerular epithelial cell hypertrophy. AMPK is a heterotrimeric protein comnposed of α, β and γ subunits, which is activated by binding of AMP and inhibited by binding of ATP to the γ subunit. Full activation requires additional phosphorylation of Thr172 of the α subunit [81]. AMPK activity is stimulated in energy-deficient states resulting in stimulation of energy-generating reactions and inhibition of energy-consuming reactions [82]. Incubation of glomerular epithelial cells with high glucose reduced phosphorylation of AMPKα on Thr172 and decreased its kinase activity [80]. Pharmacological stimulation of AMPK with metformin or AICAR attenuated protein synthesis induced by high glucose. In rats with streptozotocin-induced type 1 diabetes, renal hypertrophy was associated with activation of the Akt-mTOR-p70S6K pathway and inactivation of 4E-BP1 in renal cortical homogenates. Administration of metformin and AICAR to diabetic rats attenuated renal hypertrophy without reducing the plasma glucose levels [80]. Stimulation of AMPK with metformin and AICAR reversed high glucose-induced inactivation of 4E-BP1 and activation of eEF2, both in vivo and in vitro, suggesting that AMPK regulated both the initiation and elongation phases of mRNA translation. The cross-talk between AMPK and the Akt-mTOR pathway was studied in glomerular epithelial cells. High glucose activated phosphatidylinositol-3 kinase (PI3K) and increased generation of phosphatidylinositol-3,4,5-trisphosphate (PtdInsP3). This led to activation of the Akt-mTOR pathway, resulting in phosphorylation of 4E-BP1 and p70S6K. Stimulation of AMPK by metformin and AICAR reduced mTOR activation by diabetes and high glucose without affecting Akt activation, suggesting that AMPK acts between Akt and mTOR in the renal cells [80]. How does AMPK inhibit mTOR activation? mTOR is activated by a small G protein called Rheb, in its GTP-bound state [83], and the GTP loading of Rheb is under the control of hamartin/tuberin complex (TSC1/TSC2), which functions as a GTPase activating protein for Rheb [84]. This TSC1/TSC2 complex is inactivated through phosphorylation of TSC2 on Thr1462 by Akt [85] and activated by phosphorylation of Thr1227 and Thr1345 by AMPK [83]. Therefore, AMPK prevents mTOR activation by deactivating Rheb, through TSC2-dependent hydrolysis of bound GTP. Studies in non-renal cells have shown that Akt inhibits AMPK signaling [86]. In renal cells, inhibition of AMPK by Akt relieves the inhibition of mTOR activity, and stimulates the initiation and elongation phases of translation by phosphorylation of 4E-BP1 and p70S6K, respectively [80]. It is important to note that mTOR-mediated phosphorylation and inactivation of 4E-BP1 is also important for compensatory kidney hypertrophy induced by uninephrectomy [87].

Another compound has raised considerable interest in the past few years is resveratrol, a phytophenol present in grapes, which possesses cancer chemopreventive, cardioprotective, and neuroprotective activities [88]. Lee et al. have shown that reseveratrol activated AMPK and inhibited high glucose-induced protein synthesis in the glomerular epithelial cells and renal hypertrophy in mice with streptozotocin-induced type 1 diabetes [89]. AMPK activation is dependent on phosphorylation of the α subunit on Thr172 by LKB1 [90]. In glomerular epithelial cells, high glucose inhibited LKB1 activity and reduced AMPKα phosphorylation on Thr172; LKB1 inhibition was associated with its acetylation. Resveratrol restored LKB1 activity and reversed its acetylation. Resveratrol is known to activate the deacetylase Sirt1 [91]; however, Sirt1 did not appear to be involved in resveratrol-induced deacetylation of LKB1 in glomerular epithelial cells [89]. Activation of AMPK by resveratrol resulted in reversal of high glucose-induced eEF2 activation, and in inhibition of protein synthesis [89], suggesting that inhibition of protein synthesis by resveratrol involved regulation of the elongation phase of mRNA translation mediated by AMPK. In vivo, administration of resveratrol to mice with streptozotocin-induced type 1 diabetes inhibited renal hypertrophy significantly, without affecting hyperglycemia; this effect was associated with restoration of AMPK activity in diabetic renal cortex [89]. Resveratrol is a promising tool to promote weight control and improve insulin sensitivity in obesity [92,93]. Further work is needed to explore if it can ameliorate long-term kidney injury in diabetes.

Adiponectin, a cytokine synthetised in the adipose tissue, also acts through AMPK. Interestingly, reduction in plasma levels of adiponectin correlates with insulin resistance [94]. Sharma et al. have recently reported that adiponectin knockout mice display podocyte injury and albuminuria, associated with disordered distribution of the tight junction protein ZO-1 in the podocyte membrane [95]. This was associated with reduction in AMPK activation and increase in oxidative stress. Pharmacologic activation of AMPK or administration of adiponectin reduced oxidative stress, ameliorated podocyte injury and albuminuria in the adiponectin-deficient mice with or without diabetes [95]. These studies show that AMPK activation by adiponectin is important for the maintenance of the podocyte structure and the selective permeability function of the glomerular capillary wall.

PI3K and PTEN

High glucose activates PI3K in glomerular epithelial cells, and pharmacological inhibition of PI3K abolished high glucose-induced inactivation of 4E-BP1 and protein synthesis [80]. Phosphatase and tensin homolog (PTEN), is an ubiquitously expressed protein and lipid phosphatase that dephosphorylates PtdInsP3 and counteracts the effect of PI3K [96]. PTEN is down-regulated in the hypertrophic renal cortex in streptozotocin-induced diabetes, and in mesangial cell in culture, high glucose or TGFβ reduce PTEN expression and activity. PTEN inhibition is accompanied by mesangial cell hypertrophy, which is prevented by restoration of the PTEN gene expression [97]. These data show that the balance between PI3K and PTEN regulates diabetes-induced renal hypertrophy.

Angiotensin II in Diabetic Nephropathy

The importance of the renin-angiotensin-aldosterone system in the pathogenesis of diabetic nephropathy has been established [98,99], and antagonists of these proteins ameliorate clinical manifestations of diabetic nephropathy [100]. In addition to its direct actions on the hemodynamics of the kidney and on renal cells, Ang II has been shown to upregulate other mediators of kidney injury, such as TGFβ and connective tissue growth factor [101]. Increased expression of VEGF in kidneys from mice with both type 1 and type 2 diabetes [74] is relevant to diabetic nephropathy since clinical indices of kidney injury in diabetic rodents are improved by neutralizing antibodies against VEGF [102,103]. Feliers et al. have examined if VEGF synthesis is also under the control of Ang II in the diabetic kidney. Physiologic concentrations of Ang II (1 nM) rapidly increased synthesis and secretion of VEGF by proximal tubular epithelial cells, starting at 5 min and lasting for up to 1 h, through a non-transcriptional mechanism [104]. Analysis of the polysomal distribution of VEGF mRNA showed that Ang II increased the amount of ribosomes associated with VEGF mRNA, providing direct evidence of increase in efficiency of initiation phase of translation. This was associated with rapid inactivating inactivation of 4E-BP1 (Thr37/46 hyperphosphorylation), which required activation of the PI3K-Akt signaling pathway. Experiments performed in cells stably overexpressing a inactivation-resistant mutant of 4E-BP1 showed that inactivation of 4E-BP1 was indispensable for this process [104]. The rapid induction of VEGF mRNA translation by Ang II was found to be dependent on generation of reactive oxygen species by an NAD(P)H oxidase but not by the mitochondria [105].

Feliers et al. explored whether events occurring at the 3' UTR also played role in Ang II induction of VEGF mRNA translation, and focused on the role of heterogeneous nuclear ribonucleoprotein K (hnRNP K), which is known to bind the 3' UTR of mRNA and generally repress mRNA translation [106]. Surprsingly, stimulation of VEGF mRNA translation by Ang II was accompanied with binding of hnRNP K to VEGF mRNA [107]. Down-regulation hnRNP K by RNA interference reduced but did not prevent Ang II-stimualted VEGF mRNA translation, suggesting that hnRNP K contributes but is not essential to this process. Ang II stimulated phosphorylation of hnRNP K on tyrosine and serine residues; however, only the serine phosphorylation correlated temporally with increased binding to VEGF mRNA [107]. Src, a nonreceptor tyrosine kinase, was activated by Ang II and was required for hnRNP K phosphorylation on both tyrosine and serine residues, indicating that Src activated another, serine/threonine kinase, responsible for hnRNP K serine phosphorylation. In a subsequent study, these investigators identified the kinase as PKCδ. These studies have revealed that events occurring at both the 5' and 3' UTRs of the mRNA play regulatory role in VEGF mRNA translation induced by Ang II.

Extracellular Matrix Accumulation in Diabetic Nephropathy

Prolonged and uncontrolled diabetes leads to gradual accumulation of proteins in glomerular (glomerulosclerosis) and tubulointerstitial extracellular matrices (tubulointerstitial fibrosis) [108]. Although hyperglycemia is an obvious pathogenic factor, we have also examined the role of hyperinsulinemia in renal fibrosis in type 2 diabetes, since elevation of plasma insulin levels precedes hyperglycemia and persists following the onset of hyperglycemia in both rodent models and humans with type 2 diabetes [109,110]. In the db/db mouse model of type 2 diabetes, insulin resistance accompanies obesity and precedes appearance of type 2 diabetes, similar to humans [111]. Insulin resistance and hyperinsulinemia coincide with the onset of hypertrophy and matrix accumulation in the kidney [112]. In vitro, insulin activates the PI3K-Akt-mTOR and ERK signaling pathways and stimulates protein synthesis [113]. In the early (4 weeks) and established (3 to 4 months) stages of type 2 diabetes in the db/db mouse, increased tyrosine phosphorylation of the insulin receptor β chain and of insulin receptor substrate 2 (IRS2, a docking protein required for insulin signaling in the kidney), increased insulin receptor tyrosine kinase activity and increased PI3K activity associated with the insulin receptor show that contrary to the liver, the kidney is not insulin-resistant [114]. Therefore, the kidney is susceptible to pathologic effects of hyperinsulinemia in type 2 diabetes. Insulin receptor activation has also been reported in the retina and the vessel wall in a state of insulin resistance [115] and in type 2 diabetes [116]. Renal fibrosis in type 2 diabetes has been studied through regulation of laminin, a heterotrimeric protein with distinct chain composition in each of the extracellular matrix compartments of the kidney [117]. Accumulation of laminin β1, γ1 and α5 chains in the renal cortex of db/db mice occurred without corresponding increase in their mRNA content [112], which could be due to increased efficiency of translation of the mRNA and/or decreased degradation of the protein. The former possibility was further examined. Incubation of proximal tubular epithelial cells with 1 nM insulin or 30 mM glucose, levels seen in db/db mice [112], alone or in combination, resulted in a rapid increase in laminin β1 expression without changes in its mRNA content [118]. This was abolished by cycloheximide, a translation inhibitor, but not actinomycin D, a transcription inhibitor, suggesting increased mRNA translation. High glucose- and high insulin-induced laminin β1 synthesis require inactivation of 4E-BP1, dissociation of the eIF4E/4E-BP1 complex and formation of the eIF4E/eIF4G complex, two rate-limiting events in the initiation phase of mRNA translation. This was mediated by the PI3K-Akt-mTOR signaling pathway [118].

Both the initiation and elongation phases of mRNA translation are under the control of mTOR, whose activity is found in two functionally distinct complexes. mTOR complex1 (mTORC1) contains mTOR, raptor and GβL, and mTORC2 contains mTOR, rictor and GβL [119]. The two complexes differ by their sensitivity to rapamycin: short-term incubation with rapamycin inhibits mTORC1 but not mTORC2. The numerous substrates of mTORC1 include 4E-BP1 and p70^{S6K}, which are involved in the regulation of protein synthesis. Although the function of mTORC2 is not fully understood, it includes reorganization of the actin cytoskeleton [119] as well as activation of Akt [120]. Crosstalk between mTORC2 and mTORC1 signaling pathways has been studied in mesangial cells; inhibition of Rictor by RNA interference inactivated mTORC2 and activated mTORC1, as judged by increased phosphorylation of its substrates, 4E-BP1 and p70^{S6K}. These data suggest that mTORC2 may impose a tonic inhibition of activity of mTORC1 in unstimulated cells [121].

Sataranatarajan and associates examined the regulation of elongation phase of mRNA translation by conditions encountered in type 2 diabetes. They found that high glucose and high insulin activated eEF2, through Thr56 dephosphorylation, an effect that was inhibited by rapamycin, a mTOR inhibitor [122]. Inactivating phosphorylation of Thr56 is carried out by eEF2K, which is active in its hypophosphorylated form [45]. $p70^{S6K}$, activated by mTOR phosphorylates eEF2K on Ser366 and inactivates it [45]. Because phosphorylation is a covalent modification, inhibiting the upstream kinase is not sufficient to achieve dephosphorylation of a substrate; that requires a phosphatase. Protein phosphatase 2A (PP2A) has been shown to dephosphorylate eEF2 [43]. Whether PP2A is activated by high glucose and insulin in renal cells remains to be determined, as insulin has been shown to down-regulate PP2A expression in skeletal muscles [123] and there are conflicting reports about the effects of glucose on PP2A activity in pancreatic β cells [124,125].

The same group studied the effect of rapamycin on renal fibrosis in diabetes and focused on laminin accumulation in db/db mice [122]. Administration of rapamycin for 2 weeks inhibited renal hypertrophy and laminin accumulation in both glomeruli and tubules of diabetic mice, without affecting plasma glucose levels in either the control or diabetic mice. This amelioration was associated with reversal of diabetes-induced activation of the elongation phase of mRNA translation: activation of eEF2 (Thr56 dephosphorylation), inactivation of eEF2K (Ser366 phosphorylation) and activation of mTOR [122]. Previous report had shown that rapamycin improves renal disease in rodents with type 1 diabetes or type 2 diabetes [126,127], but the underlying mechanisms were not studied in depth. The studies of Sataranatarajan et al. provide a mechanistic basis for these observations. Taken together, these studies suggest mTOR is a potential therapeutic target for treatment of diabetic nephropathy.

The identification of activated signaling pathways could yield other potential sites for intervention in diabetic nephropathy. We have examined the role of glycogen synthase kinase 3 β (GSK3β), which regulates pathways involved in glycogen metabolism [128], cytoskeletal regulation [129], cell cycle progression [130] and cell survival. GSK3β regulates protein synthesis by modifying the activity of eIF2B [131]. During the initiation phase of mRNA translation, activation of eIF2α, a constituent of the 43S PIC, requires exchange of the associated GDP for GTP, a step catalyzed by eIF2B, a guanidine nucleotide exchange factor consisting of five subunits [132]. In resting cells, active GSK3β phosphorylates and inactivates eIF2B, thus putting a brake on protein synthesis [133]. Mariappan et al. studied the role of GSK3β in diabetes-induced laminin β1 synthesis [134]. Stimulation of laminin β1 synthesis by high glucose and/or insulin was associated with the inactivation of GSK3β, and reduced phosphorylation of eIF2Bε on Ser539, a direct target of GSK3β. Dephosphorylation of eIF2Bε would activate eIF2B, which in turn would activate eIF2α and stimulate the initiation phase of mRNA translation. Accordingly, this was associated with inactivation of 4E-BP1 and activation of eEF2, important regulatory steps in the initiation and elongation phases of translation, respectively [134]. GSK3β inactivation was under the control of the PI3K-Akt-mTOR and ERK signaling pathways. In renal cortices of db/db mice with type 2 diabetes, inactivation of GSK3β (Ser9 phosphorylation) and activation of eIF2Bε (Ser539 phosphorylation) were evident during the phase of renal hypertrophy and at a time when laminin β1 synthesis is increased. These data suggest that GSK3β inactivation is important in renal hypertrophy and matrix accumulation in the kidney in type 2 diabetes. Since Akt activity is increased in renal cortex at this time [114], it is likely that Akt is responsible for phosphorylation of GSK3β on Ser9, as reported in non-renal cells. These data by Mariappan et al. suggest that GSK3β activators could be used in the treatment of diabetic nephropathy. However, systemic stimulation of GSK3β is not desirable in type 2 diabetes as it would further inhibit glycogen synthesis and promote more resistance to insulin; thus, agent that selectively stimulate GSK3β in the kidney will have to be developed.

Role of miRNAs in Diabetic Nephropathy

General differences in miRNA expression as well as in the proteome profile have been shown in the rat renal medulla and in the renal cortex region using the microRNA microarray [135], suggesting that miRNAs could play different roles in the control of normal and pathogenic renal functions. Podocyte-specific deletion of Dicer demonstrated a critical role for miRNA regulation in the progression of glomerular and tubular damage, and therefore the development of proteinuria [136]. Dicer deletion in podocytes led to podocyte apoptosis and depletion; proteinuria was significant 3 weeks after birth in mouse models. Also the rapid progression of glomerular and tubular injury was prominent at week 3, and culminated in death several weeks later. Based on altered gene expression profile in podocyte-specific Dicer knock-down glomeruli, especially the miR-30 family has been highlighted as candidates participating in podocyte homestasis and pathogenesis of kidney diseases of podocyte origin. In another study with the podocyte-specific Dicer knock-out mice, it was noticed that expression of slit diaphragm proteins nephrin [135] and podocin [136] was decreased [137]. In this study, mmu-miR-23b, mmu-miR24 and mmu-miR26a were implicated as critical to maintain the glomerular filtration barrier [137].

Recently, a correlation between elevated Notch signalling pathway gene expression and diabetic nephropathy has been shown, in concert with Gremlin, the gene associated with tubulointerstinal fibrosis in diabetic nephropathy [138]. Interestingly, distinct miRNAs, such as miR-7, miR-4, miR-79, miR-2 and miR-11, appear to modify Notch pathways in Drosophila melanogaster with an effect in signalling cascades determining cell specification and development [139]; however, it remains to be determined whether these miRNAs regulate Notch signalling in diabetic nephropathy. miR-15 and miR-16, which are expressed in the kidney, have been proposed to control the Wnt/β-catenin signalling pathway during the embryonal stage [140]. Wnt/β-catenin signalling regulates the early events of nephrogenic induction during mouse kidney development [141] and β-catenin seems to be critical for the development of renal carcinoma and polycystic kidney disease [142]. These studies underscore the potential importance of miRNAs in the development of various kidney diseases.

Conclusions - Perspective

Protein synthesis is a very complex process that involves coordinated activation/inactivation of numerous proteins. Activation of gene transcription is coupled to activation of mRNA translation in order to regulate the levels of the gene product, the protein. However, regulation of mRNA translation as an independent mechanism of protein expression has only recently received attention. The rapidity with which translation can be stimulated allows regulation of protein expression within minutes, instead of hours for transcriptional mechanisms. In this regard, it is important to note that many mRNAs are stored in granules at specific locations inside the cell, and can be mobilized for translation within minutes by various hormones and growth factors [143-145]. Recent investigations have revealed that increased mRNA translation is an important mechanism of synthesis of growth factors and extracellular matrix proteins in the kidney relevant to compensatory renal growth, diabetic nephropathy, and glomerulonephritis. It is almost certain that in the future we will find more examples of regulation by mRNA translation in a wide variety of physiological and pathological states of the kidney. One simple guideline for considering mRNA translation as an independent mechanism of protein synthesis is to measure protein and mRNA levels simultaneously: dissociation of these levels (i.e. increased protein without change in mRNA) indicates regulation at the level of mRNA translation; additionally, decreased degradation could also contribute to increase in protein content. Although difficult to study, it is important to note that synthesis of a single protein may be regulated at the level of both transcription and translation, the focus of regulation changing with the duration of stimulus application [118,146].

As increased protein synthesis is an important contributing factor in the pathogenesis of diabetic nephropathy, control of that process represents a legitimate therapeutic target. Protein levels can be reduced by interfering with either gene transcription or mRNA translation. Although inhibition of gene transcription would lead to reduction in protein synthesis, it should be noted that this entails a lag period during which the existing mRNAs can still be translated. On the other hand, inhibiting mRNA translation would result in nearly immediate cessation of protein synthesis [147]. This can be achieved by RNA silencing via siRNA or miRNA, by targeting individual steps in initiation or elongation stage of translation, or, by modulating signaling pathways. Whereas the use of siRNA or microRNA can lend specificity in terms of protein target, other steps may inhibit general protein synthesis in the kidney and may be useful in blocking general renal hypertrophy. Thus, translation can be an attractive additional site of therapeutic intervention in diabetic nephropathy.

Acknowledgments

Studies were supported by grants from the NIH- DK061597 (O'Brien Kidney Research Center, BSK), NIH-DK077295 (BSK), American Diabetes Association—7-05-RA-60 (BSK), VA Research Service (BSK), Juvenile Diabetes Research Foundation—3-2007-245 (MMM/BSK), NIH—DK050190 (GGC), and American Heart Association SDG 0630283N (DF).

Bibliography

[1] Nygard, O. and Westermann, P., Specific interaction of one subunit of eukaryotic initiation factor eIF-3 with 18S ribosomal RNA within the binary complex, eIF-3 small ribosomal subunit, as shown by cross-linking experiments. *Nucleic Acids Res*, 1982. 10: 1327-34.

[2] Westermann, P. and Nygard, O., The spatial arrangement of the complex between eukaryotic initiation factor eIF-3 and 40 S ribosomal subunit. Cross-linking between factor and ribosomal proteins. *Biochim Biophys Acta*, 1983. 741: 103-8.

[3] Tolan, D.R., Hershey, J.W. and Traut, R.T., Crosslinking of eukaryotic initiation factor eIF3 to the 40S ribosomal subunit from rabbit reticulocytes. *Biochimie*, 1983. 65: 427-36.

[4] Emanuilov, I., Sabatini, D.D., Lake, J.A., and Freienstein, C., Localization of eukaryotic initiation factor 3 on native small ribosomal subunits. *Proc Natl Acad Sci U S A*, 1978. 75: 1389-93.

[5] Safer, B., Adams, S.L., Kemper, W.M., Berry, K.W., Lloyd, M., and Merrick, W.C., Purification and characterization of two initiation factors required for maximal activity of a highly fractionated globin mRNA translation system. *Proc Natl Acad Sci U S A*, 1976. 73: 2584-8.

[6] Seal, S.N., Schmidt, A. and Marcus, A., A heat-stable protein synthesis initiation factor from wheat germ. *J Biol Chem*, 1982. 257: 8634-7.

[7] Moldave, K., Eukaryotic protein synthesis. *Annu Rev Biochem*, 1985. 54: 1109-49.

[8] Korneeva, N.L., Lamphear, B.J., Hennigan, F.L., and Rhoads, R.E., Mutually cooperative binding of eukaryotic translation initiation factor (eIF) 3 and eIF4A to human eIF4G-1. *J Biol Chem*, 2000. 275: 41369-76.

[9] Mangus, D.A., Evans, M.C. and Jacobson, A., Poly(A)-binding proteins: multifunctional scaffolds for the post-transcriptional control of gene expression. *Genome Biol*, 2003. 4: 223.

[10] von Der Haar, T., Gross, J.D., Wagner, G., and McCarthy, J.E., The mRNA cap-binding protein eIF4E in post-transcriptional gene expression. *Nat Struct Mol Biol*, 2004. 11: 503-11.

[11] Rogers, G.W., Jr., Komar, A.A. and Merrick, W.C., eIF4A: the godfather of the DEAD box helicases. *Prog Nucleic Acid Res Mol Biol*, 2002. 72: 307-31.

[12] Methot, N., Song, M.S. and Sonenberg, N., A region rich in aspartic acid, arginine, tyrosine, and glycine (DRYG) mediates eukaryotic initiation factor 4B (eIF4B) self-association and interaction with eIF3. *Mol Cell Biol*, 1996. 16: 5328-34.

[13] Le, H., Tanguay, R.L., Balasta, M.L., Wei, C.C., Browning, K.S., Metz, A.M., Goss, D.J., and Gallie, D.R., Translation initiation factors eIF-iso4G and eIF-4B interact with the poly(A)-binding protein and increase its RNA binding activity. *J Biol Chem*, 1997. 272: 16247-55.

[14] Rogers, G.W., Jr., Richter, N.J., Lima, W.F., and Merrick, W.C., Modulation of the helicase activity of eIF4A by eIF4B, eIF4H, and eIF4F. *J Biol Chem*, 2001. 276: 30914-22.

[15] Pestova, T.V., Borukhov, S.I. and Hellen, C.U., Eukaryotic ribosomes require initiation factors 1 and 1A to locate initiation codons. *Nature*, 1998. 394: 854-9.

[16] Das, S., Ghosh, R. and Maitra, U., Eukaryotic translation initiation factor 5 functions as a GTPase-activating protein. *J Biol Chem*, 2001. 276: 6720-6.

[17] Bandyopadhyay, A. and Maitra, U., Cloning and characterization of the p42 subunit of mammalian translation initiation factor 3 (eIF3): demonstration that eIF3 interacts with eIF5 in mammalian cells. *Nucleic Acids Res*, 1999. 27: 1331-7.

[18] Chakrabarti, A. and Maitra, U., Function of eukaryotic initiation factor 5 in the formation of an 80 S ribosomal polypeptide chain initiation complex. *J Biol Chem*, 1991. 266: 14039-45.

[19] Huang, H.K., Yoon, H., Hannig, E.M., and Donahue, T.F., GTP hydrolysis controls stringent selection of the AUG start codon during translation initiation in Saccharomyces cerevisiae. *Genes Dev*, 1997. 11: 2396-413.

[20] Asano, K., Shalev, A., Phan, L., Nielsen, K., Clayton, J., Valasek, L., Donahue, T.F., and Hinnebusch, A.G., Multiple roles for the C-terminal domain of eIF5 in translation initiation complex assembly and GTPase activation. *EMBO J*, 2001. 20: 2326-37.

[21] Thornton, S., Anand, N., Purcell, D., and Lee, J., Not just for housekeeping: protein initiation and elongation factors in cell growth and tumorigenesis. *J Mol Med*, 2003. 81: 536-48.

[22] Heurgue-Hamard, V., Karimi, R., Mora, L., MacDougall, J., Leboeuf, C., Grentzmann, G., Ehrenberg, M., and Buckingham, R.H., Ribosome release factor RF4 and termination factor RF3 are involved in dissociation of peptidyl-tRNA from the ribosome. *EMBO J*, 1998. 17: 808-16.

[23] Dong, Z. and Zhang, J.T., Initiation factor eIF3 and regulation of mRNA translation, cell growth, and cancer. *Crit Rev Oncol Hematol*, 2006. 59: 169-80.

[24] Marcotrigiano, J., Gingras, A.C., Sonenberg, N., and Burley, S.K., Cap-dependent translation initiation in eukaryotes is regulated by a molecular mimic of eIF4G. *Mol Cell*, 1999. 3: 707-16.

[25] Gingras, A.C., Raught, B., Gygi, S.P., Niedzwiecka, A., Miron, M., Burley, S.K., Polakiewicz, R.D., Wyslouch-Cieszynska, A., Aebersold, R., and Sonenberg, N., Hierarchical phosphorylation of the translation inhibitor 4E-BP1. *Genes Dev*, 2001. 15: 2852-64.

[26] Holz, M.K., Ballif, B.A., Gygi, S.P., and Blenis, J., mTOR and S6K1 mediate assembly of the translation preinitiation complex through dynamic protein interchange and ordered phosphorylation events. *Cell*, 2005. 123: 569-80.

[27] Yang, H.S., Jansen, A.P., Komar, A.A., Zheng, X., Merrick, W.C., Costes, S., Lockett, S.J., Sonenberg, N., and Colburn, N.H., The transformation suppressor Pdcd4 is a novel eukaryotic translation initiation factor 4A binding protein that inhibits translation. *Mol Cell Biol*, 2003. 23: 26-37.

[28] Dorrello, N.V., Peschiaroli, A., Guardavaccaro, D., Colburn, N.H., Sherman, N.E., and Pagano, M., S6K1- and betaTRCP-mediated degradation of PDCD4 promotes protein translation and cell growth. *Science*, 2006. 314: 467-71.

[29] Jang, S.K., Krausslich, H.G., Nicklin, M.J., Duke, G.M., Palmenberg, A.C., and Wimmer, E., A segment of the 5' nontranslated region of encephalomyocarditis virus RNA directs internal entry of ribosomes during in vitro translation. *J Virol*, 1988. 62: 2636-43.

[30] Pelletier, J., Kaplan, G., Racaniello, V.R., and Sonenberg, N., Cap-independent translation of poliovirus mRNA is conferred by sequence elements within the 5' noncoding region. *Mol Cell Biol*, 1988. 8: 1103-12.

[31] Sonenberg, N. and Hinnebusch, A.G., Regulation of translation initiation in eukaryotes: mechanisms and biological targets. *Cell*, 2009. 136: 731-45.

[32] Sonenberg, N. and Pelletier, J., Poliovirus translation: a paradigm for a novel initiation mechanism. *Bioessays*, 1989. 11: 128-32.

[33] Martinez-Salas, E., Pacheco, A., Serrano, P., and Fernandez, N., New insights into internal ribosome entry site elements relevant for viral gene expression. *J Gen Virol*, 2008. 89: 611-26.

[34] Pestova, T.V., de Breyne, S., Pisarev, A.V., Abaeva, I.S., and Hellen, C.U., eIF2-dependent and eIF2-independent modes of initiation on the CSFV IRES: a common role of domain II. *EMBO J*, 2008. 27: 1060-72.

[35] Terenin, I.M., Dmitriev, S.E., Andreev, D.E., and Shatsky, I.N., Eukaryotic translation initiation machinery can operate in a bacterial-like mode without eIF2. *Nat Struct Mol Biol*, 2008. 15: 836-41.

[36] Komar, A.A. and Hatzoglou, M., Internal ribosome entry sites in cellular mRNAs: mystery of their existence. *J Biol Chem*, 2005. 280: 23425-8.

[37] Bushell, M., Stoneley, M., Kong, Y.W., Hamilton, T.L., Spriggs, K.A., Dobbyn, H.C., Qin, X., Sarnow, P., and Willis, A.E., Polypyrimidine tract binding protein regulates IRES-mediated gene expression during apoptosis. *Mol Cell*, 2006. 23: 401-12.

[38] Janzen, D.M., Frolova, L. and Geballe, A.P., Inhibition of translation termination mediated by an interaction of eukaryotic release factor 1 with a nascent peptidyl-tRNA. *Mol Cell Biol*, 2002. 22: 8562-70.

[39] Hinnebusch, A.G. and Natarajan, K., Gcn4p, a master regulator of gene expression, is controlled at multiple levels by diverse signals of starvation and stress. *Eukaryot Cell*, 2002. 1: 22-32.

[40] Wek, R.C., Jiang, H.Y. and Anthony, T.G., Coping with stress: eIF2 kinases and translational control. *Biochem Soc Trans*, 2006. 34: 7-11.

[41] Ibuki, F. and Moldave, K., The effect of guanosine triphosphate, other nucleotides, and aminoacyl transfer ribonucleic acid on the activity of transferase I and on its binding to ribosomes. *J Biol Chem*, 1968. 243: 44-50.

[42] Nairn, A.C. and Palfrey, H.C., Identification of the major Mr 100,000 substrate for calmodulin-dependent protein kinase III in mammalian cells as elongation factor-2. *J Biol Chem*, 1987. 262: 17299-303.

[43] Redpath, N.T. and Proud, C.G., The tumour promoter okadaic acid inhibits reticulocyte-lysate protein synthesis by increasing the net phosphorylation of elongation factor 2. *Biochem J*, 1989. 262: 69-75.

[44] Eichhorn, P.J., Creyghton, M.P. and Bernards, R., Protein phosphatase 2A regulatory subunits and cancer. *Biochim Biophys Acta*, 2009. 1795: 1-15.

[45] Wang, X., Li, W., Williams, M., Terada, N., Alessi, D.R., and Proud, C.G., Regulation of elongation factor 2 kinase by p90(RSK1) and p70 S6 kinase. *EMBO J*, 2001. 20: 4370-9.

[46] Diggle, T.A., Subkhankulova, T., Lilley, K.S., Shikotra, N., Willis, A.E., and Redpath, N.T., Phosphorylation of elongation factor-2 kinase on serine 499 by cAMP-dependent protein kinase induces Ca2+/calmodulin-independent activity. *Biochem J*, 2001. 353: 621-6.

[47] Knebel, A., Morrice, N. and Cohen, P., A novel method to identify protein kinase substrates: eEF2 kinase is phosphorylated and inhibited by SAPK4/p38delta. *EMBO J*, 2001. 20: 4360-9.

[48] Kim, V.N., MicroRNA biogenesis: coordinated cropping and dicing. *Nat Rev Mol Cell Biol*, 2005. 6: 376-85.

[49] Bartel, D.P., MicroRNAs: genomics, biogenesis, mechanism, and function. *Cell*, 2004. 116: 281-97.
[50] Lee, Y., Ahn, C., Han, J., Choi, H., Kim, J., Yim, J., Lee, J., Provost, P., Radmark, O., Kim, S., and Kim, V.N., The nuclear RNase III Drosha initiates microRNA processing. *Nature*, 2003. 425: 415-9.
[51] Chendrimada, T.P., Gregory, R.I., Kumaraswamy, E., Norman, J., Cooch, N., Nishikura, K., and Shiekhattar, R., TRBP recruits the Dicer complex to Ago2 for microRNA processing and gene silencing. *Nature*, 2005. 436: 740-4.
[52] Meister, G., Landthaler, M., Peters, L., Chen, P.Y., Urlaub, H., Luhrmann, R., and Tuschl, T., Identification of novel argonaute-associated proteins. *Curr Biol*, 2005. 15: 2149-55.
[53] Weinmann, L., Hock, J., Ivacevic, T., Ohrt, T., Mutze, J., Schwille, P., Kremmer, E., Benes, V., Urlaub, H., and Meister, G., Importin 8 is a gene silencing factor that targets argonaute proteins to distinct mRNAs. *Cell*, 2009. 136: 496-507.
[54] Liu, J., Rivas, F.V., Wohlschlegel, J., Yates, J.R., 3rd, Parker, R., and Hannon, G.J., A role for the P-body component GW182 in microRNA function. *Nat Cell Biol*, 2005. 7: 1261-6.
[55] Till, S., Lejeune, E., Thermann, R., Bortfeld, M., Hothorn, M., Enderle, D., Heinrich, C., Hentze, M.W., and Ladurner, A.G., A conserved motif in Argonaute-interacting proteins mediates functional interactions through the Argonaute PIWI domain. *Nat Struct Mol Biol*, 2007. 14: 897-903.
[56] Jakymiw, A., Lian, S., Eystathioy, T., Li, S., Satoh, M., Hamel, J.C., Fritzler, M.J., and Chan, E.K., Disruption of GW bodies impairs mammalian RNA interference. *Nat Cell Biol*, 2005. 7: 1267-74.
[57] Eulalio, A., Huntzinger, E. and Izaurralde, E., GW182 interaction with Argonaute is essential for miRNA-mediated translational repression and mRNA decay. *Nat Struct Mol Biol*, 2008. 15: 346-53.
[58] Li, X. and Carthew, R.W., A microRNA mediates EGF receptor signaling and promotes photoreceptor differentiation in the Drosophila eye. *Cell*, 2005. 123: 1267-77.
[59] Humphreys, D.T., Westman, B.J., Martin, D.I., and Preiss, T., MicroRNAs control translation initiation by inhibiting eukaryotic initiation factor 4E/cap and poly(A) tail function. *Proc Natl Acad Sci U S A*, 2005. 102: 16961-6.
[60] Pillai, R.S., Bhattacharyya, S.N., Artus, C.G., Zoller, T., Cougot, N., Basyuk, E., Bertrand, E., and Filipowicz, W., Inhibition of translational initiation by Let-7 MicroRNA in human cells. *Science*, 2005. 309: 1573-6.
[61] Kiriakidou, M., Tan, G.S., Lamprinaki, S., De Planell-Saguer, M., Nelson, P.T., and Mourelatos, Z., An mRNA m7G cap binding-like motif within human Ago2 represses translation. *Cell*, 2007. 129: 1141-51.
[62] Mathonnet, G., Fabian, M.R., Svitkin, Y.V., Parsyan, A., Huck, L., Murata, T., Biffo, S., Merrick, W.C., Darzynkiewicz, E., Pillai, R.S., Filipowicz, W., Duchaine, T.F., and Sonenberg, N., MicroRNA inhibition of translation initiation in vitro by targeting the cap-binding complex eIF4F. *Science*, 2007. 317: 1764-7.
[63] Wakiyama, M., Takimoto, K., Ohara, O., and Yokoyama, S., Let-7 microRNA-mediated mRNA deadenylation and translational repression in a mammalian cell-free system. *Genes Dev*, 2007. 21: 1857-62.

[64] Seggerson, K., Tang, L. and Moss, E.G., Two genetic circuits repress the Caenorhabditis elegans heterochronic gene lin-28 after translation initiation. *Dev Biol*, 2002. 243: 215-25.

[65] Maroney, P.A., Yu, Y., Fisher, J., and Nilsen, T.W., Evidence that microRNAs are associated with translating messenger RNAs in human cells. *Nat Struct Mol Biol*, 2006. 13: 1102-7.

[66] Nottrott, S., Simard, M.J. and Richter, J.D., Human let-7a miRNA blocks protein production on actively translating polyribosomes. *Nat Struct Mol Biol*, 2006. 13: 1108-14.

[67] Petersen, C.P., Bordeleau, M.E., Pelletier, J., and Sharp, P.A., Short RNAs repress translation after initiation in mammalian cells. *Mol Cell*, 2006. 21: 533-42.

[68] Behm-Ansmant, I., Rehwinkel, J., Doerks, T., Stark, A., Bork, P., and Izaurralde, E., mRNA degradation by miRNAs and GW182 requires both CCR4:NOT deadenylase and DCP1:DCP2 decapping complexes. *Genes Dev*, 2006. 20: 1885-98.

[69] Chendrimada, T.P., Finn, K.J., Ji, X., Baillat, D., Gregory, R.I., Liebhaber, S.A., Pasquinelli, A.E., and Shiekhattar, R., MicroRNA silencing through RISC recruitment of eIF6. *Nature*, 2007. 447: 823-8.

[70] Rasch, R. and Norgaard, J.O., Renal enlargement: comparative autoradiographic studies of 3H-thymidine uptake in diabetic and uninephrectomized rats. *Diabetologia*, 1983. 25: 280-7.

[71] Hostetter, T.H., Progression of renal disease and renal hypertrophy. *Annu Rev Physiol*, 1995. 57: 263-78.

[72] Huang, H.C. and Preisig, P.A., G1 kinases and transforming growth factor-beta signaling are associated with a growth pattern switch in diabetes-induced renal growth. *Kidney Int*, 2000. 58: 162-72.

[73] Satriano, J., Kidney growth, hypertrophy and the unifying mechanism of diabetic complications. *Amino Acids*, 2007. 33: 331-9.

[74] Senthil, D., Choudhury, G.G., McLaurin, C., and Kasinath, B.S., Vascular endothelial growth factor induces protein synthesis in renal epithelial cells: A potential role in diabetic nephropathy. *Kidney Int*, 2003. 64: 468-79.

[75] Baserga, R., Is cell size important? *Cell Cycle*, 2007. 6: 814-6.

[76] Bloom, J. and Cross, F.R., Multiple levels of cyclin specificity in cell-cycle control. *Nat Rev Mol Cell Biol*, 2007. 8: 149-60.

[77] Feliers, D., Frank, M.A. and Riley, D.J., Activation of cyclin D1-Cdk4 and Cdk4-directed phosphorylation of RB protein in diabetic mesangial hypertrophy. *Diabetes*, 2002. 51: 3290-9.

[78] Awazu, M., Omori, S., Ishikura, K., Hida, M., and Fujita, H., The Lack of Cyclin Kinase Inhibitor p27^{Kip1} Ameliorates Progression of Diabetic Nephropathy. *J Am Soc Nephrol*, 2003. 14: 699-708.

[79] Wolf, G., Schanze, A., Stahl, R.A., Shankland, S.J., and Amann, K., p27 knockout mice are protected from diabetic nephropathy: Evidence for p27 haplotype insufficiency. *Kidney Int*, 2005. 68: 1583-9.

[80] Lee, M.J., Feliers, D., Mariappan, M.M., Sataranatarajan, K., Mahimainathan, L., Musi, N., Foretz, M., Viollet, B., Weinberg, J.M., Choudhury, G.G., and Kasinath, B.S., A role for AMP-activated protein kinase in diabetes-induced renal hypertrophy. *Am J Physiol Renal Physiol*, 2007. 292: F617-27.

[81] Hardie, D.G., The AMP-activated protein kinase pathway--new players upstream and downstream. *J Cell Sci*, 2004. 117: 5479-87.

[82] Viollet, B., Andreelli, F., Jorgensen, S.B., Perrin, C., Flamez, D., Mu, J., Wojtaszewski, J.F., Schuit, F.C., Birnbaum, M., Richter, E., Burcelin, R., and Vaulont, S., Physiological role of AMP-activated protein kinase (AMPK): insights from knockout mouse models. *Biochem Soc Trans*, 2003. 31: 216-9.

[83] Inoki, K., Zhu, T. and Guan, K.L., TSC2 mediates cellular energy response to control cell growth and survival. *Cell*, 2003. 115: 577-90.

[84] Jozwiak, J., Hamartin and tuberin: working together for tumour suppression. *Int J Cancer*, 2006. 118: 1-5.

[85] Manning, B.D., Tee, A.R., Logsdon, M.N., Blenis, J., and Cantley, L.C., Identification of the tuberous sclerosis complex-2 tumor suppressor gene product tuberin as a target of the phosphoinositide 3-kinase/akt pathway. *Mol Cell*, 2002. 10: 151-62.

[86] Kovacic, S., Soltys, C.L., Barr, A.J., Shiojima, I., Walsh, K., and Dyck, J.R., Akt activity negatively regulates phosphorylation of AMP-activated protein kinase in the heart. *J Biol Chem*, 2003. 278: 39422-7.

[87] Chen, J.K., Chen, J., Neilson, E.G., and Harris, R.C., Role of mammalian target of rapamycin signaling in compensatory renal hypertrophy. *J Am Soc Nephrol*, 2005. 16: 1384-91.

[88] Pervaiz, S., Resveratrol: from grapevines to mammalian biology. *FASEB J*, 2003. 17: 1975-85.

[89] Lee, M.J., Mariappan, M.M., Sataranatarajan, K., Li, M., Feliers, D., Ghosh Choudhury, G., and Kasinath, B.S., Resveratrol ameliorates renal hypertrophy in diabetic mice. *J Am Soc Nephrol*, 2007. 18: 170A.

[90] Hong, S.P., Leiper, F.C., Woods, A., Carling, D., and Carlson, M., Activation of yeast Snf1 and mammalian AMP-activated protein kinase by upstream kinases. *Proc Natl Acad Sci U S A*, 2003. 100: 8839-43.

[91] Howitz, K.T., Bitterman, K.J., Cohen, H.Y., Lamming, D.W., Lavu, S., Wood, J.G., Zipkin, R.E., Chung, P., Kisielewski, A., Zhang, L.L., Scherer, B., and Sinclair, D.A., Small molecule activators of sirtuins extend Saccharomyces cerevisiae lifespan. *Nature*, 2003. 425: 191-6.

[92] Baur, J.A., Pearson, K.J., Price, N.L., Jamieson, H.A., Lerin, C., Kalra, A., Prabhu, V.V., Allard, J.S., Lopez-Lluch, G., Lewis, K., Pistell, P.J., Poosala, S., Becker, K.G., Boss, O., Gwinn, D., Wang, M., Ramaswamy, S., Fishbein, K.W., Spencer, R.G., Lakatta, E.G., Le Couteur, D., Shaw, R.J., Navas, P., Puigserver, P., Ingram, D.K., de Cabo, R., and Sinclair, D.A., Resveratrol improves health and survival of mice on a high-calorie diet. *Nature*, 2006. 444: 337-42.

[93] Lagouge, M., Argmann, C., Gerhart-Hines, Z., Meziane, H., Lerin, C., Daussin, F., Messadeq, N., Milne, J., Lambert, P., Elliott, P., Geny, B., Laakso, M., Puigserver, P., and Auwerx, J., Resveratrol improves mitochondrial function and protects against metabolic disease by activating SIRT1 and PGC-1alpha. *Cell*, 2006. 127: 1109-22.

[94] Matsuzawa, Y., Therapy Insight: adipocytokines in metabolic syndrome and related cardiovascular disease. *Nat Clin Pract Cardiovasc Med*, 2006. 3: 35-42.

[95] Sharma, K., Ramachandrarao, S., Qiu, G., Usui, H.K., Zhu, Y., Dunn, S.R., Ouedraogo, R., Hough, K., McCue, P., Chan, L., Falkner, B., and Goldstein, B.J., Adiponectin regulates albuminuria and podocyte function in mice. *J Clin Invest*, 2008. 118: 1645-56.

[96] Lee, J.O., Yang, H., Georgescu, M.M., Di Cristofano, A., Maehama, T., Shi, Y., Dixon, J.E., Pandolfi, P., and Pavletich, N.P., Crystal structure of the PTEN tumor suppressor: implications for its phosphoinositide phosphatase activity and membrane association. *Cell*, 1999. 99: 323-34.

[97] Mahimainathan, L., Das, F., Venkatesan, B., and Choudhury, G.G., Mesangial cell hypertrophy by high glucose is mediated by downregulation of the tumor suppressor PTEN. *Diabetes*, 2006. 55: 2115-25.

[98] Burns, K.D., Angiotensin II and its receptors in the diabetic kidney. *Am J Kidney Dis*, 2000. 36: 449-67.

[99] Leehey, D.J., Singh, A.K., Alavi, N., and Singh, R., Role of angiotensin II in diabetic nephropathy. *Kidney Int Suppl*, 2000. 77: S93-8.

[100] Lewis, E.J., Hunsicker, L.G., Bain, R.P., and Rohde, R.D., The effect of angiotensin-converting-enzyme inhibition on diabetic nephropathy. The Collaborative Study Group. *N Engl J Med*, 1993. 329: 1456-62.

[101] Kagami, S., Border, W.A., Miller, D.E., and Noble, N.A., Angiotensin II stimulates extracellular matrix protein synthesis through induction of transforming growth factor-beta expression in rat glomerular mesangial cells. *J Clin Invest*, 1994. 93: 2431-7.

[102] Flyvbjerg, A., Dagnaes-Hansen, F., De Vriese, A.S., Schrijvers, B.F., Tilton, R.G., and Rasch, R., Amelioration of long-term renal changes in obese type 2 diabetic mice by a neutralizing vascular endothelial growth factor antibody. *Diabetes*, 2002. 51: 3090-4.

[103] de Vriese, A.S., Tilton, R.G., Elger, M., Stephan, C.C., Kriz, W., and Lameire, N.H., Antibodies against vascular endothelial growth factor improve early renal dysfunction in experimental diabetes. *J Am Soc Nephrol*, 2001. 12: 993-1000.

[104] Feliers, D., Duraisamy, S., Barnes, J.L., Ghosh-Choudhury, G., and Kasinath, B.S., Translational regulation of vascular endothelial growth factor expression in renal epithelial cells by angiotensin II. *Am J Physiol Renal Physiol*, 2005. 288: F521-9.

[105] Feliers, D., Gorin, Y., Ghosh-Choudhury, G., Abboud, H.E., and Kasinath, B.S., Angiotensin II stimulation of VEGF mRNA translation requires production of reactive oxygen species. *Am J Physiol Renal Physiol*, 2006. 290: F927-36.

[106] Ostareck, D.H., Ostareck-Lederer, A., Wilm, M., Thiele, B.J., Mann, M., and Hentze, M.W., mRNA silencing in erythroid differentiation: hnRNP K and hnRNP E1 regulate 15-lipoxygenase translation from the 3' end. *Cell*, 1997. 89: 597-606.

[107] Feliers, D., Lee, M.J., Ghosh-Choudhury, G., Bomsztyk, K., and Kasinath, B.S., Heterogeneous nuclear ribonucleoprotein K contributes to angiotensin II stimulation of vascular endothelial growth factor mRNA translation. *Am J Physiol Renal Physiol*, 2007. 293: F607-15.

[108] Mason, R.M. and Wahab, N.A., Extracellular matrix metabolism in diabetic nephropathy. *J Am Soc Nephrol*, 2003. 14: 1358-73.

[109] Saltiel, A.R. and Kahn, C.R., Insulin signalling and the regulation of glucose and lipid metabolism. *Nature*, 2001. 414: 799-806.

[110] Shanik, M.H., Xu, Y., Skrha, J., Dankner, R., Zick, Y., and Roth, J., Insulin resistance and hyperinsulinemia: is hyperinsulinemia the cart or the horse? *Diabetes Care*, 2008. 31 Suppl 2: S262-8.

[111] Hummel, K.P., Dickie, M.M. and Coleman, D.L., Diabetes, a new mutation in the mouse. *Science*, 1966. 153: 1127-8.

[112] Ha, T.S., Barnes, J.L., Stewart, J.L., Ko, C.W., Miner, J.H., Abrahamson, D.R., Sanes, J.R., and Kasinath, B.S., Regulation of renal laminin in mice with type II diabetes. *J Am Soc Nephrol*, 1999. 10: 1931-9.

[113] Bhandari, B.K., Feliers, D., Duraisamy, S., Stewart, J.L., Gingras, A.C., Abboud, H.E., Choudhury, G.G., Sonenberg, N., and Kasinath, B.S., Insulin regulation of protein translation repressor 4E-BP1, an eIF4E-binding protein, in renal epithelial cells. *Kidney Int*, 2001. 59: 866-75.

[114] Feliers, D., Duraisamy, S., Faulkner, J.L., Duch, J., Lee, A.V., Abboud, H.E., Choudhury, G.G., and Kasinath, B.S., Activation of renal signaling pathways in db/db mice with type 2 diabetes. *Kidney Int*, 2001. 60: 495-504.

[115] Zecchin, H.G., Bezerra, R.M., Carvalheira, J.B., Carvalho-Filho, M.A., Metze, K., Franchini, K.G., and Saad, M.J., Insulin signalling pathways in aorta and muscle from two animal models of insulin resistance--the obese middle-aged and the spontaneously hypertensive rats. *Diabetologia*, 2003. 46: 479-91.

[116] Kondo, T. and Kahn, C.R., Altered insulin signaling in retinal tissue in diabetic states. *J Biol Chem*, 2004. 279: 37997-8006.

[117] Miner, J.H., Patton, B.L., Lentz, S.I., Gilbert, D.J., Snider, W.D., Jenkins, N.A., Copeland, N.G., and Sanes, J.R., The laminin alpha chains: expression, developmental transitions, and chromosomal locations of alpha1-5, identification of heterotrimeric laminins 8-11, and cloning of a novel alpha3 isoform. *J Cell Biol*, 1997. 137: 685-701.

[118] Mariappan, M.M., Feliers, D., Mummidi, S., Choudhury, G.G., and Kasinath, B.S., High glucose, high insulin, and their combination rapidly induce laminin-beta1 synthesis by regulation of mRNA translation in renal epithelial cells. *Diabetes*, 2007. 56: 476-85.

[119] Wullschleger, S., Loewith, R. and Hall, M.N., TOR signaling in growth and metabolism. *Cell*, 2006. 124: 471-84.

[120] Sarbassov, D.D., Guertin, D.A., Ali, S.M., and Sabatini, D.M., Phosphorylation and regulation of Akt/PKB by the rictor-mTOR complex. *Science*, 2005. 307: 1098-101.

[121] Das, F., Ghosh-Choudhury, N., Mahimainathan, L., Venkatesan, B., Feliers, D., Riley, D.J., Kasinath, B.S., and Choudhury, G.G., Raptor-rictor axis in TGFbeta-induced protein synthesis. *Cell Signal*, 2008. 20: 409-23.

[122] Sataranatarajan, K., Mariappan, M.M., Lee, M.J., Feliers, D., Choudhury, G.G., Barnes, J.L., and Kasinath, B.S., Regulation of elongation phase of mRNA translation in diabetic nephropathy: amelioration by rapamycin. *Am J Pathol*, 2007. 171: 1733-42.

[123] Hojlund, K., Poulsen, M., Staehr, P., Brusgaard, K., and Beck-Nielsen, H., Effect of insulin on protein phosphatase 2A expression in muscle in type 2 diabetes. *Eur J Clin Invest*, 2002. 32: 918-23.

[124] Palanivel, R., Veluthakal, R. and Kowluru, A., Regulation by glucose and calcium of the carboxylmethylation of the catalytic subunit of protein phosphatase 2A in insulin-secreting INS-1 cells. *Am J Physiol Endocrinol Metab*, 2004. 286: E1032-41.

[125] Ravnskjaer, K., Boergesen, M., Dalgaard, L.T., and Mandrup, S., Glucose-induced repression of PPARalpha gene expression in pancreatic beta-cells involves PP2A activation and AMPK inactivation. *J Mol Endocrinol*, 2006. 36: 289-99.

[126] Lloberas, N., Cruzado, J.M., Franquesa, M., Herrero-Fresneda, I., Torras, J., Alperovich, G., Rama, I., Vidal, A., and Grinyo, J.M., Mammalian target of rapamycin

pathway blockade slows progression of diabetic kidney disease in rats. *J Am Soc Nephrol*, 2006. 17: 1395-404.

[127] Sakaguchi, M., Isono, M., Isshiki, K., Sugimoto, T., Koya, D., and Kashiwagi, A., Inhibition of mTOR signaling with rapamycin attenuates renal hypertrophy in the early diabetic mice. *Biochem Biophys Res Commun*, 2006. 340: 296-301.

[128] Embi, N., Rylatt, D.B. and Cohen, P., Glycogen synthase kinase-3 from rabbit skeletal muscle. Separation from cyclic-AMP-dependent protein kinase and phosphorylase kinase. *Eur J Biochem*, 1980. 107: 519-27.

[129] Hanger, D.P., Hughes, K., Woodgett, J.R., Brion, J.P., and Anderton, B.H., Glycogen synthase kinase-3 induces Alzheimer's disease-like phosphorylation of tau: generation of paired helical filament epitopes and neuronal localisation of the kinase. *Neurosci Lett*, 1992. 147: 58-62.

[130] Cui, H., Meng, Y. and Bulleit, R.F., Inhibition of glycogen synthase kinase 3beta activity regulates proliferation of cultured cerebellar granule cells. *Brain Res Dev Brain Res*, 1998. 111: 177-88.

[131] Welsh, G.I., Miller, C.M., Loughlin, A.J., Price, N.T., and Proud, C.G., Regulation of eukaryotic initiation factor eIF2B: glycogen synthase kinase-3 phosphorylates a conserved serine which undergoes dephosphorylation in response to insulin. *FEBS Lett*, 1998. 421: 125-30.

[132] Alone, P.V. and Dever, T.E., Direct binding of translation initiation factor eIF2gamma-G domain to its GTPase-activating and GDP-GTP exchange factors eIF5 and eIF2B epsilon. *J Biol Chem*, 2006. 281: 12636-44.

[133] Kerkela, R., Woulfe, K. and Force, T., Glycogen synthase kinase-3beta -- actively inhibiting hypertrophy. *Trends Cardiovasc Med*, 2007. 17: 91-6.

[134] Mariappan, M.M., Ghosh Choudhury, G. and Kasinath, B.S., Role of GSK3 beta (GSK3β) inactivation in high glucose (HG)- and high insulin (HI)-induced extracellular matrix protein synthesis in proximal tubular epithelial (MCT) cells. *J Am Soc Nephrol*, 2007. 18: 651A.

[135] [135] Harvey, S.J., Jarad, G., Cunningham, J., Goldberg, S., Schermer, B., Harfe, B.D., McManus, M.T., Benzing, T., Miner, J.H., Podocyte-specific deletion of dicer alters cytoskeletal dynamics and causes glomerular disease. *J Am Soc Nephrol,* 2008. 19: 2150-8.

[136] Holzman, L.B., St John, P.L., Kovari, I.A., Verma, R., Holthofer, H., and Abrahamson, D.R., Nephrin localizes to the slit pore of the glomerular epithelial cell. *Kidney Int*, 1999. 56: 1481-91.

[137] Roselli, S., Gribouval, O., Boute, N., Sich, M., Benessy, F., Attie, T., Gubler, M.C., and Antignac, C., Podocin localizes in the kidney to the slit diaphragm area. *Am J Pathol*, 2002. 160: 131-9.

[138] Ho, J., Ng, K.H., Rosen, S., Dostal, A., Gregory, R.I., and Kreidberg, J.A., Podocyte-specific loss of functional microRNAs leads to rapid glomerular and tubular injury. *J Am Soc Nephrol*, 2008. 19: 2069-75.

[139] Dolan, V., Murphy, M., Sadlier, D., Lappin, D., Doran, P., Godson, C., Martin, F., O'Meara, Y., Schmid, H., Henger, A., Kretzler, M., Droguett, A., Mezzano, S., and Brady, H.R., Expression of gremlin, a bone morphogenetic protein antagonist, in human diabetic nephropathy. *Am J Kidney Dis*, 2005. 45: 1034-9.

[140] Lai, E.C., Tam, B. and Rubin, G.M., Pervasive regulation of Drosophila Notch target genes by GY-box-, Brd-box-, and K-box-class microRNAs. *Genes Dev*, 2005. 19: 1067-80.

[141] Martello, G., Zacchigna, L., Inui, M., Montagner, M., Adorno, M., Mamidi, A., Morsut, L., Soligo, S., Tran, U., Dupont, S., Cordenonsi, M., Wessely, O., and Piccolo, S., MicroRNA control of Nodal signalling. *Nature*, 2007. 449: 183-8.

[142] Park, S., Bivona, B.J. and Harrison-Bernard, L.M., Compromised renal microvascular reactivity of angiotensin type 1 double null mice. *Am J Physiol Renal Physiol*, 2007. 293: F60-7.

[143] Peruzzi, B. and Bottaro, D.P., Beta-catenin signaling: linking renal cell carcinoma and polycystic kidney disease. *Cell Cycle*, 2006. 5: 2839-41.

[144] Anderson, P. and Kedersha, N., RNA granules: post-transcriptional and epigenetic modulators of gene expression. *Nat Rev Mol Cell Biol*, 2009. 10: 430-6.

[145] Martin, K.C. and Ephrussi, A., mRNA localization: gene expression in the spatial dimension. *Cell*, 2009. 136: 719-30.

[146] Parker, R. and Sheth, U., P bodies and the control of mRNA translation and degradation. *Mol Cell*, 2007. 25: 635-46.

[147] Mariappan, M.M., Shetty, M., Sataranatarajan, K., Choudhury, G.G., and Kasinath, B.S., Glycogen synthase kinase 3beta is a novel regulator of high glucose- and high insulin-induced extracellular matrix protein synthesis in renal proximal tubular epithelial cells. *J Biol Chem*, 2008. 283: 30566-75.

[148] Grosshans, H. and Filipowicz, W., Molecular biology: the expanding world of small RNAs. *Nature*, 2008. 451: 414-6.

In: Advances in Pathogenesis of Diabetic Nephropathy
Editor: Sharma S. Prabhakar

ISBN: 978-1-61122-134-3
© 2012 Nova Science Publishers, Inc.

Chapter XIV

Genetics of Diabetic Nephropathy

Barbara C. Pence and Wyatt McMahon
Texas Tech University Health Sciences Center, Lubbock, Texas 79430, US

Abstract

Accumulated evidence from family studies as well as the natural history of the development of diabetic nephropathy (DN) indicates a role for genetic determinants in overall susceptibility. However, since DN does not appear to be a monogenic disease, the search for genetic markers has been complicated. The research has included family linkage studies, candidate gene studies and more recently case-control genome-wide association studies. While the accumulated genomic data have not yielded a predictive test to this point, there are a number of promising genetic markers that will provide not only future research directions in search of a diagnostic test, but also new directions in terms of the pathogenesis of this disease.

Introduction

Diabetes mellitus is a major cause of renal morbidity and mortality, and diabetic nephropathy (DN) is one of the leading causes of chronic kidney failure in the United States [1]. Approximately 30% to 40% of both Type 1 and Type 2 diabetics will develop advanced or end-stage kidney disease, although a considerably smaller fraction of patients with Type 2 diabetes progress to end-stage renal disease (ESRD). Because it is not a universal complication of diabetes, it has become obvious that other factors are involved in its etiology, especially genetic factors. This is especially evident when examining the frequency of DN: Native Americans, Hispanic and African Americans have a greater risk of developing ESRD than do non-Hispanic whites with Type 2 diabetes [2]. For these and other reasons, the search for genetic causes for DN have been ongoing for a number of years (see Figure 1). The types of approaches taken in the search for genetic associations with DN can be divided into two different strategies: the candidate gene approach and the genome-wide association approach, which is based upon a case-control comparison of genome scans of up to one million single nucleotide polymorphisms (SNPs) leading to new hypotheses and mechanisms for the development of the disease.

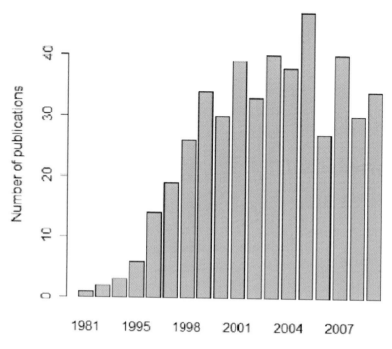

Figure 1. Studies for identification of diabetic nephropathy susceptibility/protection alleles.ISI Web of Science was searched for the words "diabetic nephropathy" AND allele. The number of articles published is shown for each year involving searches for DN alleles.

Pathogenesis

The pathological entity known as DN is applied to the continuum of lesions that often occur concurrently in the diabetic kidney and is characterized by primarily glomerular involvement resulting in three distinct clinical syndromes: non-nephrotic proteinuria (< 3.5 g/day), nephrotic syndrome (> 3.5 g/day), and chronic renal failure [2].Morphological changes in the glomeruli include capillary basement membrane thickening, diffuse mesangial sclerosis, and nodular glomerulosclerosis.

Pathogenesis stems from the insulin deficiency driven hyperglycemia which causes biochemical alterations in the glomerular basement membrane, including increases in collagen type IV and fibronectin and decreased heparan sulfate proteoglycan. These changes are also associated with increased presence of reactive oxygen species which may inflict further damage on the glomerular filter apparatus [2]. Another contributing factor in the pathogenesis of DN is the presence of advanced glycosylation end products (AGE) which are generated by the non-enzymatic glycosylation of proteins which occurs in diabetics [1]. These biochemical and structural changes result in hemodynamic changes which lead to an increased glomerular filtration rate, increased glomerular capillary pressure, and glomerular hypertrophy [2].Thus DN appears to be caused by the interaction of the metabolic defect that produces AGE and the hemodynamic effect resulting from the glomerular hypertrophy.The pathological features of DN may reflect some of the genetic factors which drive the development of the disease.

Clinically, the earliest manifestation of DN is microalbuminuria, low amounts of albumin in the urine (>30 mg/day).Without specific interventions, approximately 80% of Type 1 diabetics and 20% to 40% of Type 2 diabetics will develop overt nephropathy with macroalbuminuria (>300 mg of urinary albumin per day) [2]. The progression to end-stage renal disease is highly variable and may be genetically determined. After 20 years of diabetes, over 75% of Type 1 diabetics and about 20% of Type 2 diabetics with overt nephropathy will develop ESRD [2]. As with the pathogenesis susceptibility, the progression of DN to ESRD is likely to be genetically determined.

Genome-Wide Linkage Studies in DN

Identification of genetic variants that predispose an individual to DN is challenging, because it is apparently not a monogenic disorder in which a single gene has a rare mutation that confers a very high risk of developing the disease [3]. Familial clustering of DN may result from shared susceptibility genes, common environmental exposures, or a complex interaction between the two. There have been many observations that DN and diabetic ESRD cluster in families, mostly independent of blood glucose concentration [4]. After adjusting for a number of confounding covariates [5], the conclusion suggests the likelihood of the existence of DN-susceptibility genes. The largest familial aggregation study to date [6] screened almost 26,000 U.S. dialysis patients from more than 450 dialysis clinics for a family history of ESRD. Nearly 32% of black women and 27% of black men, compared with 15% and 12% of European American women and men, respectively, reported having relatives with ESRD [6]. Another recent US population-based sample for C-reactive protein and family history of ESRD confirmed the effects of ethnicity, gender, and family history as a cause of renal disease [7].

Linkage studies based on family clustering of disease traits discovered polymorphic markers that are associated with disease and are relatively uniformly distributed throughout the genome [8]. SNPs are now commonly used to identify chromosomal regions that are linked with DN and may presumably contain DN susceptibility genes.There are limitations to the conduct of such linkage studies in that one must recruit large numbers of affected families and the analyses are often difficult, expensive, and time-consuming [8]. However, linkage studies in families have contributed significantly to our knowledge of candidate genes that may be associated with susceptibility of DN in both Type 1 and Type 2 diabetes.

Candidate Genes in DN

A Genetics Primer

Genetics is a complex field with a terminology that most physicians deal with only rarely; therefore, the authors thought it convenient to give a short primer of the methods and terminology used in genetics before delving into the role of genetics in DN susceptibility.

Probably the most important concept in genetics is something with which most practicing physicians are painfully familiar – the concept that all people are different. While in patients this may manifest as differences in symptomolgy or response to a given therapy, in genetics differences are expressed in terms of *polymorphic markers*. A polymorphic marker is a sequence of DNA with a known location (called a locus).While the marker itself is often present in almost all humans, it occurs in different forms in different people (thus making it "polymorphic"). For example, a marker may contain a restriction enzyme cut site in some individuals, while others lack the cut site (this is an example of a restriction fragment length polymorphism) or there may be 12 copies of a CA repeat in the intronic sequence of one individual but other individuals may have 14 copies. Extensive previous research has uncovered thousands of polymorphic markers within the human genome and geneticists use these markers to associate a particular form of the marker (called an *allele*) with a characteristic (for example, increased susceptibility to DN). Ultimately, it is the purpose of genetics to attempt to associate alleles with a trait, and there are multiple ways to achieve this goal.

Genetics studies basically break down into two types: linkage and association. Linkage studies involve trying to associate a given allele with the appearance of a trait within related individuals. Using DN susceptibility as an example, geneticists may find that many members of a family that are diabetic and have nephropathy have allele A in locus 1, while most family members that are diabetic but have no evidence of nephropathy have allele B in locus 1. This would suggest that allele A is linked to DN susceptibility. In order to have the power necessary to link allele A with DN susceptibility, it would be necessary to genotype many families with a high incidence of diabetes containing relatives both with and without DN. Linkage studies are particularly helpful in traits that involve only one gene (monogenic traits) such as Huntington's chorea, because it is relatively straightforward to determine which patients have the disease and which patients do not.

In contrast to Huntington's chorea, DN susceptibility is a *quantitative trait:* a multitude of alleles within an individual's genome each contributes a small amount to DN susceptibility. Because of the relatively small contribution each allele makes to the overall phenotype, it can be difficult to use linkage analysis to identify DN susceptibility genes; however, linkage studies have proven very powerful in identifying a number of alleles linked to DN (see below).

The other type of genetic study is the *association study*. These studies are case-control studies: a large number of individuals with the affliction (in this case DN) are collected and the controls are the unafflicted (in good DN genetics studies – diabetic patients living with diabetes for >10 years but who have not developed nephropathy).Association studies – as opposed to linkage studies – do not require the study subjects to be related, making recruitment much simpler. However, because unrelated individuals are less similar genetically, association studies have an inherently high "noise" level – alleles that predispose to DN will be present in unaffected individuals and those that protect from DN will be present in patients without DN. While these sorts of disparities also occur in linkage studies, because of the decreased heterogeneity that exists when studying related individuals, these disparities occur with lower frequency.

Having established the different types of studies that are common, it is important to distinguish between the methods of allele selection for genotyping. When selecting which alleles to use for either a linkage or association study, an investigator must choose to use either a *candidate gene approach* or a *scan approach*. The candidate gene approach involves the *a priori* selection of a subset of alleles within or near genes that the investigators believe are likely to contribute to DN susceptibility based on previous evidence that the gene may be associated with DN. This evidence could come in the form of previous studies indicating that alleles for that gene were associated with a predisposition for other vascular complications in diabetes (as in the case of aldose reductase – see below).Alternatively, studies may indicate a central role for some protein in the pathogenesis of DN, which would lead investigators to study the association/linkage of an allele with DN (as in the case of the angiotensin converting enzyme gene ACE).

In contrast, a scan approach does not require the investigators to limit their search to a small subset of alleles for genotyping: instead, investigators take advantage of the large number of polymorphic markers that have already been identified and screen a large number of them for association or linkage with DN susceptibility. The markers selected could be from the entire genome, or they could be from a limited (although still very large) chromosomal region that previous studies had suggested might be linked/associated with DN susceptibility.

Until recently, the candidate gene approach has been by far the most popular means of identifying susceptibility genes for any disease, including DN.There are multiple reasons for this. First of all, the candidate gene approach is much less expensive. Because a subset of alleles is selected in the candidate gene approach, the materials needed to perform the genotyping are more limited and often technically more straightforward. Additionally, because of the small number of markers being assayed, another advantage to the candidate gene approach is that a smaller sample size is needed, leading to more power. Because of the multiple testing problem, large sample sizes are required for genome wide (or chromosome-wide) scans in order to have sufficient power to identify alleles that make small contributions to DN susceptibility. For these reasons, the candidate gene approach is the most common method for identifying susceptibility genes.

Results from Candidate Gene Studies

We will now begin a discussion of the various genes that contain alleles that have been implicated in DN susceptibility. Thus far, >30 different genes have been implicated in various studies – however, few have been independently replicated. Therefore, we have chosen to discuss in detail the various genes that have been found associated with DN in multiple studies – and are therefore the most reliable – and are of particular interest. For other genes for which there is no definitive replication, we will simply mention these in a table (Table 1): it is possible that in future studies these findings will be replicated. While every effort was made to report all genes that have thus far been shown to contain DN-predisposing alleles, it is possible that some less well known alleles have escaped our attention.

ACE

Alleles within the angiotensin converting enzyme (ACE) gene are the first to be definitively associated with DN susceptibility [9-11]. ACE encodes a protein that is responsible for the conversion of angiotensin I to angiotensin II (Ang II) [11]. Ang II is a powerful vasoconstricting hormone that is elevated in DN and plays an important role in the pathogenesis of DN, both by hemodynamic effects and by signaling within the glomerulus which can lead to mesangial cell and smooth muscle cell proliferation, matrix expansion, and others and together these effects lead to increased glomerulosclerosis and progressive loss of renal function [12]. Therefore, the levels of Ang II play a key role in the development and progression of DN. Furthermore, the most common treatment for DN is blockade of the renin-angiotensin system (RAS) either by inhibiting Ang II binding of receptors (this class of drugs is known as angiotensin receptor blockers or ARBs) or by directly blocking the conversion of renin to angiotensin through the use of ACE inhibitors (ACEi) [13]. Together, these data highlight the central role that Ang II levels play in the development and progression of DN.

It was therefore both predictable and exciting when alleles of the ACE gene were shown to be associated with a predisposition for developing DN [9, 10]. Intron 16 contains an insertion/deletion polymorphism (I/D) of approximately 300 base pairs, which is the most commonly studied polymorphism in the ACE gene. Numerous studies in a wide array of populations have indicated that the I allele of the I/D polymorphism is highly protective against DN. Interestingly, this polymorphism was known to control levels of the ACE protein, both in the plasma and at the tissue level. In some studies, the only covariate that was associated with DN risk as well as the I/D genotype was ACE plasma levels, indicating that a significant proportion of the risk provided or protection by the I/D polymorphism was in the regulation of plasma ACE levels [14]. This provided a functional explanation to the ACE I/D association with DN. Numerous studies have supported the hypothesis that the I allele is associated with protection, although not all. It is important to note, though, that the studies could not find evidence for the protective effects of the I allele were typically smaller than those that could, and meta-analyses of many studies indicate that the I allele is indeed protective against DN [15].

Given that the most common pharmacological treatment for DN is blockade of the renin-angiotensin pathway [13], it is interesting to note that the ACE genotype appears to dictate at least to some degree the ability of DN patients to respond to inhibition of this pathway. In fact, multiple studies have found that patients with two copies of the I allele were more like to respond favorably to ACEi treatment than patients with only one copy of the I allele or two copies of the D allele [16-18]. Therefore, not only is the I allele protective against DN, but amongst patients with DN, homozygous for the I allele respond better to treatment. This indicates a significant role for the I allele in the development and treatment of DN, and underscores the key role that this pathway plays in the pathophysiology of this disease.

TGF-β pathway

Another key component to the pathophysiology of DN is the transforming growth factor-β (TGF-β).

Table 1. Genes that have been implicated in DN pathogenesis in candidate gene studies

Gene symbol	Gene name	Gene Product Function	Population(s)	Diabetes type
ACE	Angiotensin converting enzyme	Convert angiotensin I to Ang II - regulate vascular tone	Numerous	I and II
ADIPOQ	adiponectin q	adipose-specific protein regulates obesity	African American	II
AGER	Receptor of advanced glycosylation end products	binds extracellular glycosylation products	Caucasian	I
AGTR1	angiotensin II receptor, type I	mediates the major cardiovascular effects of Ang II	Caucasians	I
AKR1B1	Aldose reductase	reduction of glucose to sorbitol	Chinese, Caucasian African American,	II
APOE	apolipoprotein E	Lipid metabolism	Caucasian	I, II
AQP1	aquaporin 1	water channel protein; expressed in renal tubules	Caucasians	I
BCL2	B-cell CLL/Lymphoma 2	blocks apoptotic cell death	Caucasians	I
CALD1	caldesmon	actin-binding protein	Northern Ireland	I
CAT	catalase	combats oxidative stress	Caucasians	I
CCR5	chemokine receptor 5	differentiation, inflammation, receptor for HIV	Asian Indians	II
COL4A1	collagen, type IV, alpha1	collagen member of basement membranes	Caucasians	I
CYBA	cytochrome b-245, alpha polypeptide	oxidase system	Caucasians	I
GFPT2	glutamine:fructose-6-phosphate	associated with insulin resistance	African-Americans	II
GLUT1	glucose transporter 1	transports glucose into the cell	Chinese, Caucasian	I, II
GNB3	guanine nucleotide binding protein (G protein) beta polypeptide 3	associated with essential hypertension and obesity	Europeans	II
GPX1	glutathione peroxidase 1	detoxification of hydrogen peroxide	Caucasians	I
HNF1B	HNF1 homeobox B	nephron and pancreas development	Caucasians	I
IGF1	insulin-like growth factor 1	similar to insulin; mediates growth and development	Caucasians	I
IGFBP1	Insulin-like growth factor binding protein 1	prolongs the life of inslulin-like growth factors	Europeans	II
LAMA4	laminin, alpha 4	constituent of basement membrane	Caucasians	I
LAMC1	laminin, gamma 1	constituent of basement membrane	Caucasians	I

Table 1. (Continued)

Gene symbol	Gene name	Gene Product Function	Population(s)	Diabetes type
L	lipoprotein lipase	lipoprotein uptake	Caucasians	I
MMP9	matrix metalloproteinase 9	breakdown of extracellular matrix	Japanese	II
NOS3	endothelial nitric oxide synthase	synthesizes nitric oxide, causes relaxation of blood vessels	Caucasian	I
NRP1	neuropilin 1	tyrosine kinase receptor for VEGF and semaphorin	Caucasians	I
PPARG2	Peroxisome Proliferator-activated receptor gamma 2	various aspects of fat metabolism - adipocyte differentiation	Caucasians, Aboriginal Canadians	II
PRKCB1	protein kinase C, beta	Apoptosis induction, endothelial cell proliferation, sugar absorption	Europeans	I
SMAD3	Mothers against decapentaplegic homolog 3	Downstream effector of TGF-b	Caucasian	I
SOD2	Mitochondrial manganese superoxide dismutase	Remove reactive oxidative species	Japanese, Koreans, Finnish, Swedish	I, II
TGFB1	Transforming growth factor-b	Inflammatory cytokine	Chinese, Danish	II
TGFBR2	TGF-b receptor 2	receptor of TGF-b; inflammation	Caucasians	I
TGFBR3	TGF-b receptor 3	receptor of TGF-b; inflammation	Caucasians	I
TIMP3	TIMP metallopeptidase inhibitor 3	inhibitor of matrix metalloproteinase	Caucasians	I
TSC22D1	TGF-b induced clone 22	Downstream effector of TGF-b	Caucasians, Japanese, Europeans	II
USF1	upstream transcription factor 1	transcription factor	Caucasians	I
VEGFA	vascular endothelial growth factor A	angiogenesis	Europeans	

This cytokine is expressed at elevated levels in the diabetic kidney and has been implicated primarily in the accumulation of extracellular matrix (ECM) and thereby the development of glomerulosclerosis [19]. However, TGF-β has also been suggested to regulate the expression of other cytokines, including vascular endothelial growth factor (VEGF), as well as regulating intracellular glucose levels, indicating that it likely has multiple functions within the diabetic kidney[19].

Despite the central role that TGF-β plays in DN pathophysiology, evidence for alleles of TGFB1 (which encodes the TGF-β protein) playing an important role in DN have been limited. Some studies were unable to associate TGFB1 alleles with a predisposition for development of DN [20, 21]. In type II diabetics, Chinese patients with the T869C allele were shown to be at an elevated risk for developing DN [22]. This allele leads to an alanine-to-proline change within the signaling peptide of TGF-β, and it is suggested that this change leads to an increased expression of TGF- β. This has also been replicated in a group of type I diabetic Caucasians [23]. Another study found a separate allele associated with DN in the TGFB1, but this particular association has not been replicated to the authors' knowledge [24]. Therefore, despite the clear role for the TGF- β peptides in DN, a clear role for alleles influencing susceptibility are more controversial.

TGF- β – being a cytokine – requires the activities of other proteins in order to carry out its activity (receptors, signaling molecules, downstream transcription factors, etc.).Therefore, it is important to note that polymorphisms in genes encoding other members of the TGF-β pathway have also been shown to contribute to DN. One of these includes the TGF-β stimulated clone 22 (TSC-22) - which was cloned based on its increased expression following TGF-β treatment and is a transcription factor that works to upregulate genes that are induced by TGF- β [25]. Two independent studies have indicated that polymorphisms in the promoter of this gene were associated with DN susceptibility [24, 26]. In addition, in a screen of 115 candidate genes, Ewens et al., found that two polymorphisms within different TGF- β receptors and SMAD3 – another transcription factor that activates TGF- β -regulated genes – were associated with DN susceptibility [21], although it should be noted that both of these genes have only been implicated in one study, and therefore further investigation will be necessary. However, given the observation that multiple alleles in genes encoding members of the TGF- β signaling pathway have been implicated in DN pathogenesis, it is likely that alleles in genes encoding members of this pathway plays an important role in DN susceptibility.

Aldose Reductase

As mentioned, hyperglycemia is the major factor involved in predisposing individuals to developing DN. Aldose reductase, the protein responsible for converting glucose into sorbitol –elevated levels of which have been implicated in DN pathogenesis [27] - is therefore a prominent candidate gene in predisposing to DN. The aldose reductase gene (AKR1B1) contains a stretch of CA dinucleotide repeats within the promoter with several variants in the number of repeats (21, 22, 23, 24, 25, 26, and 27 called alleles Z-6, Z-4, Z-2, Z, Z+2, Z+4, and Z+6, respectively). Patients with at least one copy of the Z+2 allele are possibly as much as 7 fold less likely to develop DN than other diabetics, indicating pronounced protection from this allele [28-30].This allele has been associated specifically with decreased renal matrix production in diabetics and even with decreased diabetic retinopathy [31], suggesting that this allele is a key protective allele in multiple diabetic complications. With this functional evidence, it is clear that AKR1B1 alleles play a very important role in DN susceptibility.

GLUT1

Glucose is transported into the cell via numerous glucose-transporting proteins, the most noted of which if the GLUT4 protein.Glut4 is expressed in muscle cells and therefore plays an important role in maintaining blood glucose concentrations. However, within the kidney, the major glucose transporter is GLUT1. Numerous studies have suggested that polymorphisms in the gene encoding GLUT1 are nominally associated with DN susceptibility [28, 32, 33]. Not all studies have found a correlation between GLUT1 polymorphism and DN [34], but at least some of these discrepancies appear to be explainable by poor experimental design and small sample sizes. However, meta-analyses of various studies have suggested a true association between GLUT1 alleles and DN. It is therefore reasonable to suggest that GLUT1 alleles contribute to DN susceptibility.

SOD2

One of the major factors contributing to the pathogenesis of DN is oxidative stress. Excess free radicals generated by the mitochondria as a result of increased metabolic activity are known to contribute to multiple forms of renal damage, including glomerulosclerosis and cell death, not to mention the molecular effects of increased DNA damage and oxidation of proteins/lipids that lead to other dysfunction [35, 36]. It is therefore interesting that alleles in the mitochondrial manganese superoxide dismutase (MnSOD – encoded by SOD2) have been repeatedly shown to contribute to susceptibility to DN [37-39]. The susceptibility allele (called V16A) causes a change in the signal peptide for the encoded protein that leads to increased targeting to the mitochondria. Individuals with the V16A polymorphism are at an increased risk of developing DN.

Importantly, this association has been replicated in Caucasian, Korean, and Japanese populations, indicating that this allele is predisposing to DN in numerous ethnicities.

Interestingly, one study found that the disease-causing SOD2 genotype, in diabetics who have ever smoked, led to the highest risk group for the study, suggesting that smoking and the SOD2 genotype interact [38].This is worth highlighting because it demonstrates how genotype interacts with environmental factors other than diabetes to predispose to DN development.

eNOS

The endothelial nitric oxide synthase (eNOS) has been implicated in numerous aspects of DN pathophysiology [40].These include maintenance of intraglomerular pressure, glomerular permeability, and oxidative stress, among others. Underscoring a role for eNOS in the pathogenesis of DN, multiple polymorphisms within the promoter and intronic sequences of the gene encoding encoding eNOS (NOS3) have been associated with DN [21, 41, 42]. This, however, has been controversial as some investigators have been unable to replicate these findings. Despite these inconsistencies, the fact that these findings could be replicated at all suggests that polymorphisms in the NOS3 gene contribute to an individual's susceptibility to DN.

PPARG2

The peroxisome proliferator-activator receptor gamma2 (PPAR-γ2 – encoded by PPARG2) is a transcription factor involved in regulating various aspects of metabolism including glucose and lipid metabolism, fatty acid transport, and even adipocyte differentiation. The Pro12Ala polymorphism – which has been associated with insulin sensitivity and is protective for type II diabetes – was shown to play a role in susceptibility to DN. Specifically, the Ala12 allele (which encodes the alanine in position 12 of the PPAR-γ2 protein) was shown to be protective against DN in Caucasians [43]. A second study confirmed these findings but in aboriginal Canadians [44]. Therefore, alleles of the PPARG2 gene seem to protect not only against diabetes, but also against DN, although the mechanism of PPARG2 protection is not known.

ApoE

A particularly intriguing polymorphism occurs in the gene encoding apolipoprotein E (ApoE), a protein that binds cholesterol and facilitates its uptake into the cell. Numerous studies have supported a DN susceptibility allele with the ε2 allele in ApoE (which leads to elevated triglyceride levels), and one study actually performed both an association and transmission/disequilibrium test, thereby validating their results themselves [45-48]. Additionally, the ε4 allele (associated with elevated HDL and lower triglyceride levels) appears to be protective against DN [49]. One study found that the odds ratio for the ε2 allele was a startling 10, while the odds ratio for the ε4 allele was 0.13 indicating an extraordinarily powerful susceptibility and protective effect for these alleles [49]. Other studies have been unable to validate these findings, and larger studies have yielded more moderate results, indicating that the effect of these alleles might be less powerful that previously suggested [50]. However, one study suggested that ApoE alleles were associated with differential susceptibility to chronic kidney disease independent of diabetes, indicating that ApoE may regulate kidney disease more generally rather than DN *per se* [50]. Regardless, it is clear that ApoE genotype can have a profound effect on an individual's ability to develop DN.

The candidate gene approach has clearly led to the identification of multiple genes involved in DN susceptibility, and this common approach will certainly be used extensively in the future. As understanding of genomic polymorphisms continues to grow and our understanding of DN pathogenesis continues to increase, it is sure that more investigations into specific genes involved in DN susceptibility will increase.

Genome-Wide Association Studies

A more recent approach to the identification of genetic regions that are associated with the disease of interest (e.g., DN) is to perform an association study in unrelated cases and controls, instead of families. In these studies one can examine the entire genome using high throughput technology that allows the evaluation of up to 1 million gene SNPs per individual sample. These so-called genome-wide association studies (GWAS) then generate odds ratios (OR) that reflect the detection of modest effects of the presence of specific SNPs, usually in the range of an OR of 1.2 to 1.5. However, the success of these GWAS approaches is dependent on the presence in the cases of a relatively common risk allele. This is known as the "common disease, common variant" hypothesis [51]. This hypothesis, which postulates that in common diseases such as diabetes and its associated DN, there are a small number of common alleles that are responsible for the disease [51]. This popular hypothesis proposes that most of the genetic risk for common, complex diseases such as DN, is due to one or perhaps a small number of common variant alleles at the disease loci, and that association mapping in GWAS should be able to detect them. Thus, the common disease – common variant hypothesis suggests that these susceptibility variants have low to medium penetrance in populations, and are probably not subject to strong selection, so although they may represent a small fraction of the total number of disease alleles, they may contribute disproportionately to the total population risk [51]. These assumptions form the basis for the use of large sample sizes in case-control comparisons in the association studies scanning the entire genome.

Another confounding limitation of the GWAS approach is the problem of population stratification. Population stratification occurs when there are major differences in the genetic SNPs due to different ethnic ancestry, and not due to specific disease SNPs. Thus, the detection of modest effect risk alleles can be overshadowed by the presence of strong population stratification. More recent GWAS analyses have chosen to minimize population stratification by using a homogeneous ethnic group or by defining the ancestry-based markers and eliminating the bias a priori in the analysis [4]. A recent approach is called mapping by admixture disequilibrium (MALD), and this tests for SNP association of ethnic-specific genetic markers that are more common in a particular ethnic group that are disproportionately transmitted into affected members in another ethnic group. This analysis is particularly useful when there are ethnic differences in disease incidence existing in recently admixed populations (e.g., Mexican-Americans and non-Hispanic whites) [8].

Accurate phenotyping of the cases and controls is also essential to the success of GWAS because any misclassification will increase the noise level and reduce the power of the study [3]. A specific issue in the study of DN, is the need for recruiting control patients with diabetes, but who have no evidence of microalbuminuria, even after 15 years of diabetes, and are therefore assumed to be of very low risk of development of DN [3].

A final requirement for accurate assessment of genome-wide association with disease susceptibility genes involves the need for setting statistical significance at a very stringent level, such as P < 1.0 X 10-7 or greater. This is required due to the potential for detection of 'false positive' associations due strictly to the large number of multiple comparisons that occur when one is assessing the presence of 0.5 to 1 million SNPs in a large number (100's to 10,000's) of subjects.

Genome-Wide Association Studies in DN

A small number of genome-wide association studies have been conducted to examine the common genetic variants associated with DN from both Type 1 and Type 2 diabetes. A recent GWAS for DN susceptibility genes in Type 1 diabetes patients was conducted in participants of the Diabetes Control and Complications Trial (DCCT)/Epidemiology of Diabetes Interventions and Complications (EDIC) study, a long-term prospective investigation of the development of diabetes-associated complications[52]. This study genotyped ~ 360,000 SNPs in 820 case subjects (284 with proteinuria and 536 with ESRD) and 885 controls, all with Type 1 diabetes. Thirteen SNPs located in four loci were found to be associated with DN[52]. The strongest association was at the *FRMD3* locus with an OR of 1.45, and a P value of 5.0 X 10^{-7}. Another strong association was identified at the *CARS* locus (OR = 1.36, P = 3.1 X 10^{-6}). Two other loci that were strongly associated with DN in this study were *CPVL*, a carboxypeptidase that is highly expressed in the kidney proximal tubules, and multiple SNPs within a 33 kb haplotype block on chromosome 13q, a region associated with linkage to congenital renal abnormalities [52]. These gene associations represent new and previously unidentified pathways in the pathogenesis of DN in Type 1 diabetes.

In a GWAS conducted in Type 2 diabetic patients in a Japanese population, Maeda et al. [53] examined SNPs. They also specifically focused on specific SNPs within the genes encoding for the renin-angiotensin system that have been considered as candidate genes for DN susceptibility, and also those SNPs within the TCF7L2 (transcription factor 7-like 2) as a candidate gene for Type 2 diabetes. The genome-wide scan also identified SLC12A3 (which encodes the thiazide-sensitive NaCl co-transporter expressed in the apical membrane of the distal convoluted tubule of the kidney [54]) and the engulfment and cell motility 1 gene (ELMO1) as new candidates for DN [53]. They further discovered that the genes encoding the angiotensin-converting enzyme, angiotensinogen, and angiotensin II type I receptor had a significant interactive effect on susceptibility to DN [53]. These findings need to be further validated in replication studies.

In a follow-up study to the above GWAS [52], Pezzolesi et al. [55] further analyzed polymorphisms in the *ELMO1* locus in Type 1 diabetes and in two additional ethnically diverse Type 2 populations. A GWAS using the GoKinD study collection was analyzed for associations across the *ELMO1* locus using 118 SNPs and 1705 individuals of European ancestry. The strongest association in ELMO1 occurred at SNPs rs11769038 (OR = 1.24, P + 1.7 X 10^{-3}) and rs1882080 (OR = 1.23 X 10^{-3}) in intron 16 [55]. No evidence of variants previous reported for Type 2 DN was observed in this collection. This is the third report of associations in *ELMO1* with DN in multiple ethnic backgrounds [55].

In a related study in ESRD patients, Hanson et al. [56] conducted a GWAS of 115,352 SNPs in a sample of 105 unrelated case subjects with ESRD and Type 2 diabetes, and 102 controls with Type 2 diabetes who had not developed microalbuminuria in over 10 years. They reported strong associations with SNP rs2720709, which is located in the plasmacytoma variant translocation gene (*PVT1*) along with rs2648875 which maps to intron 8 of the same gene [56]. The mechanism of pathogenesis associated with these SNPs remains to be elucidated.

Biological Mechanisms of Genomic Associations

In the GWAS discussed in the previous section there have been several genes reported to have strong associations with the susceptibility to development of DN. These genes include *FRMD*, *CARS*, *CVPL*, *SLC12A3*, *ELMO1*, and *PVT1*. While there is no complete mechanistic assessment of how these all might be involved in susceptibility to DN in either Type 1 or Type 2 diabetes, the potential biological associations of these genes with DN will be reviewed.

The *FRMD3* gene encodes the 4.10 protein, which is a structural protein with a currently unknown function, which is a member of the 4.1 family of proteins [52]. This protein family has roles as cytoskeletal proteins, which maintain both cellular shape and form in a number of cell types and the data of Pezzolesi et al. [52] have extended the expression profile of *FRMD3* to include mesangial and proximal tubule cells. They have reported that among 18 genes that contain FERM domains, which are modules which maintain cell integrity through interactions with transmembrane proteins and actin filaments [52], many of these are seen in DN. They have further identified nominally significant associations with DN for SNPs located in eight of these FERM domain genes [52]. These findings require further study, including replication in other populations, but the data are provocative and may involve new pathways in the pathogenesis of DN.

The *CARS* gene encodes the enzyme, cysteinyl-tRNA synthetase, which is one of several aminoacyl-tRNA synthetases (ARSs) that have been identified in humans [52]. The ARS are important regulators of intracellular amino acid concentrations and protein biosynthesis, and *CARS* has specifically been implicated in cystinosis, an autosomal recessive renal tubule disorder, caused by accumulation of free cystine in cellular lysosomes [52]. In the Pezzolesi et al. [52] GWAS, all of the SNPs seen to be associated with DN, were associated primarily with ESRD, which is also a prominent feature of cystinosis. Future research is needed in the role of the *CARS* pathway in ESRD in diabetes and DN.

Another gene associated with DN in the Pezzolesi et al. [52] GWAS is the *CPVL* gene, which is a carboxypeptidase that is highly expressed in kidney, especially in proximal tubules. Other carboxypeptidases, such as ACE and bradykinin, have previously been implicated in the pathogenesis of DN [57].

SCL12A3 is a gene that codes for the thiazide-sensitive NaCl co-transporter expressed in the apical membrane of the distal convoluted tubule of the kidney [54]. Maeda et al. [53] identified this gene in a GWAS in Type 2 diabetics. This is the cotransporter believed to be the principal mediator of sodium and chloride reabsorption in this nephron segment, accounting for a significant fraction of net renal sodium reabsorption.

Table 2. Gene Associations with DN reported from GWAS

Gene	SNPs	OR	Function	Population	Phenotype	Reference
FRMD3	rs10868025	1.45	4.1 family of cytoskeletal proteins	820 DN cases/885 controls European	Type 1	Pezzolesi et al. [52]
	rs1888747	1.45				
CARS	rs451041	1.36	cysteinyl-aminoacyl-tRNA synthetase			
	rs739401	1.36				
CPVL	rs39059	1.39	Carboxypeptidase			
	rs39075	1.43				
SLC12A3	rs2289116	ND	thiazide-sensitive NaCl co-transporter	94 DN cases/94 controls Japanese	Type 2	Maeda et al. [53]
ELMO1	rs11769038	1.24	engulfment and cell motility 1	820 DN cases/885 controls, European	Type 1	Pezzolesi [55]
	others	<1.24				
	intron18+9170	2.67		640 patients Japanese	Type 2	Shimazaki et al. [61]
	multiple	ND		577 ESRD cases/ 596 non-diabetic controls African-American	Type 2	Leak et al. [59]
	rs741301	ND		94 DN cases/94 controls Japanese	Type 2	Maeda et al. [53]

DN = diabetic nephropathy; GWAS = genome-wide association studies; SNPs = single nucleotide polymorphisms; OR = odds ratio; ESRD = end-stage renal disease; ND = not determined.

This cotransporter is the target of thiazide diuretics used in the treatment of high blood pressure [58]. Mutations in the gene appear to be responsible for Gitelman's syndrome, but its mechanism in the pathogenesis of DN remains to be elucidated.

ELMO1 has recently been confirmed in the GoKinD collection as a susceptibility gene in DN in 1705 individuals of European ancestry with Type 1 diabetes [55]. The *ELMO1* gene codes for a soluble cytoplasmic protein that functionally cooperates with other genes to mediate cytoskeletal rearrangements during mammalian phagocytosis of apoptotic cells and cell motility in mammalian cells [59]. Functional studies of *ELMO1* revealed that increased levels were observed in COS cells cultured at high glucose concentration, with loss of cell adhesion properties and enhanced synthesis of collagen and fibronectin in *ELMO1* transfected cells, all suggestive of a pathological role in diabetic kidney disease [60]. Indeed, the pathology of DN as described in [2] shows increased collagen type IV and fibronectin in the glomerular basement membrane, demonstrating a functional role for this gene in the pathogenesis of DN. Variants of *ELMO1* have been documented as associated with Type 2 diabetes DN in a Japanese cohort [61] and most recently in African-American Type 2 diabetes patients with ESRD [59].

Conclusion

The authors have reviewed all of the pertinent genetic variations that have been reported to date that are associated with DN, either by candidate gene function or by statistical genetics resulting from a GWAS. No definitive genetic determinant has emerged from all of the studies that were reviewed by the authors. Future directions for research into the genetic determinants of susceptibility of either Type 1 or Type 1 diabetes-associated DN should follow two strategies: 1) to further replicate the current findings in other ethnic populations, especially Mexican-American; and 2) to work out the functional significance of the gene variants discovered. The first strategy should focus on validating the presence of the already discovered gene variants associated with DN in populations that are at increased risk to determine if there are similar genetic associations across ethnically diverse groups of individuals. Thus far, GWAS have established a link of certain genetic variants to DN in African Americans [59], European ancestry cohorts [52, 53], and Japanese [60, 61]. Mexican-Americans are a large subset at increased risk for diabetes and likely increased risk as well for DN.

The second future research strategy should focus on examining the functional significance of the gene variants which should also be validated in clinical populations. Is susceptibility increased by specific alleles alone, or in combination, and does copy number variation impact DN susceptibility with the known gene variants? Additionally, establishing the mechanism of genetic dysfunction associated with gene variants in DN could lead to development of new therapeutic modalities based upon the new pathways. The future holds many discovery possibilities for increasing our understanding of the pathogenesis and treatment of DN.

References

[1] Kumar V, Abbas A, Fausto N, Aster J. In: *Robbins and Kotran Pathologic Basis of Disease*. 8th ed: Saunders; 2010. pp. 934-935.

[2] Kumar V, Abbas A, Fausto N, Aster J. Robbins and Kotran Pathologic Basis of Disease. In. 8th ed; 2010. pp. 1141.

[3] Conway BR, Maxwell AP. Genetics of Diabetic Nephropathy: Are There Clues to the Understanding of Common Kidney Diseases? *Nephron Clinical Practice* 2009,112:C213-C220.

[4] Satko SG, Sedor JR, Iyengar SK, Freedman BI. Familial clustering of chronic kidney disease. *Seminars in Dialysis* 2007,20:229-236.

[5] Lei HH, Perneger TV, Klag MJ, Whelton PK, Coresh J. Familial aggregation of renal disease in a population-based case-control study. *Journal of the American Society of Nephrology* 1998,9:1270-1276.

[6] Freedman BI, Volkova NV, Satko SG, Krisher J, Jurkovitz C, Soucie JM, *et al.* Population-based screening for family history of end-stage renal disease among incident dialysis patients. *American Journal of Nephrology* 2005,25:529-535.

[7] McClellan W, Speckman R, McClure L, Howard V, Campbell RC, Cushman M, *et al.* Prevalence and characteristics of a family history of EndStage renal disease among adults in the United States population: Reasons for Geographic and Racial Differences in Stroke (REGARDS) renal cohort study. *Journal of the American Society of Nephrology* 2007,18:1344-1352.

[8] Freedman BI, Bostrom M, Daeihagh P, Bowden DW. Genetic factors in diabetic nephropathy. *Clinical Journal of the American Society of Nephrology* 2007,2:1306-1316.

[9] Doria A, Warram JH, Krolewski AS. Genetic predisposition to diabetic nephropathy - evidence for a role of the angiotensin i-converting enzyme gene. *Diabetes* 1994,43:690-695.

[10] Marre M, Bernadet P, Gallois Y, Savagner F, Guyene TT, Hallab M, *et al.* Relationships between angiotensin-i converting-enzyme gene polymorphism, plasma-levels, and diabetic retinal and renal complications. *Diabetes* 1994,43:384-388.

[11] McMahon W, Iznaola O, Prabhakar S. Angiotensin-Nitric Oxide Interactions. In: *Angiotensin Research Progress*. Edited by Miurna H, Sasaki Y. Hauppauge, NY: Nova Publishers; 2008.

[12] Mehta PK, Griendling KK. Angiotensin II cell signaling: physiological and pathological effects in the cardiovascular system. *American Journal of Physiology-Cell Physiology* 2007,292:C82-C97.

[13] Brenner BM, Cooper ME, de Zeeuw D, Keane WF, Mitch WE, Parving HH, *et al.* Effects of losartan on renal and cardiovascular outcomes in patients with type 2 diabetes and nephropathy. *New England Journal of Medicine* 2001,345:861-869.

[14] Wang Y, Ma RC, Ng MCY, Chow CC, So WY, Cockram CS, *et al.* Prognostic effect of insertion/deletion polymorphism of the ACE gene on renal and cardiovascular clinical outcomes in Chinese patients with type 2 diabetes. *Diabetes Care* 2005,28:348-354.

[15] Ng DPK, Tai BC, Lim XL. Is the presence of retinopathy of practical value in defining cases of diabetic nephropathy in genetic association studies? The experience with the

ACE insertion/deletion polymorphism in 53 studies comprising 17,791 subjects. *Diabetes* 2008,57:2541-2546.

[16] Penno G, Chaturvedi N, Talmud PJ, Cotroneo P, Manto A, Nannipieri M, *et al.* Effect of angiotensin-converting enzyme (ACE) gene polymorphism on progression of renal disease and the influence of ACE inhibition in IDDM patients - Findings from the EUCLID randomized controlled trial. *Diabetes* 1998,47:1507-1511.

[17] Jacobsen P, Rossing K, Rossing P, Tarnow L, Mallet C, Poirier O, *et al.* Angiotensin converting enzyme gene polymorphism and ACE inhibition in diabetic nephropathy. *Kidney International* 1998,53:1002-1006.

[18] Jacobsen P, Tarnow L, Carstensen B, Hovind P, Poirier O, Parving HH. Genetic variation in the renin-angiotensin system and progression of diabetic nephropathy. *Journal of the American Society of Nephrology* 2003,14:2843-2850.

[19] McGowan TA, Zhu Y, Sharma K. Transforming growth factor-beta: a clinical target for the treatment of diabetic nephropathy. *Curr Diab Rep* 2004,4:447-454.

[20] Prasad P, Tiwari AK, Kumar KMP, Ammini AC, Gupta A, Gupta R, *et al.* Association of TGF beta 1, TNF alpha, CCR2 and CCR5 gene polymorphisms in type-2 diabetes and renal insufficiency among Asian Indians. *Bmc Medical Genetics* 2007,8.

[21] Ewens KG, George RA, Sharma K, Ziyadeh FN, Spielman RS. Assessment of 115 candidate genes for diabetic nephropathy by transmission/disequilibrium test. *Diabetes* 2005,54:3305-3318.

[22] Wong TYH, Poon P, Chow KM, Szeto CC, Cheung MK, Li PKT. Association of transforming growth factor-beta (TGF-beta) T869C (Leu 10Pro) gene polymorphisms with type 2 diabetic nephropathy in Chinese. *Kidney International* 2003,63:1831-1835.

[23] Patel A, Scott WR, Lympany PA, Rippin JD, Gill GV, Barnett AH, *et al.* The TGF-beta 1 gene codon 10 polymorphism contributes to the genetic predisposition to nephropathy in Type 1 diabetes. *Diabetic Medicine* 2005,22:69-73.

[24] Buraczynska M, Baranowicz-Gaszczyk I, Borowicz E, Ksiazek A. TGF-beta 1 and TSC-22 gene Polymorphisms and susceptibility to microvascular complications in type 2 diabetes. *Nephron Physiology* 2007,106:69-75.

[25] Choi SJ, Moon JH, Ahn YW, Ahn JH, Kim DU, Han TH. Tsc-22 enhances TGF-ss signaling by associating with Smad4 and induces erythroid cell differentiation. *Molecular and Cellular Biochemistry* 2005,271:23-28.

[26] Sugawara F, Yamada Y, Watanabe R, Ban N, Miyawaki K, Kuroe A, *et al.* The role of the TSC-22 (-396) A/G variant in the development of diabetic nephropathy. *Diabetes Research and Clinical Practice* 2003,60:191-197.

[27] Kinoshita JH, Nishimura C. The involvement of aldose reductase in diabetic complications. *Diabetes Metab Rev* 1988,4:323-337.

[28] Hodgkinson AD, Sondergaard KL, Yang BM, Cross DF, Millward BA, Demaine AG. Aldose reductase expression is induced by hyperglycemia in diabetic nephropathy. *Kidney International* 2001,60:211-218.

[29] Neamat-Allah M, Feeney SA, Savage DA, Maxwell AP, Hanson RL, Knowler WC, *et al.* Analysis of the association between diabetic nephropathy and polymorphisms in the aldose reductase gene in Type 1 and Type 2 diabetes mellitus. *Diabetic Medicine* 2001,18:906-914.

[30] Makiishi T, Araki S, Koya D, Maeda S, Kashiwagi A, Haneda M. C-106T polymorphism of AKR1B1 is associated with diabetic nephropathy and erythrocyte aldose reductase content in Japanese subjects with type 2 diabetes mellitus. *American Journal of Kidney Diseases* 2003,42:943-951.

[31] Kao YL, Donaghue K, Chan A, Knight J, Silink M. A novel polymorphism in the aldose reductase gene promoter region is strongly associated with diabetic retinopathy in adolescents with type 1 diabetes. *Diabetes* 1999,48:1338-1340.

[32] Liu ZH, Guan TJ, Chen ZH, Li LS. Glucose transporter (GLUT1) allele (XbaI-) associated with nephropathy in non-insulin-dependent diabetes mellitus. *Kidney International* 1999,55:1843-1848.

[33] Ng DPK, Canani L, Araki S, Smiles A, Moczulski D, Warram JH, *et al*. Minor effect of GLUT1 polymorphisms on susceptibility to diabetic nephropathy in type 1 diabetes. *Diabetes* 2002,51:2264-2269.

[34] Gutierrez C, Vendrell J, Pastor R, Broch M, Aguilar C, Llor C, *et al*. GLUT1 gene polymorphism in non-insulin-dependent diabetes mellitus: genetic susceptibility relationship with cardiovascular risk factors and microangiopathic complications in a Mediterranean population. *Diabetes Research and Clinical Practice* 1998,41:113-120.

[35] Prabhakar S, Starnes J, Shi S, Lonis B, Tran R. Diabetic nephropathy is associated with oxidative stress and decreased renal nitric oxide production. *Journal of the American Society of Nephrology* 2007,18:2945-2952.

[36] Brenner BM, Meyer TW, Hostetter TH. Dietary protein intake and the progressive nature of kidney disease: the role of hemodynamically mediated glomerular injury in the pathogenesis of progressive glomerular sclerosis in aging, renal ablation, and intrinsic renal disease. *N Engl J Med* 1982,307:652-659.

[37] Nomiyama T, Tanaka Y, Piao L, Nagasaka K, Sakai K, Ogihara T, *et al*. The polymorphism of manganese superoxide dismutase is associated with diabetic nephropathy in Japanese type 2 diabetic patients. *Journal of Human Genetics* 2003,48:138-141.

[38] Mollsten A, Marklund SL, Wessman M, Svensson M, Forsblom C, Parkkonen M, *et al*. A functional polymorphism in the manganese superoxide dismutase gene and diabetic nephropathy. *Diabetes* 2007,56:265-269.

[39] Lee SJ, Choi MG, Kim DS, Kim TW. Manganese superoxide dismutase gene polymorphism (V16A) is associated with stages of albuminuria in Korean type 2 diabetic patients. *Metabolism-Clinical and Experimental* 2006,55:1-7.

[40] Prabhakar SS. Role of nitric oxide in diabetic nephropathy. *Seminars in Nephrology* 2004,24:333-344.

[41] Noiri E, Satoh H, Taguchi J, Brodsky SV, Nakao A, Ogawa Y, *et al*. Association of eNOS Glu298Asp polymorphism with end-stage renal disease. *Hypertension* 2002,40:535-540.

[42] Zanchi A, Moczulski DK, Hanna LS, Wantman M, Warram JH, Krolewski AS. Risk of advanced diabetic nephropathy in type 1 diabetes is associated with endothelial nitric oxide synthase gene polymorphism. *Kidney International* 2000,57:405-413.

[43] Caramori ML, Canani LH, Costa LA, Gross JL. The human peroxisome proliferator-activated receptor gamma 2 (PPAR gamma 2) Pro12Ala polymorphism is associated with decreased risk of diabetic nephropathy in patients with type 2 diabetes. *Diabetes* 2003,52:3010-3013.

[44] Pollex RL, Mamakeesick M, Zinman B, Harris SB, Hegele RA, Hanley AJG. Peroxisome proliferator-activated receptor gamma polymorphism Pro12Ala is associated with nephropathy in type 2 diabetes. *Journal of Diabetes and Its Complications* 2007,21:166-171.

[45] Liberopoulos E, Siamopoulos K, Elisaf M. Apolipoprotein E and renal disease. *American Journal of Kidney Diseases* 2004,43:223-233.

[46] Eto M, Horita K, Morikawa A, Nakata H, Okada M, Saito M, *et al*. Increased frequency of apolipoprotein epsilon 2 allele in non-insulin dependent diabetic (NIDDM) patients with nephropathy. *Clinical Genetics* 1995,48:288-292.

[47] Araki S, Moczulski DK, Hanna L, Scott LJ, Warram JH, Krolewski AS. APOE polymorphisms and the development of diabetic nephropathy in type 1 diabetes - Results of case-control and family-based studies. *Diabetes* 2000,49:2190-2195.

[48] Leiva E, Mujica V, Elematore I, Orrego R, Diaz G, Prieto M, *et al*. Relationship between Apolipoprotein E polymorphism and nephropathy in type-2 diabetic patients. *Diabetes Research and Clinical Practice* 2007,78:196-201.

[49] Eto M, Saito M, Okada M, Kume Y, Kawasaki F, Matsuda M, *et al*. Apolipoprotein E genetic polymorphism, remnant lipoproteins, and nephropathy in type 2 diabetic patients. *American Journal of Kidney Diseases* 2002,40:243-251.

[50] Hsu CC, Kao WHL, Coresh J, Pankow JS, Marsh-Manzi J, Boerwinkle E, *et al*. Apolipoprotein E and progression of chronic kidney disease. *Jama-Journal of the American Medical Association* 2005,293:2892-2899.

[51] Pritchard JK, Cox NJ. The allelic architecture of human disease genes: common disease - common variant ... or not? *Human Molecular Genetics* 2002,11:2417-2423.

[52] Pezzolesi MG, Poznik GD, Mychaleckyj JC, Paterson AD, Barati MT, Klein JB, *et al*. Genome-Wide Association Scan for Diabetic Nephropathy Susceptibility Genes in Type 1 Diabetes. *Diabetes* 2009,58:1403-1410.

[53] Maeda S, Osawa N, Hayashi T, Tsukada S, Kobayashi M, Kikkawa R. Genetic variations associated with diabetic nephropathy and type II diabetes in a Japanese population. *Kidney International* 2007,72:S43-S48.

[54] Syrén M-L, Tedeschi S, Cesareo L, Bellantuono R, Colussi G, Procaccio M, *et al*. Identification of fifteen novel mutations in the SLC12A3 gene encoding the Na-Cl Co-transporter in Italian patients with Gitelman syndrome %J *Human Mutation*. 2002,20:78.

[55] Pezzolesi MG, Katavetin P, Kure M, Poznik GD, Skupien J, Mychaleckyj JC, *et al*. confirmation of genetic associations at ELMO1 in the GoKinD collection supports its role as a susceptibility gene in diabetic nephropathy. *Diabetes* 2009,58:2698-2702.

[56] Hanson RL, Craig DW, Millis MP, Yeatts KA, Kobes S, Pearson JV, *et al*. Identification of PVT1 as a candidate gene for end-stage renal disease in type 2 diabetes using a pooling-based genonte-wide single nucleotide polymorphism association study. *Diabetes* 2007,56:975-983.

[57] Adler S. Diabetic nephropathy: Linking histology, cell biology, and genetics. *Kidney International* 2004,66:2095-2106.

[58] Simon DB, NelsonWilliams C, Bia MJ, Ellison D, Karet FE, Molina AM, *et al*. Gitelman's variant of Bartter's syndrome, inherited hypokalaemic alkalosis, is caused by mutations in the thiazide-sensitive Na-Cl cotransporter. *Nature Genetics* 1996,12:24-30.

[59] Leak TS, Perlegas PS, Smith SG, Keene KL, Hicks PJ, Langefeld CD, *et al.* Variants in Intron 13 of the ELMO1 Gene are Associated with Diabetic Nephropathy in African Americans. *Annals of Human Genetics* 2009,73:152-159.

[60] Shimazaki A, Tanaka Y, Shinosaki T, Ikeda M, Watada H, Hirose T, *et al.* ELMO1 increases expression of extracellular matrix proteins and inhibits cell adhesion to ECMs. *Kidney International* 2006,70:1769-1776.

[61] Shimazaki A, Kawamura Y, Kanazawa A, Sekine A, Saito S, Tsunoda T, *et al.* Genetic variations in the gene encoding ELM01 are associated with susceptibility to diabetic nephropathy. *Diabetes* 2005,54:1171-1178.

Index

#

20th century, 21
21st century, 200

A

acetic acid, 202
acetylation, 254, 298
acetylcholine, 240, 241, 245, 251
acid, 6, 8, 9, 23, 42, 78, 88, 155, 188, 200, 201, 212, 216, 253, 267, 270, 290, 291, 306, 325
acidosis, 42, 47
acromegaly, 156
active type, 114
acute infection, 14
acute renal failure, 26
adenine, 200, 206, 207, 240
adenosine, 108, 208, 214, 240, 251
adenosine triphosphate, 108, 208, 240
adhesion, 11, 57, 72, 79, 86, 95, 114, 124, 126, 149, 239, 248, 264, 281, 282, 287, 330, 335
adhesion properties, 330
adhesive interaction, 285
adipocyte, 322, 325
adiponectin, 253, 268, 298, 321
adipose, 298
adipose tissue, 298
adolescents, 81, 82, 83, 132, 154, 156, 284, 333
ADP, 78, 89, 91, 225, 251
adrenal glands, 166
adverse effects, 72, 77, 82
age-related diseases, 107
aggregation, 317, 331
agonist, 241
alanine, 212, 323, 325

albumin, 5, 11, 23, 31, 33, 46, 53, 54, 57, 96, 97, 104, 105, 112, 117, 118, 121, 131, 132, 133, 134, 140, 141, 146, 148, 149, 156, 177, 178, 179, 197, 217, 242, 257, 265, 273, 276, 279, 280, 284, 287, 317
albuminuria, 1, 5, 22, 30, 41, 47, 54, 56, 57, 58, 66, 71, 72, 74, 75, 76, 78, 79, 82, 86, 96, 97, 101, 102, 112, 115, 116, 117, 118, 123, 125, 127, 130, 132, 133, 134, 135, 136, 140, 152, 162, 163, 164, 186, 213, 215, 228, 229, 235, 244, 246, 247, 248, 249, 251, 258, 259, 264, 279, 280, 284, 298, 309, 333
aldehydes, 94
aldosterone, 21, 34, 40, 41, 42, 46, 47, 57, 65, 79, 91, 111, 127, 151, 184, 221, 299
alkalosis, 334
allele, 56, 175, 222, 243, 316, 318, 320, 323, 324, 325, 326, 333, 334
alpha-tocopherol, 156, 211
ALT, 106
alters, 72, 89, 99, 294, 312
American Heart Association, 180, 303
amines, 214
amino, 77, 94, 113, 122, 127, 172, 202, 204, 241, 252, 289, 291, 292, 293, 328
amino acid, 77, 94, 113, 123, 127, 172, 202, 204, 252, 289, 292, 293, 328
amino acids, 94, 113, 123, 127, 202, 204
amino groups, 94, 204
amputation, 22
amyloidosis, 5, 15
analgesic, 14
anchorage, 274
anchoring, 281
androgen, 194
angiogenesis, 76, 89, 152, 155, 227, 254, 280, 322
angiotensin converting enzyme, 37, 38, 39, 46, 73, 77, 79, 81, 117, 162, 189, 200, 215, 284, 319

angiotensin II, 44, 58, 64, 66, 79, 87, 89, 105, 110, 119, 134, 142, 143, 144, 145, 146, 161, 162, 163, 165, 166, 168, 170, 172, 173, 177, 178, 180, 181, 182, 183, 184, 185, 186, 187, 188, 189, 190, 191, 192, 196, 205, 210, 223, 229, 235, 241, 251, 263, 265, 267, 296, 310, 320, 321, 327
angiotensin receptor blockers, 40, 41, 100, 225, 320
animal disease, 64
antagonism, 47, 130, 136, 140, 144, 151, 156, 187
antibody, 11, 36, 76, 77, 116, 117, 121, 123, 124, 130, 139, 140, 153, 216, 222, 278, 280, 282, 287, 310
anticoagulation, 224
antigen, 192, 286
antihypertensive agents, 39
antioxidant, 67, 78, 86, 94, 102, 103, 110, 178, 199, 200, 201, 203, 205, 209, 210, 212, 213, 225
aorta, 73, 144, 172, 241, 245, 246, 268, 271, 311
aortic valve, 250, 265
APC, 72
apoptosis, 47, 51, 69, 72, 74, 75, 78, 84, 86, 87, 91, 92, 95, 105, 113, 124, 134, 135, 149, 155, 157, 158, 204, 208, 212, 214, 223, 227, 232, 247, 254, 263, 267, 273, 275, 278, 279, 280, 281, 285, 286, 288, 293, 294, 302, 306
arginine, 123, 165, 223, 225, 226, 230, 232, 241, 252, 257, 258, 267, 304
arterial hypertension, 216
arteries, 10, 52, 64, 99, 119, 136, 189, 240
arterioles, 10, 16, 23, 24, 25, 26, 29, 52, 79, 164, 165, 168, 183, 243, 247, 263
arteriosclerosis, 10, 16, 139, 200
arteritis, 56
artery, 2, 27, 88, 117, 245
aspartate, 207
aspartic acid, 304
assessment, 180, 327, 328
ataxia, 217, 218
atherogenesis, 288
atherosclerosis, 56, 57, 98, 104, 107, 132, 154, 240, 264
atherosclerotic vascular disease, 226
ATP, 78, 99, 182, 208, 209, 240, 251, 255, 291, 297
atrophy, 10, 23, 42, 51, 56, 124, 134, 200, 277
attachment, 204, 209, 275, 277, 278, 290
authorities, viii, 2
autonomic nervous system, 165
autooxidation, 200
autopsy, 14, 23
autosomal recessive, 328
azotemia, 2, 23

B

backcross, 246
basal lamina, 134
base pair, 76, 291, 295, 320
basement membrane, 6, 7, 10, 11, 12, 13, 18, 23, 24, 25, 39, 43, 45, 53, 54, 59, 66, 73, 85, 96, 102, 114, 116, 117, 130, 134, 142, 162, 200, 273, 274, 275, 283, 285, 316, 321, 330
beneficial effect, 41, 80, 101, 119, 168, 176, 226
bicarbonate, 42
bihydrobiopterin (BH4), 206, 241, 253, 257
bioavailability, 165, 223, 224, 230, 235, 239, 240, 241, 245, 251, 253, 255
biological activities, 254
biological activity, 99
biological responses, 247
biomarkers, 191, 256
biopsy, 5, 10, 14, 15, 16, 18, 23, 52, 117, 277
biosynthesis, 35, 36, 37, 120, 144, 146, 192, 221, 328
birefringence, 15
blood flow, 21, 24, 81, 98, 117, 119, 164, 165, 183, 222, 224, 231, 244, 247
blood pressure, 2, 31, 38, 39, 41, 73, 81, 82, 87, 118, 154, 163, 176, 177, 178, 186, 187, 195, 221, 227, 229, 233, 235, 247, 249, 254, 263
blood pressure reduction, 176
blood urea nitrogen, 116
blood vessels, 35, 280, 322
body weight, 27, 32
bonds, 113
bone, 36, 92, 124, 127, 151, 152, 312
bradykinin, 79, 90, 240, 251, 328
breakdown, 96, 102, 106, 215, 224, 322

C

Ca^{2+}, 213, 306
calcification, 57
calcium, 36, 40, 41, 72, 75, 182, 186, 208, 251, 294, 311
calcium channel blocker, 40
caloric restriction, 203, 269
cancer, 124, 152, 298, 305, 306
cancer cells, 152
candidates, 302, 327
capillary, 5, 6, 7, 9, 10, 11, 12, 16, 17, 18, 26, 27, 28, 29, 38, 39, 40, 41, 42, 44, 72, 95, 119, 128, 132, 143, 149, 164, 202, 227, 248, 250, 262, 265, 274, 298, 316
capsular drop, 6, 9

capsule, 9, 277, 281
carcinoma, 302
cardiac catheterization, 117
cardiac muscle, 281
cardiomyopathy, 106, 209
cardiovascular disease, 23, 98, 162, 182, 188, 191, 232, 240, 257, 258, 270, 309
cardiovascular morbidity, 22, 193, 258
cardiovascular risk, 229, 333
cardiovascular system, 331
carnosine, 100, 110
catabolism, 102, 109, 151, 252
cathepsin G, 166
cell biology, 84, 103, 145, 214, 231, 257, 277, 334
cell body, 274, 276
cell culture, 49, 50, 51, 52, 113, 124, 125, 147, 244, 278, 280
cell cycle, 71, 90, 114, 124, 240, 278, 281, 301
cell death, 74, 75, 209, 321, 324
cell differentiation, 114, 332
cell line, 50, 72, 77, 78, 175, 273, 278, 282, 286
cell lines, 50, 72, 78, 273, 278, 282, 286
cell membranes, 203
cell signaling, 221, 264, 274, 331
cell size, 173, 308
cell surface, 94, 128, 215, 248
cellular homeostasis, 288
cellular signaling pathway, 94, 292
central nervous system, 84
chemokine receptor, 321
chemokines, 69, 124, 150, 173
childhood, 43, 85, 132, 154
children, 81, 82, 83, 84, 89, 90, 101, 109, 132, 154, 156, 208, 218, 233
chitosan, 96
cholesterol, 57, 66, 207, 240, 325
chorea, 318
chromosome, 37, 243, 319, 327
chronic diseases, 98
chronic kidney failure, 315
chronic renal failure, 11, 18, 22, 23, 24, 34, 38, 101, 109, 175, 277, 316
chymotrypsin, 172
circulation, 26, 96, 97, 117, 202, 222, 232
citrulline, 241, 244
clinical application, 207
clinical disorders, 50
clinical presentation, 15
clinical syndrome, 316
clinical trials, 40, 76, 100, 101, 111, 163, 200, 229, 280
clone, 322, 323
cloning, 137, 311

clustering, 118, 317, 331
coding, 124
codon, 118, 141, 289, 291, 292, 293, 305, 332
coenzyme, 208
collaboration, 37
collage, 287
collagen, 35, 36, 72, 76, 79, 85, 89, 94, 95, 96, 99, 103, 104, 109, 112, 114, 116, 117, 134, 139, 141, 144, 145, 149, 150, 155, 157, 158, 159, 213, 214, 242, 276, 279, 280, 286, 316, 321, 330
collateral, 152
combination therapy, 100, 103
complications, viii, 2, 14, 21, 39, 46, 50, 51, 58, 67, 70, 81, 88, 89, 93, 94, 99, 103, 104, 105, 108, 109, 141, 145, 154, 155, 156, 159, 173, 181, 190, 193, 194, 200, 201, 203, 204, 208, 211, 212, 214, 220, 221, 224, 227, 229, 231, 232, 234, 235, 236, 239, 240, 241, 254, 257, 258, 259, 263, 266, 308, 319, 324, 327, 331, 332, 333
composition, 114, 134, 300
compounds, 2, 94, 97, 98, 100, 101, 102, 103, 107
conduction, 214
configuration, 290, 291
confounding variables, 132
congenital malformations, 84
connective tissue, 66, 69, 76, 87, 88, 125, 147, 148, 150, 151, 296, 299
control group, 28, 30, 122
controversial, 2, 122, 124, 201, 208, 277, 323, 325
controversies, 220
corepressor, 158
coronary arteries, 241
coronary artery disease, 2
coronary heart disease, 189
correlation, 18, 63, 99, 112, 118, 132, 134, 224, 236, 277, 302, 324
correlations, 18, 139, 183, 224
cortex, 24, 40, 42, 78, 92, 96, 115, 144, 167, 169, 171, 173, 183, 244, 247, 261, 296, 298, 300, 301, 302
covalent bond, 122
creatinine, 40, 96, 97, 113, 116, 132, 133, 144, 176, 179
crescentic glomerulonephritis, 14
cross sectional study, 277
culture, 35, 49, 50, 54, 63, 112, 113, 119, 124, 134, 135, 157, 185, 208, 254, 278, 296, 298
curcumin, 58, 225
cycles, 45, 119
cyclooxygenase, 73, 85, 217, 236, 237
cysteine, 71, 75, 113, 125, 137
cystine, 328
cytochrome, 74, 99, 108, 241, 321

cytokines, vii, 3, 34, 45, 69, 81, 113, 115, 125, 136, 157, 165, 166, 173, 181, 192, 205, 220, 233, 241, 248, 264, 280, 323
cytoplasm, 73, 275, 294
cytosine, 133
cytoskeleton, 85, 189, 274, 276, 282, 286, 300

D

deacetylation, 254, 298
decomposition, 204
defects, 199, 207, 208, 212, 245, 250, 265
deficiencies, 200, 203
deficiency, 22, 42, 73, 77, 92, 156, 165, 172, 183, 207, 208, 217, 223, 224, 226, 230, 241, 245, 246, 247, 248, 249, 250, 251, 256, 263, 316
degradation, 74, 76, 94, 95, 102, 110, 120, 127, 144, 166, 170, 172, 204, 251, 292, 295, 300, 303, 305, 308, 313
dephosphorylation, 114, 297, 300, 301, 312
derivatives, 94, 98, 229
destruction, 22, 30, 37
detachment, 135, 250, 265, 278
detectable, 27, 82
detection, 326, 327
detoxification, 201, 205, 215, 321
diabetic glomerulopathy, 5, 6, 17, 44, 53, 90, 140, 143, 145, 163, 182, 287
diabetic glomerulosclerosis, 6, 15, 16, 18, 140, 150, 281
diabetic kidney disease, xi, 45, 52, 65, 69, 81, 84, 86, 111, 112, 114, 115, 116, 119, 122, 124, 126, 131, 135, 138, 148, 152, 157, 181, 199, 208, 233, 240, 312, 330
diabetic neuropathy, 204, 205, 214, 218
diabetic patients, 2, 7, 14, 17, 18, 22, 39, 40, 82, 89, 103, 104, 108, 112, 114, 117, 118, 131, 132, 133, 142, 144, 154, 156, 175, 176, 177, 178, 179, 183, 193, 200, 201, 205, 212, 217, 231, 233, 234, 236, 241, 242, 248, 251, 256, 257, 260, 264, 267, 268, 269, 277, 284, 318, 327, 333, 334
diabetic retinopathy, 14, 136, 154, 218, 232, 233, 260, 324, 333
diacylglycerol, 173, 174, 251
dialysis, 22, 39, 162, 176, 317, 331
diaphragm, 134, 135, 273, 274, 275, 277, 279, 282, 283, 284, 302, 312
diet, 2, 38, 42, 58, 66, 97, 98, 99, 100, 101, 107, 108, 193, 213, 271, 288, 296, 309
dietary fat, 207
dietary supplementation, 212
differential diagnosis, viii, 15
diffuse lesion, 6, 16

dimerization, 128, 241
direct action, 299
direct measure, 168
disease gene, 334
disease model, 115
disease progression, 170
diseases, 6, 9, 13, 16, 18, 41, 59, 81, 101, 116, 132, 134, 140, 153, 161, 173, 177, 185, 196, 204, 208, 218, 236, 259, 269, 284, 302, 326
disequilibrium, 28, 141, 175, 325, 326, 332
disorder, 5, 14, 15, 22, 24, 37, 135, 200, 208, 210, 239, 240, 317, 328
dissociation, 116, 132, 147, 295, 300, 303, 305
distribution, 126, 150, 167, 169, 189, 298, 299
diuretic, 41
DNA, 44, 54, 118, 141, 250, 278, 281, 294, 296, 318, 324
DNA damage, 44, 250, 324
DNA repair, 281
donors, 15, 18, 207
down-regulation, 94, 97, 114, 150, 208, 248, 267
Drosophila, 137, 295, 302, 307, 313
drug action, 41
drug discovery, 65
drug therapy, 40
drugs, 39, 40, 41, 67, 100, 103, 163, 170, 201, 254, 320
dyslipidemia, 58, 215
dysplasia, 265

E

ECM, 35, 114, 115, 117, 119, 122, 127, 128, 174, 323
ECM degradation, 114
eIF4A, 290, 291, 292, 304
electron, 5, 6, 12, 13, 78, 120, 130, 205, 206, 207, 208, 241, 277, 279, 283
electron microscopy, 5, 6, 130
electrons, 203, 208, 209, 240
ELISA, 54, 177, 196, 222
elongation, 70, 289, 292, 294, 297, 298, 300, 301, 303, 305, 306, 311
elucidation, 135
embryology, 126
embryonic stem cells, 54
emission, 190
encoding, 214, 293, 323, 324, 325, 327, 334, 335
end stage renal disease worldwide, 1
endocrine, 162
endothelial (eNOS), viii, xi, 7, 25, 30, 34, 35, 37, 45, 51, 57, 64, 65, 69, 72, 77, 78, 79, 81, 82, 84, 85, 86, 87, 88, 89, 90, 91, 95, 98, 108, 113, 114, 115,

119, 120, 121, 123, 124, 127, 128, 129, 132, 134, 135, 141, 142, 143, 146, 147, 152, 153, 154, 155, 156, 159, 164, 165, 171, 173, 182, 202, 205, 206, 207, 209, 210, 213, 214, 215, 216, 217, 218, 219, 220, 221, 222, 223, 224, 226, 227, 228, 229, 230, 231, 232, 233, 234, 235, 239, 240, 241, 242, 243, 244, 245, 246, 247, 248, 249, 250, 251, 252, 253, 254, 255, 256, 257, 259, 260, 261, 262, 263, 264, 265, 266, 267, 268, 269, 270, 271, 280, 287, 288, 308, 310, 322, 323, 325, 333
endothelial cells, 7, 34, 51, 64, 72, 77, 78, 79, 85, 88, 91, 95, 99, 119, 121, 123, 124, 132, 134, 135, 146, 147, 159, 171, 173, 182, 202, 205, 209, 214, 215, 218, 223, 244, 248, 249, 251, 252, 253, 254, 255, 257, 261, 263, 264, 266, 267, 268, 269, 280
endothelial dysfunction, viii, xi, 51, 57, 65, 78, 81, 82, 88, 89, 91, 99, 134, 143, 165, 217, 220, 221, 223, 224, 227, 228, 235, 239, 240, 241, 242, 247, 251, 252, 253, 254, 255, 256, 257, 267, 270, 288
endothelial NO synthase, 240, 265, 269
endothelium, 64, 72, 87, 98, 108, 134, 170, 181, 217, 220, 221, 222, 226, 227, 232, 239, 240, 241, 242, 243, 245, 249, 250, 252, 253, 254, 258, 261, 262, 266, 267, 269
end-stage renal disease, 45, 93, 161, 166, 175, 231, 239, 259, 260, 315, 317, 329, 331, 333, 334
enzymatic activity, 73, 172, 251, 294
enzyme, 46, 47, 64, 67, 71, 74, 77, 78, 85, 87, 110, 120, 137, 142, 144, 145, 146, 170, 174, 177, 181, 185, 187, 188, 189, 190, 191, 193, 194, 201, 203, 205, 206, 207, 211, 212, 224, 228, 240, 241, 243, 252, 253, 294, 310, 321, 327, 328, 331, 332
enzyme inhibitors, 110, 137, 142, 191
enzymes, 114, 120, 166, 189, 201, 205, 208, 264, 276, 281
epithelial cells, 10, 12, 51, 69, 71, 73, 74, 77, 78, 84, 85, 86, 104, 110, 114, 115, 120, 121, 122, 123, 124, 125, 127, 148, 149, 157, 172, 202, 214, 244, 250, 264, 273, 278, 282, 283, 285, 296, 297, 298, 299, 300, 308, 310, 311, 313
epithelium, 76, 91
erythropoietin, 113, 159
ester, 165, 190, 292
estrogen, 251, 253
ethnic background, 118, 133, 327
ethnicity, 22, 317
etiology, 49, 259, 315
eukaryotic, 70, 292, 303, 304, 305, 306, 307, 312
excretion, 23, 31, 32, 33, 36, 39, 40, 42, 46, 51, 53, 54, 57, 81, 82, 96, 100, 102, 106, 112, 130, 131, 132, 133, 140, 142, 154, 156, 157, 158, 164, 177, 179, 196, 197, 217, 223, 228, 229, 230, 242, 244, 257, 277, 279, 284, 285

exons, 116, 127, 128
experimental design, 129, 324
experimentaldiabetic nephropathy, 205
exposure, 69, 71, 72, 73, 74, 75, 78, 79, 89, 93, 104, 123, 125, 163, 203, 228, 251, 264, 279
extracellular matrix, 12, 35, 36, 45, 72, 73, 74, 76, 77, 79, 81, 94, 95, 102, 114, 115, 139, 142, 145, 146, 148, 151, 163, 172, 173, 174, 191, 279, 285, 295, 300, 303, 310, 312, 313, 322, 323, 335
extraction, 252
extracts, 117, 172

F

FAD, 206, 240
false positive, 327
fat, 66, 101, 107, 288, 322
fatty acids, 64, 73, 87, 181, 207, 241, 251, 267
femoral artery, 27, 117
ferritin, 248
fetal development, 84
fibrin, 7, 9, 74, 246
fibrinogen, 11
fibroblast growth factor, 91, 147, 158
fibroblasts, 91, 119, 120, 123, 124, 141, 145, 146, 205
fibrocytes, 124
fibrogenesis, 151
fibrosis, 11, 16, 23, 30, 33, 36, 41, 52, 53, 59, 64, 69, 73, 74, 76, 77, 81, 84, 96, 106, 112, 113, 114, 115, 123, 124, 125, 127, 139, 140, 145, 147, 149, 150, 151, 162, 166, 170, 173, 200, 215, 225, 227, 231, 234, 246, 277, 280, 295, 299, 301, 302
filament, 73, 312
filtration, 6, 21, 23, 24, 25, 26, 28, 29, 72, 81, 84, 92, 95, 97, 119, 122, 127, 135, 155, 156, 157, 162, 182, 243, 257, 273, 274, 277, 296, 302, 316
flavinmononucleotide (FMN), 206, 241
flexibility, 59, 137
fluctuations, 202
fluid, 44, 119, 164, 166, 168, 185
focal segmental glomerulosclerosis, 9, 15, 27, 170, 246, 276, 283
free radicals, 143, 200, 324
fructose, 120, 146, 203, 321
functional changes, 56, 104, 161, 228, 229, 278
fusion, 38, 130

G

gastroparesis, 23
Gcn4p, 306

GDP, 293, 301, 312
gene expression, 72, 73, 84, 85, 86, 94, 105, 120, 139, 140, 141, 145, 146, 148, 151, 153, 174, 175, 190, 192, 193, 217, 236, 251, 264, 266, 284, 286, 289, 293, 295, 298, 302, 304, 306, 311, 313
gene promoter, 192, 267, 333
gene silencing, 252, 307
gene therapy, 112, 158
gene transfer, 241, 257
genes, vii, 3, 37, 52, 53, 54, 63, 75, 87, 113, 114, 116, 118, 123, 131, 141, 148, 193, 195, 240, 246, 250, 270, 285, 289, 294, 296, 313, 317, 318, 319, 323, 326, 327, 328, 330, 332
genetic background, 93, 182, 249
genetic defect, 208
genetic factors, 1, 118, 221, 315, 317
genetic marker, 315, 326
genetic predisposition, 141, 163, 332
genetic traits, 195
genetics, ix, xi, 37, 50, 67, 84, 131, 154, 317, 318, 330, 334
genome, 54, 55, 56, 72, 86, 315, 317, 318, 319, 326, 327, 329
genomics, 63, 307
genotype, 175, 193, 222, 318, 320, 324, 325
genotyping, 318, 319
gestation, 84
gestational diabetes, 22
glomerular capillary, 5, 7, 11, 18, 26, 28, 38, 39, 40, 41, 42, 44, 95, 119, 132, 143, 164, 248, 250, 262, 265, 298, 316
glomeruli, 6, 10, 15, 16, 35, 43, 50, 52, 56, 59, 70, 74, 77, 87, 97, 115, 123, 125, 126, 127, 130, 131, 132, 138, 139, 140, 142, 146, 149, 152, 153, 157, 158, 166, 168, 169, 174, 190, 191, 196, 200, 202, 228, 236, 244, 245, 247, 248, 250, 251, 253, 255, 258, 261, 279, 280, 285, 286, 287, 301, 302, 316
glomerulonephritis, 5, 14, 15, 26, 260, 283, 285, 303
glomerulonephropathy, 6, 7, 9, 14, 15
glomerulus, 11, 12, 15, 17, 24, 25, 26, 36, 38, 74, 115, 119, 126, 155, 168, 171, 243, 249, 274, 276, 277, 278, 279, 283, 284, 320
glucagon, 119
glucose oxidase, 120
glucose tolerance, 269
GLUT, 30, 34, 51, 74, 79, 202, 223
GLUT4, 281, 324
glutamine, 120, 146, 321
glutathione, 203, 212, 321
glycerol, 207
glycine, 113, 304
glycogen, 23, 73, 301, 312
glycolysis, 78, 199, 202, 204, 207, 217, 253

glycoproteins, 94, 114
glycosaminoglycans, 72, 86
glycosylated hemoglobin, 83
glycosylation, viii, 30, 34, 36, 38, 45, 71, 77, 78, 105, 106, 108, 158, 214, 215, 224, 230, 251, 266, 316, 321
granules, 25, 168, 172, 302, 313
growth arrest, 294
growth factor, vii, viii, xi, 3, 26, 34, 35, 36, 37, 42, 45, 50, 66, 69, 75, 76, 84, 87, 88, 91, 94, 103, 111, 116, 119, 121, 123, 125, 126, 127, 128, 129, 131, 134, 135, 136, 138, 139, 140, 141, 144, 145, 147, 148, 150, 151, 152, 153, 154, 155, 156, 157, 158, 166, 173, 181, 192, 205, 213, 219, 220, 223, 227, 233, 244, 264, 285, 287, 296, 299, 303, 308, 310, 321, 322, 332
growth hormone, 119, 156, 157
guanine, 293, 321

H

half-life, 266, 295
haplotypes, 259
heart disease, 56
heart failure, 41, 42, 59, 189, 250, 265
heat shock protein, 73, 74, 85, 253, 255
hematocrit, 27, 44
hematuria, 14
heme, 73, 241, 248, 264
heme oxygenase, 73, 248, 264
hemisphere, vii
hemoglobin, 16, 39, 156
hepatitis, 293
hepatocytes, 175, 192
heterogeneity, 210, 242, 318
heterozygote, 30
high blood pressure, 330
histamine, 189, 251
histology, 23, 84, 118, 127, 131, 162, 334
history, viii, 1, 17, 52, 137, 176, 315, 317
HIV, 192, 321
HIV-1, 192
homeostasis, 42, 52, 103, 166, 201, 202, 203, 224, 239, 241, 251, 253, 254, 267, 268, 269
homocysteine, 258
homozygote, 30
human genome, 318
human health, 55, 97
human subjects, 97
hyaline, 5, 7, 9, 10, 15, 16, 23, 246
hyalinosis lesions, 5, 6, 15, 17
hybridization, 131, 148, 184, 185
hydraulic transmembrane pressure, 27

Index

hydrogen, 78, 120, 174, 200, 201, 253, 321
hydrogen peroxide, 120, 174, 200, 201, 253, 321
hydrolysis, 291, 292, 293, 297, 305
hydronephrosis, 58
hydroxyl, 200, 287
hypercholesterolemia, 267
hyperglycaemia, 199, 200, 202, 203, 204, 206, 207, 208, 210
hyperglycemia, vii, viii, xi, 1, 21, 23, 30, 34, 36, 38, 44, 49, 56, 58, 59, 63, 69, 70, 71, 72, 73, 74, 75, 76, 78, 79, 80, 81, 82, 84, 85, 86, 87, 88, 91, 93, 100, 101, 111, 115, 118, 119, 120, 125, 129, 130, 131, 140, 146, 157, 170, 171, 181, 215, 217, 221, 222, 224, 225, 227, 229, 233, 246, 251, 254, 266, 269, 278, 280, 288, 298, 299, 316, 323, 332
hyperinsulinemia, 56, 221, 226, 235, 246, 249, 300, 310
hyperkalemia, 23, 39, 42
hyperlipidemia, 57, 58, 59, 63
hyperplasia, 296
hypertension, vii, 1, 3, 10, 22, 23, 27, 33, 37, 39, 40, 44, 45, 46, 47, 49, 53, 58, 59, 64, 67, 71, 75, 92, 98, 99, 110, 117, 118, 119, 132, 137, 139, 142, 143, 166, 170, 172, 173, 176, 177, 182, 183, 184, 185, 186, 189, 190, 193, 195, 196, 206, 207, 211, 221, 223, 224, 228, 229, 236, 246, 247, 252, 263, 265
hypertrophy, 30, 39, 44, 56, 70, 71, 76, 85, 87, 88, 90, 96, 114, 115, 116, 119, 124, 126, 127, 138, 139, 144, 148, 149, 152, 153, 156, 163, 164, 173, 184, 192, 200, 206, 214, 216, 218, 224, 229, 243, 244, 280, 281, 286, 287, 295, 296, 297, 298, 300, 301, 303, 308, 309, 310, 312, 316
hypothesis, 18, 24, 26, 44, 50, 131, 159, 161, 182, 184, 210, 212, 227, 229, 284, 320, 326
hypoxia, 76, 87, 113, 223, 232, 248
hypoxia-inducible factor, 87

I

ibuprofen, 229
IFN, 150
immune regulation, 221
immunofluorescence, 5, 15, 135
immunoglobulin, 11, 204
immunoglobulin superfamily, 204
immunohistochemistry, 115, 166, 185, 243, 250
immunoreactivity, 167, 169
improvements, 176, 204, 205
in situ hybridization, 115, 166
in utero, 69, 84
in vitro, viii, 35, 36, 49, 50, 51, 52, 63, 70, 71, 72, 73, 74, 77, 78, 79, 84, 95, 98, 101, 106, 110, 119, 123, 133, 135, 173, 189, 195, 201, 202, 208, 210, 219, 222, 227, 228, 230, 241, 254, 273, 279, 287, 297, 305, 307
in vivo, viii, 35, 70, 73, 79, 84, 88, 89, 106, 110, 123, 124, 126, 131, 134, 148, 156, 173, 175, 201, 202, 204, 207, 208, 209, 210, 219, 222, 228, 230, 241, 254, 266, 279, 297
inducer, 125, 248
inducible (iNOS), 51, 55, 64, 76, 87, 99, 121, 130, 149, 165, 194, 206, 207, 215, 220, 222, 223, 225, 226, 235, 243, 245, 246, 248, 260, 264, 294
inducible protein, 294
induction, 71, 77, 91, 96, 108, 121, 124, 125, 127, 130, 140, 145, 146, 148, 152, 165, 173, 185, 191, 192, 208, 224, 248, 269, 277, 281, 299, 302, 310, 322
inflammation, 10, 11, 23, 34, 51, 53, 64, 69, 76, 87, 90, 98, 104, 105, 147, 170, 173, 177, 191, 197, 206, 240, 247, 249, 256, 257, 258, 321, 322
inflammatory cells, 279
inflammatory responses, 94, 204, 221
INS, 311
insertion, 133, 162, 193, 221, 320, 331, 332
insulin, 5, 17, 18, 22, 23, 27, 28, 29, 30, 37, 43, 46, 47, 56, 58, 66, 71, 72, 75, 76, 81, 86, 91, 98, 99, 107, 108, 115, 119, 125, 129, 133, 137, 143, 152, 156, 157, 158, 168, 175, 181, 192, 193, 211, 213, 222, 226, 228, 243, 244, 247, 249, 251, 257, 265, 266, 267, 284, 296, 298, 300, 301, 311, 312, 313, 316, 321, 325, 333, 334
insulin dependent diabetes, 137
insulin resistance, 22, 30, 37, 47, 56, 58, 66, 98, 99, 192, 228, 251, 257, 265, 266, 267, 298, 300, 311, 321
insulin sensitivity, 107, 298, 325
insulin signaling, 108, 226, 250, 251, 267, 300, 311
insulin-dependent diabetes mellitus (IDDM), 5, 6, 18, 46, 158, 181, 258, 284, 332, 333
insulinoma, 27
integrin, 114, 124, 125, 147, 149, 276, 278, 282, 283, 285, 287
integrins, 122, 125, 274, 278, 281, 285
integrity, 37, 73, 97, 99, 134, 248, 328
interface, 208
interference, 75, 99, 127, 136, 299, 300, 307
interleukin-8, 192
internalization, 248
intervention, 27, 40, 96, 101, 136, 156, 202, 210, 256, 279, 301, 303
intravenously, 223
ionizing radiation, 148
iron, 208, 217
irradiation, 148

ischemia, 14, 99, 189, 206, 223, 224, 247, 252
isolation, 15
isozymes, 77

K

ketoacidosis, 23, 29
kidney failure, vii, 220
kinase activity, 113, 297, 300

L

lactoferrin, 109
L-arginine, 206, 220, 225, 226, 230, 234, 235, 241, 252, 257, 266, 267
latency, 122, 147
LDL, 121, 207, 240, 241
lead, vii, 33, 34, 38, 42, 50, 75, 78, 84, 102, 122, 123, 149, 163, 164, 165, 177, 209, 210, 225, 242, 248, 256, 281, 303, 316, 319, 320, 324, 330
leptin, 30, 56, 70, 113
lesions, 5, 6, 7, 9, 11, 13, 14, 15, 16, 17, 18, 19, 43, 45, 46, 53, 56, 58, 60, 106, 157, 215, 221, 225, 234, 246, 249, 282, 316
leucine, 293
life expectancy, 81
ligand, 75, 113, 114, 123, 125, 126, 152, 184, 204
light, 5, 15, 70, 116, 134, 155, 167, 169
light microscopy methods, 70
lipid metabolism, 152, 283, 310, 325
lipid peroxidation, 106, 173, 190
lipids, 51, 94, 99, 136, 200, 208, 324
lipooxygenase, 279
lipoproteins, 334
liposomes, 136
liver, 128, 156, 185, 300
localization, 52, 130, 167, 168, 171, 184, 185, 186, 189, 251, 313
loci, 86, 118, 326, 327
locus, 141, 195, 318, 327
longevity, 287, 288
longitudinal study, 133
low-density lipoprotein, 108
low-grade inflammation, 257
lumen, 7, 9, 166, 168, 239, 274
Luo, 88, 258
lupus, 14, 56, 283
lysine, 66, 74, 82, 94, 98, 106
lysozyme, 94, 96, 100, 101, 104, 106, 109

M

macromolecules, 34, 200, 239
macrophage inflammatory protein, 77, 89
macrophages, 7, 23, 51, 76, 114, 220
Maillard reaction, 204, 205, 214
malnutrition, 26
mammalian cells, 304, 306, 308, 330
mammalian tissues, 114
mammals, 254
manganese, 77, 201, 212, 322, 324, 333
marrow, 124
mass, 26, 33, 43, 44, 45, 117, 231
mast cells, 172, 189
matrix, 5, 6, 21, 23, 30, 33, 34, 35, 36, 39, 42, 50, 51, 58, 61, 64, 72, 74, 76, 77, 89, 91, 94, 95, 96, 99, 104, 112, 113, 114, 115, 116, 123, 125, 131, 132, 134, 140, 144, 145, 147, 152, 157, 158, 173, 229, 276, 280, 285, 286, 295, 300, 301, 310, 320, 322, 324
matrix metalloproteinase, 74, 95, 104, 322
MCP, 76, 77, 91, 92, 124, 125, 127
MCP-1, 76, 77, 91, 92, 124, 125, 127
mean arterial pressure, 27, 38, 244
measurement, 132
measurements, 27, 38, 116, 118, 244, 245
mechanical stress, 36, 74, 142, 281
mechanistic explanations, 161
media, 36, 72, 119, 122
medulla, 42, 126, 244, 261
mellitus, 5, 15, 16, 18, 21, 22, 23, 24, 30, 34, 36, 37, 39, 40, 41, 42, 70, 93, 99, 139, 143, 156, 158, 161, 162, 163, 177, 181, 183, 186, 231, 315
membranes, 6, 12, 73, 166, 168, 200, 321
membranoproliferative glomerulonephritis, 5, 14, 15, 16
membranous glomerulonephritis, 154
mesangial cells, 23, 34, 35, 36, 37, 45, 50, 64, 71, 72, 74, 75, 76, 77, 78, 79, 85, 87, 88, 92, 95, 102, 113, 119, 120, 121, 122, 123, 125, 126, 138, 139, 141, 142, 143, 144, 145, 146, 147, 148, 149, 150, 151, 152, 157, 158, 159, 168, 174, 190, 191, 202, 204, 213, 217, 220, 222, 228, 232, 236, 281, 296, 300, 310
mesangial matrix production, 51
mesangial sclerosis, 6, 16, 17, 130, 135, 316
messenger RNA, 184, 308
messengers, vii, 192, 205, 220, 228, 229
meta-analysis, 63, 175, 193, 222, 232
metabolic acidosis, 42
metabolic changes, 119
metabolic disorders, 190
metabolic pathways, 119, 223, 232

Index

metabolic syndrome, 46, 59, 99, 163, 177, 181, 228, 231, 268, 269, 309
metabolism, 44, 86, 88, 94, 142, 173, 188, 199, 201, 202, 214, 223, 224, 232, 253, 267, 294, 301, 310, 311, 321, 322, 325
metabolites, 120, 142, 164, 190, 204, 210, 214, 223, 242, 243, 252
metabolized, 230
metal ion, 205
metalloproteinase, 276
metformin, 71, 103, 254, 297
methodology, 63, 111
microaneurysms, 5, 6, 247
microcirculation, 73, 132, 165, 188, 230, 232
micrograms, 30
microRNA, 76, 149, 302, 303, 307
microspheres, 96
migration, 72, 77, 112, 128, 129, 151, 158, 227, 263
mineralocorticoid, 41, 46
miniature, 66
minimal change disease, 14, 15
minimal change nephrotic syndrome, 37
MIP, 77
mitochondria, 77, 200, 207, 208, 209, 210, 217, 236, 299, 324
mitogen, 108, 142, 146, 162, 174, 191, 192, 267, 279, 280
mitosis, 227
MMP, 95, 104
modules, 125, 328
molecular oxygen, 206, 208
molecular weight, 102, 264
molecules, 38, 71, 76, 77, 78, 79, 84, 94, 99, 113, 123, 162, 173, 190, 204, 231, 239, 240, 253, 264, 274, 276, 284, 323
momentum, ix
monoclonal antibody, 169, 186
monocyte chemoattractant protein, 76, 124, 177
monolayer, 35, 124
morbidity, 2, 3, 80, 176, 180, 229, 315
morphogenesis, 69, 84, 149
morphology, 5, 16, 17, 248, 250, 281
morphometric, 277
mortality, 2, 3, 22, 41, 45, 80, 130, 176, 180, 193, 229, 242, 252, 257, 315
mortality rate, 130
motif, 113, 123, 125, 307
mRNA, 36, 37, 71, 72, 73, 74, 76, 98, 115, 116, 117, 119, 120, 123, 125, 129, 131, 132, 139, 140, 142, 145, 146, 151, 153, 157, 166, 168, 177, 185, 186, 196, 243, 245, 251, 266, 277, 279, 289, 290, 291, 292, 293, 294, 295, 296, 297, 298, 299, 300, 301, 302, 303, 304, 305, 307, 308, 310, 311, 313

mRNAs, 168, 184, 289, 291, 292, 293, 295, 302, 303, 306, 307
multiple alleles, 323
multiple myeloma, 26, 28
multivariate analysis, 132
Munich-Wistar rats, 24, 27, 38, 44
mutant, 30, 31, 66, 121, 149, 170, 299
mutation, 56, 221, 243, 259, 310, 317
mutations, 135, 208, 334
myoblasts, 84
myofibroblasts, 124
myosin, 134, 155, 274

N

Na^+, 78, 86, 276
NaCl, 32, 327, 328, 329
NAD, 78, 199, 200, 203, 204, 205, 206, 207, 216, 233, 245, 262, 299
NADH, 203, 207, 208, 217, 218
nanoparticles, 136
National Institutes of Health, 211, 220
necrosis, 6, 14, 18, 75, 86, 205, 208, 266, 267
neovascularization, 132, 134, 153
nephrectomy, 26, 33, 214, 296
nephritic syndrome, 2, 276
nephritis, 14, 138
nephromegaly, 164
nephron, 21, 24, 25, 26, 29, 31, 33, 44, 79, 119, 141, 166, 168, 169, 183, 185, 186, 190, 231, 262, 321, 328
nephrosis, 58, 283
nephrotic syndrome, 10, 14, 15, 16, 316
nerve, 25, 66, 79, 91, 214, 216
neural function, 204
neurodegeneration, 104, 212
neuronal (nNOS), 31, 33, 165, 183, 202, 206, 217, 220, 221, 224, 243, 245, 246, 252, 262, 312
neurons, 220
neuropathy, 206, 225
neutral, 185
neutrophils, 10, 94, 205
NH2, 263
nicotinamide, 200, 207, 240
nitrates, 220
nitric oxide, viii, 30, 31, 33, 34, 50, 51, 52, 64, 65, 72, 82, 85, 87, 88, 90, 91, 92, 98, 99, 105, 108, 119, 130, 145, 155, 162, 164, 165, 182, 183, 199, 200, 206, 216, 217, 219, 220, 221, 222, 223, 227, 228, 229, 231, 232, 233, 234, 235, 236, 239, 240, 256, 257, 258, 259, 260, 261, 262, 263, 264, 265, 266, 267, 268, 269, 270, 271, 322, 325, 333

nitric oxide synthase, 30, 31, 33, 51, 64, 72, 82, 87, 88, 90, 92, 98, 105, 108, 162, 182, 183, 199, 200, 206, 216, 217, 222, 231, 232, 234, 235, 239, 256, 257, 259, 260, 261, 262, 263, 265, 266, 267, 268, 269, 271, 322, 325, 333
nitrite, 226, 235
nitrogen, 108, 201
nitrogen dioxide, 201
nitrous oxide, 201
NO synthases, 230, 260
Nobel Prize, 22, 53
nodular intercapillarv glonneruloselerosis, 6
nodules, 6, 7, 8, 13, 15, 16, 33, 53, 58, 87, 131, 250, 263
non-insulin dependent diabetes, 5, 47, 182, 211
non-insulin dependent diabetes mellitus (NIDIM), 5
norepinephrine, 29, 44
Nrf2, 52, 65, 264
NSAIDs, 229
nuclei, 116
nucleic acid, 208
nucleotides, 306
nucleus, 114, 127, 294

O

obesity, 1, 22, 30, 37, 55, 56, 58, 59, 66, 139, 162, 181, 209, 213, 252, 266, 279, 298, 300, 321
obstructive uropathy, 47
organ, 37, 47, 50, 70, 77, 84, 103, 170, 200, 201, 239
organism, 52
organs, 23, 132, 136, 189, 209
ornithine, 241
osmotic pressure, 25, 26, 28
osmotic stress, 203
osteonectin, 114
overlap, 70, 250
overproduction, 93, 95, 225, 241, 245
overweight, 254
oxidation, 64, 82, 94, 173, 200, 202, 204, 206, 207, 241, 244, 252, 253, 324
oxidative damage, 207, 209, 218, 225
oxidative stress, viii, xi, 34, 36, 47, 51, 56, 64, 73, 78, 83, 85, 86, 87, 88, 90, 91, 92, 93, 94, 98, 106, 109, 120, 122, 123, 139, 146, 148, 154, 163, 169, 173, 181, 183, 186, 191, 196, 197, 199, 200, 203, 204, 206, 210, 212, 213, 214, 222, 223, 225, 232, 234, 241, 242, 245, 250, 251, 252, 253, 261, 268, 269, 281, 287, 288, 296, 298, 321, 324, 325, 333
oxygen, 77, 85, 120, 123, 174, 190, 192, 193, 200, 203, 208, 209, 217, 223, 225, 232, 236, 292

P

p53, 213, 254
pancreas, 21, 22, 27, 30, 37, 39, 46, 222, 321
pancreas transplant, 39, 46
papillary necrosis, 14, 18
paradigm shift, 184
parenchyma, 6, 78, 226
participants, 327
pathogenesis, vii, viii, xi, 1, 2, 3, 18, 21, 31, 34, 35, 42, 44, 45, 49, 50, 51, 52, 54, 56, 57, 59, 63, 70, 78, 79, 81, 84, 89, 91, 94, 97, 105, 106, 111, 112, 113, 140, 150, 158, 161, 163, 180, 181, 182, 184, 190, 199, 206, 207, 208, 214, 215, 217, 219, 220, 225, 227, 228, 229, 231, 234, 236, 242, 247, 250, 254, 255, 261, 262, 264, 280, 286, 299, 302, 303, 315, 316, 317, 319, 320, 321, 323, 324, 325, 326, 327, 328, 330, 333
pathogens, 233
pathologist, 10
pathology, viii, 52, 117, 129, 130, 132, 208, 218, 248, 250, 330
pathophysiological, xi, 45, 50, 57, 116, 118, 172, 224, 234
pathophysiology, viii, 1, 37, 42, 49, 51, 52, 99, 126, 129, 133, 163, 170, 181, 208, 220, 223, 251, 277, 287, 320, 323, 325
pathways, 50, 52, 74, 76, 83, 93, 94, 100, 103, 108, 110, 114, 118, 120, 121, 122, 123, 124, 125, 138, 148, 161, 162, 163, 166, 170, 172, 173, 175, 189, 192, 199, 201, 203, 204, 205, 210, 212, 216, 223, 230, 239, 240, 241, 249, 251, 253, 256, 279, 301, 302, 311, 327, 328, 330
pattern recognition, 204
PCR, 117, 184
penetrance, 326
peptide, 77, 119, 122, 125, 147, 152, 169, 170, 177, 186, 289, 290, 291, 293, 323
peptides, 94, 102, 109, 113, 136, 165, 166, 172, 187, 188, 220, 252, 266, 323
perfusion, 35, 183, 244, 245, 247, 248, 249, 256, 261
peripheral blood, 270
peripheral blood mononuclear cell, 270
peripheral neuropathy, 214
peripheral vascular disease, 23
permeability, 25, 26, 45, 117, 119, 127, 128, 134, 135, 149, 153, 208, 218, 227, 248, 264, 265, 280, 287, 298, 325
permeation, 284
permission, iv, 25
permit, 293
peroxidation, 190
peroxide, 145, 174, 191, 201, 253

peroxynitrite, 201, 223, 225, 234, 241, 253
personal communication, 247
PGE, 229
PGN, 16
pH, 64, 172, 204
phagocytosis, 330
pharmacokinetics, 268
pharmacological treatment, 320
pharmacology, 41, 257
phenotype, 73, 95, 213, 247, 249, 281, 318
phenotypes, 155, 190, 281, 295
Philadelphia, 43, 153
phosphate, 78, 92, 120, 146, 200, 202, 203, 204, 207, 214, 240, 251, 265, 321
phospholipids, 266
phosphorylation, 36, 70, 74, 79, 89, 95, 104, 113, 120, 121, 125, 126, 128, 129, 130, 132, 134, 135, 137, 155, 207, 208, 210, 251, 253, 261, 266, 269, 280, 281, 292, 293, 294, 297, 298, 299, 300, 301, 305, 306, 308, 309, 312
photomicrographs, 167, 169
physical properties, 99
physicians, 317, 318
Physiological, 188, 257, 309
physiology, 44, 147, 181, 184, 220
PI3K, 71, 114, 249, 263, 280, 292, 296, 297, 298, 299, 300, 301
placebo, 40, 46, 97, 132, 176, 214
placenta, 127
plasma levels, 115, 118, 287, 298, 320
plasma membrane, 202, 276
plasma proteins, 7, 273
plasminogen, 79, 147
platelet aggregation, 240
platelet derived growth factor (PDGF), viii, 112, 157, 158, 205
platelets, 114, 122
playing, 275, 323
podocytes, viii, 36, 43, 51, 69, 71, 72, 73, 74, 75, 78, 86, 90, 91, 95, 97, 105, 112, 114, 119, 120, 123, 124, 125, 126, 131, 135, 138, 141, 142, 145, 148, 150, 151, 152, 155, 158, 168, 220, 244, 250, 274, 275, 276, 277, 278, 279, 280, 281, 282, 283, 284, 285, 286, 287, 302
point mutation, 30
polycystic kidney disease, 302, 313
polymerase, 78, 89, 91, 225, 294
polymers, 136
polymorphism, 30, 37, 118, 133, 141, 154, 155, 159, 175, 193, 195, 212, 221, 231, 243, 259, 260, 320, 324, 325, 331, 332, 333, 334

polymorphisms, 118, 133, 141, 161, 175, 201, 207, 218, 219, 221, 232, 243, 259, 260, 316, 323, 324, 325, 326, 327, 329, 332, 333, 334
polypeptide, 113, 291, 293, 305, 321
polyuria, 30
population, 3, 162, 176, 181, 260, 317, 326, 327, 331, 333, 334
positive correlation, 129, 228
positive feedback, 79, 120, 192, 253
potassium, 42, 142, 164
pressure gradient, 26
primate, 43, 58, 66
progenitor cells, 281
pro-inflammatory, 94, 98
proliferation, 27, 50, 72, 76, 88, 92, 112, 113, 114, 124, 127, 128, 129, 134, 141, 144, 149, 150, 151, 158, 159, 163, 189, 221, 224, 227, 239, 247, 254, 278, 281, 285, 287, 312, 320, 322
proline, 323
promoter, 79, 113, 120, 121, 122, 125, 133, 146, 175, 194, 195, 212, 243, 306, 323, 325
propagation, 113
propetide, 122
prostaglandins, viii, 51, 72, 165, 219, 220, 228, 229, 236
protease inhibitors, 172
protection, 41, 47, 57, 103, 163, 170, 200, 201, 202, 203, 205, 223, 249, 271, 281, 316, 320, 323, 325
protective role, 52, 65, 134, 170, 254, 257
protein family, 328
protein kinase C, 36, 37, 45, 57, 66, 87, 91, 93, 109, 119, 120, 122, 143, 146, 173, 174, 190, 210, 216, 224, 251, 258, 266, 293, 322
protein kinases, 190, 191
protein structure, 95
protein synthesis, 36, 42, 70, 141, 145, 157, 173, 191, 278, 296, 297, 298, 300, 301, 303, 304, 306, 308, 310, 311, 312, 313
proteinase, 74, 173
proteinuria, 12, 14, 15, 17, 18, 24, 27, 36, 37, 38, 40, 51, 56, 58, 59, 71, 92, 97, 113, 117, 130, 131, 133, 134, 137, 138, 141, 144, 147, 154, 157, 163, 170, 175, 176, 181, 195, 207, 224, 226, 227, 229, 237, 242, 245, 264, 270, 277, 278, 279, 280, 284, 302, 316, 327
proteoglycans, 120, 128, 248, 276
proteome, 302
proximal convoluted tubules, 166
proximal straight tubules, 166
proximal tubules, 27, 78, 125, 166, 167, 169, 188, 252, 327, 328
PTEN, 71, 75, 88, 267, 298, 310
pulmonary arteries, 172

pyelonephritis, 10, 14, 18

R

RANTES, 125
RAS blockade, 161, 179, 195, 205, 210, 211
rat kidneys, 151, 185, 243
reactive oxygen, 51, 69, 77, 79, 87, 91, 102, 108, 148, 162, 174, 186, 190, 191, 199, 200, 218, 223, 225, 230, 241, 254, 255, 269, 279, 286, 299, 310, 316
receptor sites, 143
receptors, 36, 41, 42, 66, 90, 94, 95, 113, 114, 115, 122, 126, 128, 130, 134, 136, 137, 138, 139, 141, 143, 149, 151, 152, 157, 166, 168, 169, 172, 186, 190, 205, 244, 251, 255, 265, 269, 279, 280, 285, 287, 310, 320, 323
reflux nephropathy, 9
regeneration, 273
regression, 15, 43, 45, 47, 58, 151, 170
rehydration, 109
renal cell carcinoma, 313
renal dysfunction, 6, 45, 71, 146, 153, 176, 244, 281, 287, 310
renal failure, 22, 23, 24, 33, 34, 38, 39, 49, 53, 57, 58, 59, 63, 101, 107, 131, 162, 166, 170, 177, 224, 227, 229, 242, 243, 267
renal level, 112
renal medulla, 223, 232, 302
renal replacement therapy, vii, 22, 24, 40, 93, 220
renin, vii, xi, 21, 34, 40, 41, 42, 47, 64, 65, 72, 75, 78, 79, 81, 90, 91, 92, 100, 103, 109, 111, 115, 142, 143, 144, 145, 162, 166, 168, 169, 177, 181, 183, 184, 185, 186, 187, 188, 192, 193, 194, 195, 196, 200, 211, 219, 227, 260, 283, 286, 299, 320, 327, 332
repression, 293, 295, 307, 311
repressor, 311
researchers, xi, 120, 132
residues, 128, 137, 252, 280, 292, 299
resistance, 28, 29, 41, 56, 90, 99, 107, 188, 189, 191, 235, 240, 266, 300, 302, 310
respiration, 201, 210, 213, 225, 228
response, 36, 41, 52, 71, 74, 75, 76, 77, 78, 79, 86, 87, 88, 90, 99, 109, 116, 118, 124, 125, 129, 135, 140, 148, 150, 158, 165, 171, 183, 190, 192, 199, 201, 213, 214, 221, 227, 240, 244, 245, 253, 258, 261, 269, 281, 286, 288, 289, 309, 312, 318
responsiveness, 119, 123, 142, 143, 183
restoration, 135, 165, 206, 271, 298
restriction enzyme, 318
restriction fragment length polymorphis, 318
resveratrol, 298

reticulum, 75, 266
retina, 66, 300
retinoblastoma, 296
retinopathy, 14, 23, 133, 154, 156, 224, 331
ribonucleic acid, 306
ribose, 78, 89, 91, 203, 225
ribosomal RNA, 303
ribosome, 290, 291, 292, 293, 295, 305, 306
risk, 1, 22, 46, 98, 107, 133, 154, 162, 163, 175, 181, 194, 200, 201, 211, 220, 224, 229, 231, 232, 240, 242, 243, 252, 257, 259, 260, 267, 315, 317, 320, 323, 324, 326, 330, 333
risk factors, 22, 154, 181, 220, 224, 229, 231, 242, 259
RNA, 71, 75, 290, 294, 296, 299, 300, 303, 304, 305, 307, 313
RNAs, 124, 308, 313
rodents, 57, 66, 115, 122, 168, 177, 203, 296, 299, 301

S

sclerosis, 6, 11, 14, 15, 16, 17, 35, 53, 56, 59, 63, 127, 130, 135, 224, 228, 231, 234, 282, 309, 316, 333
secretion, 37, 41, 74, 86, 99, 108, 120, 122, 124, 125, 144, 148, 184, 222, 279, 299
selectivity, 248, 264
senescence, 75, 248, 254, 264, 269
sensitivity, 14, 157, 300
sensitization, 115
serine, 36, 74, 89, 113, 137, 166, 172, 212, 292, 294, 299, 306, 312
serum, 40, 70, 71, 79, 81, 82, 83, 96, 97, 98, 99, 101, 103, 104, 106, 109, 112, 113, 132, 154, 156, 175, 176, 188, 193, 225, 229, 233, 242, 267
serum albumin, 71
severely hyperglycemic group, 29
sickle cell, 14
signal peptide, 113, 324
signal transduction, 45, 137, 173, 190, 205
signaling pathway, 3, 52, 69, 70, 71, 88, 95, 99, 105, 113, 114, 115, 120, 139, 145, 150, 152, 155, 157, 173, 191, 212, 224, 225, 229, 234, 251, 253, 261, 268, 279, 280, 286, 288, 292, 296, 299, 300, 301, 303, 311, 323
siRNA, 74, 156, 303
skeletal muscle, 99, 301, 312
skin, 96, 132, 258
smooth muscle, 37, 40, 41, 76, 88, 114, 121, 122, 123, 145, 163, 168, 172, 174, 184, 189, 205, 214, 218, 221, 222, 227, 239, 240, 254, 264, 320

smooth muscle cells, 37, 76, 88, 114, 121, 122, 123, 145, 163, 168, 172, 174, 184, 205, 214, 218, 239, 240, 254
SNP, 113, 243, 326, 328
sodium, 42, 71, 85, 89, 166, 184, 187, 237, 328
species, 42, 51, 56, 58, 59, 69, 77, 79, 85, 87, 91, 102, 108, 120, 148, 162, 174, 186, 189, 190, 191, 193, 199, 200, 217, 218, 223, 225, 230, 236, 241, 254, 255, 269, 279, 286, 294, 299, 310, 316, 322
Sprague-Dawley rats, 96, 223
Spring, 137
stability, 51, 222, 264, 290
stabilization, 264
stimulant, 108
stimulus, 42, 119, 121, 125, 148, 214, 228, 303
stratification, 326
streptozotocin (STZ), 27, 28, 29, 30, 37, 38, 44, 52, 56, 57, 58, 64, 65, 66, 71, 72, 73, 74, 75, 76, 77, 78, 79, 83, 88, 90, 96, 113, 115, 116, 126, 129, 130, 139, 140, 142, 143, 156, 159, 165, 168, 171, 186, 188, 196, 212, 215, 216, 217, 229, 232, 235, 236, 237, 243, 244, 246, 247, 248, 249, 252, 260, 261, 262, 276, 279, 280, 281, 285, 287, 297, 298
stress, 21, 35, 42, 71, 75, 77, 78, 79, 82, 84, 95, 104, 107, 108, 119, 120, 142, 199, 200, 203, 212, 213, 216, 223, 225, 231, 234, 240, 241, 250, 251, 253, 261, 266, 269, 281, 287, 293, 298, 306
structural changes, 17, 228, 277, 316
structural protein, 295, 296, 328
structure, 17, 44, 69, 70, 78, 94, 99, 113, 117, 126, 135, 224, 274, 275, 277, 284, 290, 292, 298, 310
subacute, 56
subgroups, 175
substrate, 166, 170, 177, 194, 203, 206, 241, 254, 300, 301, 306
substrates, 292, 300, 306
sulfate, 128, 248, 316
sulphur, 217
suppression, 79, 82, 154, 170, 178, 252, 258, 309
surface area, 6, 25, 26, 70, 166
surface layer, 248
susceptibility, 37, 57, 65, 86, 90, 93, 104, 118, 133, 141, 155, 161, 164, 176, 193, 221, 235, 263, 315, 316, 317, 318, 319, 323, 324, 325, 326, 327, 328, 330, 332, 333, 334, 335
syndrome, 24, 42, 132, 135, 154, 155, 330, 334
synergistic effect, 100, 210
synthesis, 35, 36, 45, 51, 69, 70, 72, 73, 74, 76, 91, 94, 104, 108, 112, 113, 119, 120, 139, 141, 142, 143, 145, 146, 148, 157, 173, 175, 183, 203, 208, 209, 214, 221, 222, 224, 228, 229, 231, 239, 240, 241, 245, 251, 258, 260, 261, 263, 266, 268, 278, 290, 291, 295, 296, 297, 298, 299, 300, 301, 302, 303, 311, 330
systemic change, 130
systolic blood pressure, 139
systolic pressure, 31

T

T cell, 174
target, 46, 52, 64, 70, 91, 101, 125, 132, 136, 157, 200, 213, 220, 250, 253, 254, 255, 256, 268, 270, 292, 296, 301, 303, 309, 311, 313, 330, 332
techniques, 24, 49, 50, 52, 244, 277
termination codon, 290, 291
testosterone, 226
TGF, viii, 36, 37, 42, 58, 74, 76, 77, 79, 82, 88, 90, 91, 92, 105, 111, 112, 113, 114, 115, 116, 117, 118, 119, 120, 121, 122, 123, 124, 125, 126, 127, 134, 136, 137, 138, 139, 140, 141, 143, 144, 145, 146, 147, 148, 149, 150, 151, 155, 158, 159, 162, 165, 173, 174, 175, 213, 219, 224, 229, 230, 246, 270, 278, 279, 280, 281, 285, 286, 287, 320, 322, 323, 332
therapeutic agents, 59, 136, 209, 256
therapeutic approaches, 239, 240, 256
therapeutic interventions, vii, 3, 93
therapeutic targets, 50, 59, 66, 77, 96, 136, 210, 253, 269, 271
therapeutic use, 264
therapeutics, 152
therapy, 22, 24, 29, 39, 40, 41, 42, 71, 81, 92, 100, 102, 106, 109, 111, 116, 122, 129, 136, 143, 151, 163, 176, 187, 193, 199, 200, 211, 212, 215, 225, 254, 255, 270, 318
thiazide, 327, 328, 329, 330, 334
thiazide diuretics, 330
threonine, 36, 75, 113, 137, 292, 294, 299
thrombin, 251, 253
thrombomodulin, 72, 242
thrombosis, 239, 240
thromboxanes, 142, 229, 230
thymine, 133
TIMP, 114, 322
tissue, 36, 41, 49, 52, 54, 72, 74, 77, 78, 90, 94, 97, 98, 100, 102, 103, 107, 119, 123, 126, 134, 142, 150, 151, 152, 166, 185, 188, 189, 200, 204, 205, 208, 215, 218, 221, 223, 241, 247, 258, 288, 311, 320
TNF, 75, 98, 125, 127, 150, 205, 266, 267, 332
TNF-alpha, 150, 266, 267
TNF-α, 125, 127
tobacco, 97
tonic, 300

toxic effect, 29, 30, 56
toxicity, 56, 57, 247
toxin, 225
transcription, 52, 71, 72, 73, 75, 76, 78, 79, 95, 105, 114, 116, 120, 122, 125, 142, 144, 175, 192, 194, 195, 225, 228, 248, 264, 281, 288, 289, 293, 294, 295, 296, 300, 302, 303, 322, 323, 325, 327
transcription factors, 228, 281, 288, 294, 323
transfection, 144
transferrin, 94
transforming growth factor, 36, 69, 86, 89, 91, 137, 138, 139, 140, 141, 142, 143, 144, 145, 146, 147, 148, 149, 150, 151, 153, 155, 162, 174, 187, 191, 192, 285, 287, 308, 310, 320, 332
transition metal, 200, 202
translation, viii, 289, 290, 291, 292, 293, 294, 295, 296, 297, 298, 299, 300, 301, 302, 303, 304, 305, 306, 307, 308, 310, 311, 312, 313
translocation, 75, 121, 255, 271, 278, 289, 291, 294, 328
transmission, 141, 325, 332
transplant, 15, 22, 39
transplantation, 3, 18, 39, 58, 66
transport, 71, 78, 113, 120, 202, 205, 207, 214, 241, 287, 325
treatment, viii, xi, 27, 39, 41, 46, 47, 49, 59, 64, 65, 71, 72, 75, 76, 78, 79, 81, 83, 90, 96, 101, 103, 110, 111, 115, 116, 117, 122, 130, 133, 134, 135, 136, 137, 140, 146, 147, 156, 159, 162, 163, 165, 168, 170, 176, 177, 178, 179, 180, 181, 193, 201, 205, 206, 209, 211, 216, 217, 220, 223, 224, 229, 230, 241, 243, 244, 246, 247, 248, 253, 254, 256, 273, 286, 301, 320, 323, 330, 332
trial, 2, 40, 46, 47, 79, 97, 102, 106, 132, 133, 137, 143, 176, 181, 193, 194, 211, 225, 332
tricarboxylic acid, 204
triggers, 69, 81, 82, 224, 295
triglycerides, 57, 207
trypsin, 166
tumor, 71, 88, 135, 251, 292, 309, 310
tumor necrosis factor, 251
tumorigenesis, 305
turnover, 94, 95, 123, 158, 204, 276
type 1 diabetes, 1, 16, 17, 43, 80, 81, 83, 85, 86, 90, 109, 115, 129, 132, 133, 137, 141, 154, 155, 156, 163, 175, 177, 179, 182, 183, 184, 191, 193, 194, 197, 206, 211, 216, 218, 232, 236, 237, 240, 242, 258, 259, 276, 279, 284, 297, 298, 301, 333, 334
type 2 diabetes, 1, 5, 13, 16, 17, 18, 44, 45, 46, 47, 66, 69, 70, 71, 77, 79, 81, 82, 84, 89, 99, 106, 107, 112, 115, 118, 130, 132, 133, 134, 139, 141, 142, 143, 146, 147, 150, 152, 153, 154, 156, 162, 163, 169, 175, 176, 177, 178, 181, 183, 194, 211, 212, 231, 232, 233, 234, 235, 236, 242, 256, 257, 258, 259, 260, 262, 266, 276, 277, 279, 283, 284, 285, 296, 299, 300, 301, 311, 331, 332, 333, 334
tyrosine, 37, 113, 122, 128, 137, 150, 174, 191, 271, 280, 299, 300, 304, 322

U

underlying mechanisms, 301
uniform, 5, 6, 7, 13, 15, 16, 17, 224
urea, 241
urea cycle, 241
uric acid, 206
urinary bladder, 27
urinary tract, 14
urine, 29, 34, 40, 43, 51, 57, 102, 115, 117, 132, 179, 188, 213, 228, 229, 242, 251, 277, 278, 317

V

validation, 59
variables, 37, 52
variations, 118, 330, 334, 335
vascular cell adhesion molecule, 108, 215
vascular endothelial growth factor (VEGF), 37, 45, 152, 153, 261, 287, 323
vascular system, 268
vasculature, 63, 86, 99, 119, 164, 166, 168, 171, 240, 245, 251, 252, 253, 255, 256
vasoconstriction, 29, 143, 173, 240, 245, 249, 268
vasodilation, 99, 119, 130, 164, 165, 224, 232, 242, 249, 262
vasodilator, 166, 170, 240, 245
vasopressor, 170
VCAM, 98, 99, 215, 242, 249
VEGF expression, 84, 129, 131, 153, 155, 248
VEGF protein, 130, 131
vein, 27, 78, 117, 269
viral gene, 306
viral vectors, 136
viruses, 293
vitamin C, 201
vitamin D, 79, 92
vitamins, 199, 202

W

water, 123, 201, 208, 277, 321
weight control, 58, 298
weight loss, 39
wheat germ, 304

work study, 130
worldwide, 1, 137, 162
wound healing, 107

X

X chromosome, 170, 293

Z

zinc, 170, 201, 241